Workbook to Accompany

Delmar's Radiographic Positioning and Procedures Volume I: Basic Positioning and Procedures

Michael Patrick Adams, PhD, RT(R)(ARRT)
Associate Dean of Health, Mathematics and Science
Pasco-Hernando Community College
New Port Richey, Florida

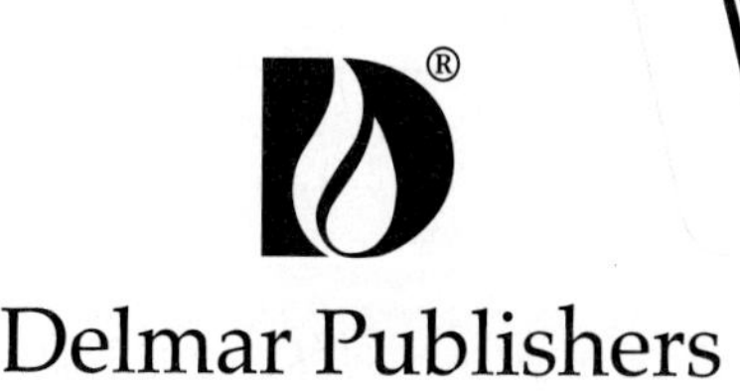

Delmar Publishers

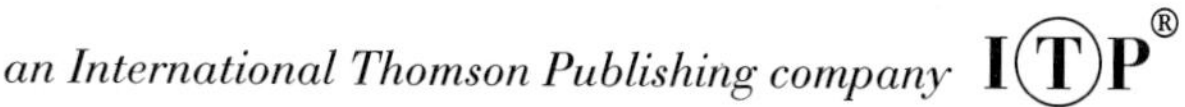

Albany • Bonn • Boston • Cincinnati • Detroit • London • Madrid
Melbourne • Mexico City • New York • Pacific Grove • Paris • San Francisco
Singapore • Tokyo • Toronto • Washington

NOTICE TO THE READER

Publisher does not warrant or guarantee any of the products described herein or perform any independent analysis in connection with any of the product information contained herein. Publisher does not assume, and expressly disclaims, any obligation to obtain and include information other than that provided to it by the manufacturer.

The reader is expressly warned to consider and adopt all safety precautions that might be indicated by the activities described herein and to avoid all potential hazards. By following the instructions contained herein, the reader willingly assumes all risks in connection with such instructions.

The publisher makes no representation or warranties of any kind, including but not limited to, the warranties of fitness for particular purpose or merchantability, nor are any such representations implied with respect to the material set forth herein, and the publisher takes no responsibility with respect to such material. The publisher shall not be liable for any special, consequential, or exemplary damages resulting, in whole or part, from the readers' use of, or reliance upon, this material.

Cover Design: Bill Finnerty

Printed in the United States of America

For more information, contact:

Delmar Publishers
3 Columbia Circle, Box 15015
Albany, New York 12212-5015

International Thomson Publishing Europe
Berkshire House 168-173
High Holborn
London, WC1V 7AA
England

Thomas Nelson Australia
102 Dodds Street
South Melbourne, 3205
Victoria, Australia

Nelson Canada
1120 Birchmount Road
Scarborough, Ontario
Canada, M1K 5G4

International Thomson Editores
Campos Eliseos 385, Piso 7
Col Polanco
11560 Mexico D F Mexico

International Thomson Publishing GmbH
Konigswinterer Strasse 418
53227 Bonn
Germany

International Thomson Publishing Asia
221 Henderson Road
#05-10 Henderson Building
Singapore 0315

International Thomson Publishing—Japan
Hirakawacho Kyowa Building, 3F
2-2-1 Hirakawacho
Chiyoda-ku, Tokyo 102
Japan

2 3 4 5 6 7 8 9 10 XXX 03 02 01 00 99 98

Library of Congress Card No: 97-43449
ISBN: 0–8273–6784–8

Contents

SECTION I INTRODUCTION TO RADIOGRAPHIC POSITIONING

Chapter 1 Introduction to Radiographic Positioning and Procedures 3

SECTION II CHEST AND ABDOMEN

Chapter 2 Chest and Upper Airway 17

Chapter 3 Abdomen 33

SECTION III LIMBS AND THORAX

Chapter 4 Upper Limb and Shoulder Girdle 51

Chapter 5 Lower Limb and Pelvis 83

Chapter 6 Ribs and Sternum 115

SECTION IV VERTEBRAL COLUMN

Chapter 7 Cervical Spine 129

Chapter 8 Thoracic Spine 141

Chapter 9 Lumbar Spine, Sacrum, and Coccyx 155

Chapter 10 Trauma Spine 175

SECTION V SKULL RADIOGRAPHY

Chapter 11 Introduction to Skull Radiography 191

Chapter 12 Basic Skull Positions/Projections 201

Chapter 13 Skull and Facial Bones 227

Chapter 14 Trauma Head Positioning 253

SECTION VI DIGESTIVE SYSTEM AND URINARY TRACT

Chapter 15 Upper Gastrointestinal Tract 265

Chapter 16 Lower Gastrointestinal Tract 281

Chapter 17 Hepatobiliary System 297

Chapter 18 Urinary System 311

SECTION VII SPECIAL RADIOGRAPHY

Chapter 19 Mobile and Intraoperative Radiography 327

CROSSWORD PUZZLE AND WORD SEARCH ACTIVITIES 335

FINAL EXAMINATION 347

Preface

The study of radiographic positioning and procedures is one of the most difficult in the radiographic sciences. The student is faced with huge numbers of facts, terms, and concepts that are presented at a rapid pace continuing over the better part of a year. The purpose of this workbook is to facilitate the learning process and to ease the student into and through this intense subject.

Questions in this workbook closely parallel material presented in Delmar's *Radiographic Positioning and Procedures, Volume 1: Basic Positioning and Procedures* by Joanne Greathouse. Although referenced to the Greathouse text, the workbook can also be used as a stand-alone review text for those preparing for certification examinations.

Several features of this workbook clearly distinguish it from other text supplements.

- Many problems in radiography are visually oriented, involving analysis of anatomic drawings and radiographs. This workbook includes more than 200 radiographs and diagrams to give the student a more visual approach to problem-solving.
- Because instructors use a variety of question types, students need to prepare for the many different styles of questions. Question types in this workbook include true/false, fill in the blank, multiple choice, and essay.
- Most workbooks test only memorization, yet radiography students are expected to apply knowledge to solve real positioning problems early in their professional careers. To help teach students how to problem solve, this workbook includes a significant number of higher level cognitive questions in each chapter. These involve applying knowledge to solve unique positioning problems and to analyze the positioning quality of radiographs. It is intended that these questions will help students leap the gap between simple memorization of facts and solving real problems in positioning.
- Many students enter the profession with poor study skills and are unprepared for the vast amount of knowledge facing them in the freshman year. The early learning of effective study and test-taking skills is essential for academic success. This workbook provides practical study tips in each chapter, which help give students the tools they need to succeed.
- Too often, each narrow topic in positioning is treated in isolation and the student rarely is shown the many interrelationships among the body areas. This workbook contains review questions that transcend a particular chapter to show relationships to topics in previous and subsequent chapters.

Each chapter will use a similar outline, beginning with the learning objectives and list of positions/projections, extracted from the Greathouse text, which will be tested in the workbook. For most chapters, questions are segregated into two sections; anatomy/physiology and radiographic procedures, analysis, and critical thinking. Each chapter concludes with review questions and a study tip.

To further test student knowledge of the content provided, crossword puzzles and word search exercises relating to specific chapters and a comprehensive final examination are provided at the end of the workbook.

Typical Chapter Outline:

Objectives

Routine and Alternative Positions/Projections

Questions

Anatomy and Physiology

Radiographic Procedures, Analysis, and Critical Thinking

Do You Remember?

Study Tip

The author genuinely hopes that this workbook will help students succeed in one of the most challenging subjects in allied health.

Acknowledgment

The author wishes to recognize Barbara Koontz, MA, RT(R)(ARRT), Robert Halenkamp, MPA, RT(R)(ARRT), and John Fleming, BA, RT(R)(ARRT) who not only contributed questions for the workbook but who also helped me form the greatest team of educators ever assembled for over a decade of excellence. Their contribution to my intellectual and humanistic growth will not be forgotten.

The author and Delmar Publishers would also like to gratefully acknowledge Mary Hagler, MHA, BA, RT(R)(N)(M)(ARRT), Connie Luna, RT(R)(M)(CT)(ARRT), and Watson Community Hospital, Watsonville, California for their assistance in obtaining radiographs for the workbook.

Dedication

This workbook is dedicated to my wife, Kim Cherie, and my daughter, Kimberly Michelle Valiance, for their love and patience and for allowing me to use the Power Mac during this long project when they really needed it. A posthumous dedication is also made to my parents, John and Shirlee Adams, for their boundless love, which continues to be felt in their absence.

SECTION I

INTRODUCTION to RADIOGRAPHIC POSITIONING

CHAPTER 1

Introduction to Radiographic Positioning and Procedures

OBJECTIVES

At the completion of this chapter, the student should be able to:

1. List and discuss patient care considerations relevant to positioning.
2. List the three primary exposure factors.
3. List specific methods of reducing patient radiation exposure.
4. Explain the 10-day rule.
5. List the three primary principles of radiation protection.
6. Define and demonstrate the anatomic position.
7. Define terms related to body planes.
8. Given diagrams, identify body planes.
9. Given topographic landmarks, list the corresponding vertebrae.
10. List and describe the characteristics of each of the four major body types.
11. Given diagrams, identify the body type illustrated.
12. Define and demonstrate given terms related to body position and body movement.
13. Define given terms related to general positioning.
14. List the three general principles of positioning.
15. List and discuss the six primary elements in radiographic positioning.

QUESTIONS

Anatomy and Physiology

For questions 1–4, identify the body habitus illustrated in Figure 1.1.

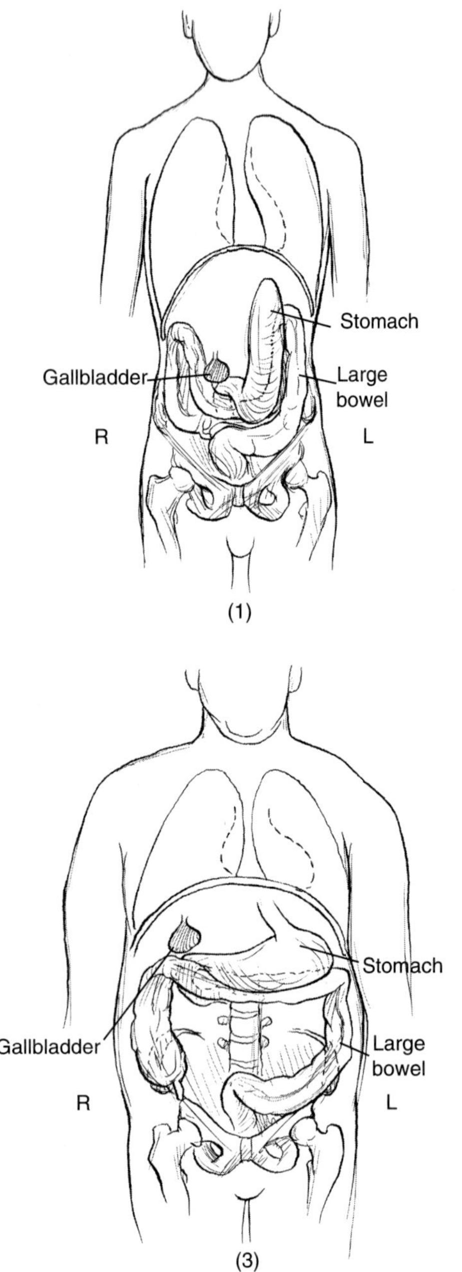

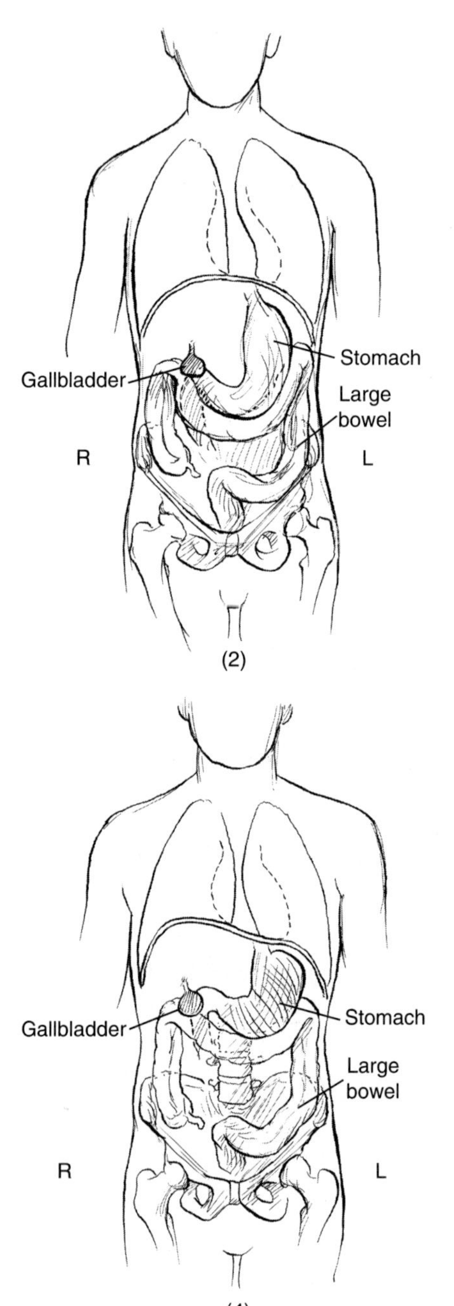

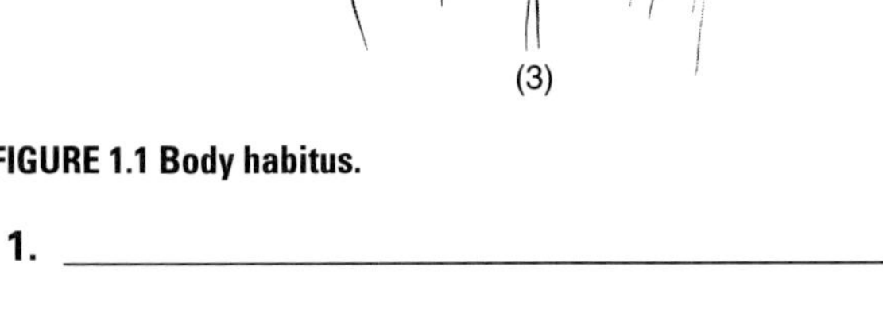

FIGURE 1.1 Body habitus.

1. ______________________________

2. ______________________________

3. ______________________________

4. ______________________________

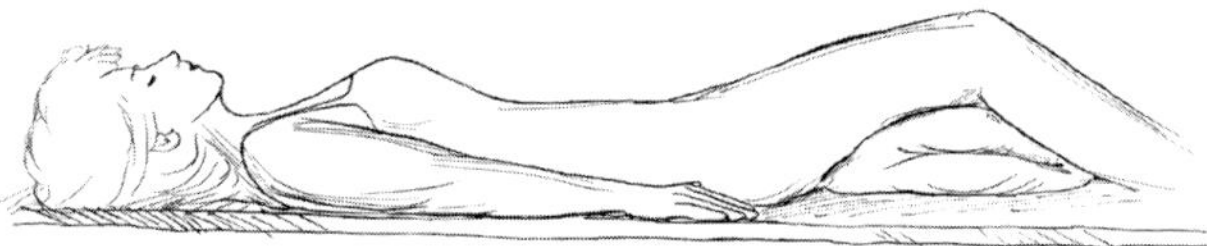

FIGURE 1.2 Body position, abdomen.

5. The position of the patient in Figure 1.2 is

______________________________.

6. The projection illustrated in Figure 1.2 is

______________________________.

7. The view illustrated in Figure 1.2 is

______________________________.

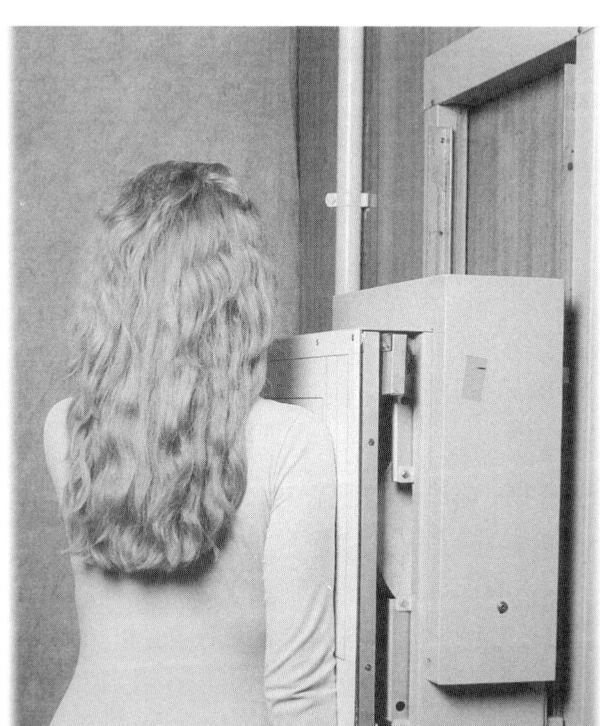

FIGURE 1.3 Body position, abdomen.

8. The position of the patient in Figure 1.3 is

______________________________.

9. The projection illustrated in Figure 1.3 is

______________________________.

10. The view illustrated in Figure 1.3 is

______________________________.

11. The three primary principles of personnel radiation protection are

______________________________,

______________________________,

and ______________________________.

For questions 12–22 match the landmark with its corresponding vertebra.

	Landmark	Vertebra(e)
12. _____	mastoid tip	**a.** C1
13. _____	manubrial notch	**b.** C2–C3
14. _____	costal margin	**c.** C5
15. _____	ASIS	**d.** C7
16. _____	thyroid cartilage	**e.** T2–T3
17. _____	sternal angle	**f.** T4–T5
18. _____	umbilicus	**g.** T7
19. _____	pubic bone	**h.** T10
20. _____	xiphoid tip	**i.** L3–L4
21. _____	iliac crest	**j.** L4
22. _____	greater trochanter	**k.** S1
		l. coccyx

23. The role of the modern radiologist is to produce and interpret the radiographic image.

a. true

b. false

24. Film badges offer reasonable protection for the radiographer from excessive exposure to radiation.

a. true

b. false

25. The transverse and sagittal planes are types of longitudinal planes.

a. true

b. false

26. Radiography can only be performed at 40- or 72-inch SID.

a. true

b. false

27. For most body parts there is only one correct positioning method for achieving an optimum film.

a. true

b. false

28. X-rays were discovered by Roentgen in:

a. 1894

b. 1985

c. 1895

d. 1896

29. The single most important factor in the prevention of pathogen transfer is:

a. handwashing

b. wearing gloves

c. wearing a mask

d. proper personal hygiene

30. Standard precautions require that:

a. hands are washed after each examination

b. the radiographer treat all patients as if they have AIDS

c. protective gear be worn for every examination

d. protective gear be worn only when exposure to body fluids is likely

31. Radiographic examination of women of childbearing age is sometimes restricted to the:

a. onset of menses to the day menses stops

b. onset of menses to the 10 days after menses stops

c. first 10 days following the onset of menses

d. first 10 days following the end of menses

32. Which plane divides the body into right and left portions?

a. sagittal

b. transverse

c. coronal

d. frontal

33. A section perpendicular to the long axis of the body dividing it into superior and inferior portions is called a:

a. sagittal plane

b. coronal plane

c. transverse plane

d. longitudinal plane

34. Which plane is parallel to the table top when the patient is placed in the lateral position?

a. transverse

b. sagittal

c. coronal

d. midaxillary

35. A patient who is facing forward with his arms at his sides and palms facing forward is in the _____ position.

a. frontal

b. anterior

c. anatomic

d. AP

36. Movement of the arm toward the central axis of the body is called:

a. flexion

b. abduction

c. extension

d. adduction

37. Turning the arm so that the palm of the hand faces forward or upward is called:

a. supination

b. extension

c. flexion

d. pronation

38. The umbilicus or navel is on the _____ surface of the body.

a. posterior

b. AP

c. supine

d. anterior

39. The head is _____ to the neck.

a. anterior

b. inferior

c. medial

d. superior

40. The elbow is _____ to the wrist.

a. anterior

b. proximal

c. posterior

d. distal

41. The ear is _____ to the nose.

a. anterior

b. superior

c. medial

d. lateral

42. Which term means the opposite of volar?

a. palmar

b. contralateral

c. plantar

d. dorsum

43. Which term is used to describe the path of the central ray?

a. projection

b. position

c. view

d. PA

44. A patient is standing with her right side against the film holder. The position of the patient is:

a. PA

b. left lateral

c. right lateral

d. right lateral decubitus

45. A decubitus position is one in which the patient is placed in a _____ position.

a. lateral

b. PA or AP

c. supine or prone

d. recumbent

46. A patient is lying on his left side and the x-ray beam is placed horizontally to exit near the umbilicus. This position is called:

a. AP left lateral decubitus

b. PA left lateral decubitus

c. AP right lateral decubitus

d. PA right lateral decubitus

47. A skull position that requires the x-ray beam to skim the surface of the cheekbone would most likely be called:

a. axial

b. tangential

c. lateral

d. decubitus

48. Which of the following is *not* a position?

a. AP

b. lateral

c. RAO

d. supine

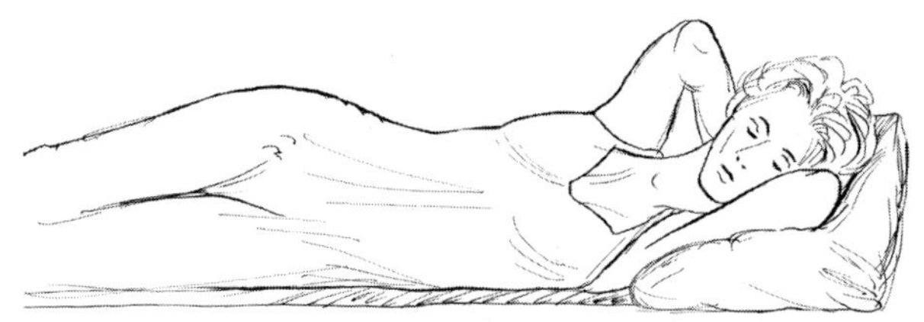

FIGURE 1.4 Body position, lateral.

49. The patient position in Figure 1.4 is best described as:

a. right lateral

b. left lateral

c. right lateral recumbent

d. left lateral recumbent

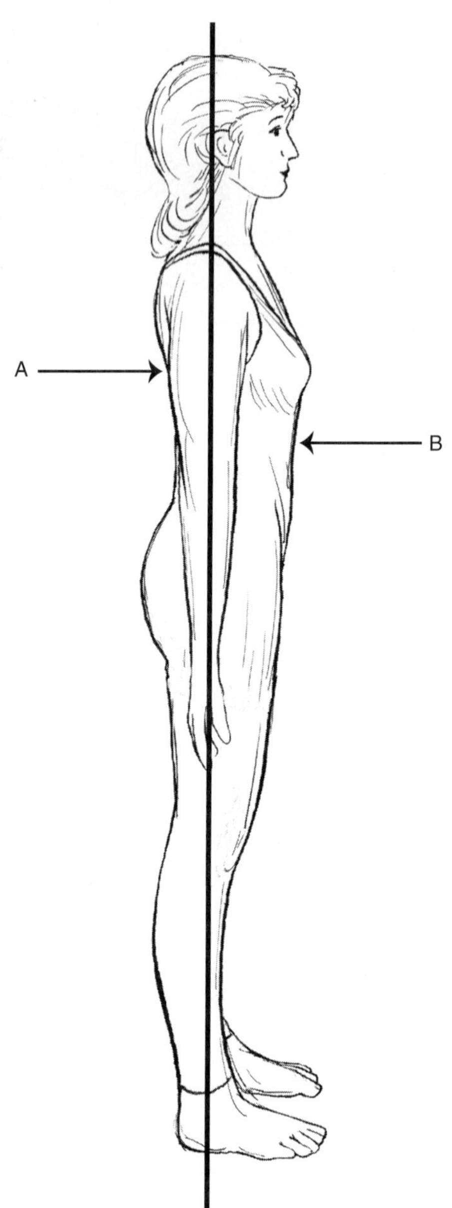

FIGURE 1.5 Body surfaces, side view.

For questions 50–52, refer to the diagram of the arm in Figure 1.5.

50. Label A refers to the _____ surface of the body.

a. anterior

b. posterior

c. lateral

d. medial

51. Label B refers to the _____ surface of the body.

a. anterior

b. posterior

c. lateral

d. medial

52. The body plane illustrated in Figure 1.5 is:

a. midsagittal

b. transverse

c. oblique

d. midcoronal

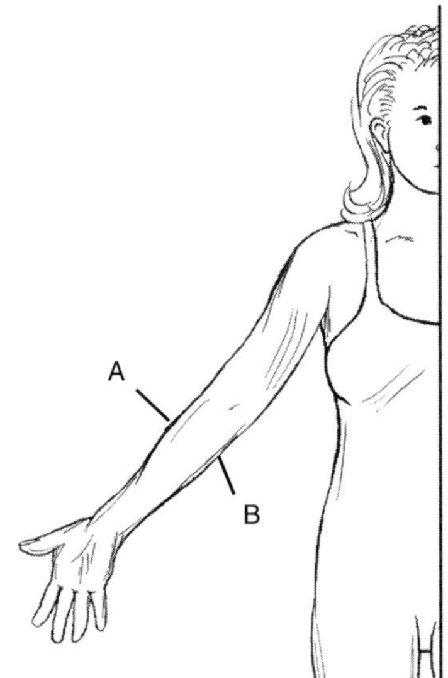

FIGURE 1.6 Body surfaces, arm.

For questions 53–55, refer to Figure 1.6.

53. Label A refers to the _____ surface of the body.

a. anterior

b. posterior

c. lateral

d. medial

54. Label B refers to the _____ surface of the body.

a. anterior

b. posterior

c. lateral

d. medial

55. The body plane illustrated in Figure 1.6 is:

a. medial

b. midcoronal

c. oblique

d. transverse

Critical Thinking

56. To accurately describe body locations it is sometimes necessary to use more than one directional term. Use at least *two* terms to describe the location of the following.

a. palm of the hand in relation to the shoulder

b. patella (kneecap) in relation to the heel of the foot

c. chin in relation to the ears

57. Explain why a satisfactory image *cannot* usually be obtained without the cooperation of the patient.

58. Why is it important for the radiographer to obtain a thorough medical history from the patient before starting the examination?

59. Give an example of how the radiographer may need to change his or her routine after receiving a medical history from the patient.

60. The ARRT Code of Ethics states that diagnosis is beyond the scope of practice of the radiographer. Explain the importance and implications of this section of the code.

61. Explain why proper patient communication/instruction is sometimes considered a means of radiation protection.

62. Explain why it is essential that the radiographer obtain at least two radiographs at right angles to each other for nearly all body parts.

STUDY TIP: LEARNING FAMILIAR SUBJECTS

(two students overheard in the hallway)

Dean: I can't believe instructor Bob spent a whole hour talking about how to study.

Briana: Me neither. Does he think we really don't know how to study? I mean, if we made it through high school and got into this program, we must know how to study.

Dean: And that part about how to take notes and when to study, what a laugh.

Briana: Yeah, let's go study our first chapter on positioning before lunch.

Dean: Nah, we have plenty of time and the test isn't until Friday. Besides, we had all this stuff in high school in medical terminology class.

Briana: You're right, let's just get together Thursday night. That should give us enough time.

Apparently instructor Bob's decision to spend valuable class time teaching study skills has not yet affected Dean and Briana. These students are making two common errors. First, they assume that because they previously studied a subject, such as anatomy or terminology, that they do not need to thoroughly restudy the subject. This leads to a false feeling of security and often causes students to perform worse in "familiar" subjects than they do in "new." Secondly, Dean and Briana are going to try an "all nighter" to cram the material into their brains. This strategy may have worked in high school and in some college courses but it rarely works in anatomy or positioning.

> Give familiar subjects or topics the same degree of attention as new subjects. Never save all your studying until the night before an examination; begin studying the material immediately after learning it in class.

SECTION II

CHEST and ABDOMEN

CHAPTER 2

Chest and Upper Airway

LEARNING OBJECTIVES

At the completion of this chapter, the student should be able to:

1. List and describe the anatomy of the chest and upper airway.
2. Given drawings and radiographs, locate anatomic structures and landmarks.
3. Explain the rationale for each projection.
4. Explain the patient preparation required for each examination.
5. Describe the positioning used to visualize anatomic structures of the chest and upper airway.
6. List or identify the central ray location and the extent of the field necessary for each projection.
7. Explain the protective measures that should be taken for each examination.
8. Recommend the technical factors for producing an acceptable radiograph for each projection.
9. State the patient instructions for each projection.
10. Given radiographs, evaluate positioning and technical factors.
11. Describe modifications of procedures for atypical or impaired patients to better demonstrate the anatomic area of interest.

Routine and Alternative Positions/Projections

Part	Routine	Alternative
Chest	PA	PA (stretcher/stool)
		Supine/semi-upright AP
		Lateral decubitus
		AP lordotic
	Lateral	Dorsal decubitus (tip: ventral decubitus)
		Lateral (stretcher/stool)
Upper airway	AP	
	Lateral	

QUESTIONS

Anatomy and Physiology

For questions 1–10, identify the anatomy of the lungs and associated structures in Figure 2.1.

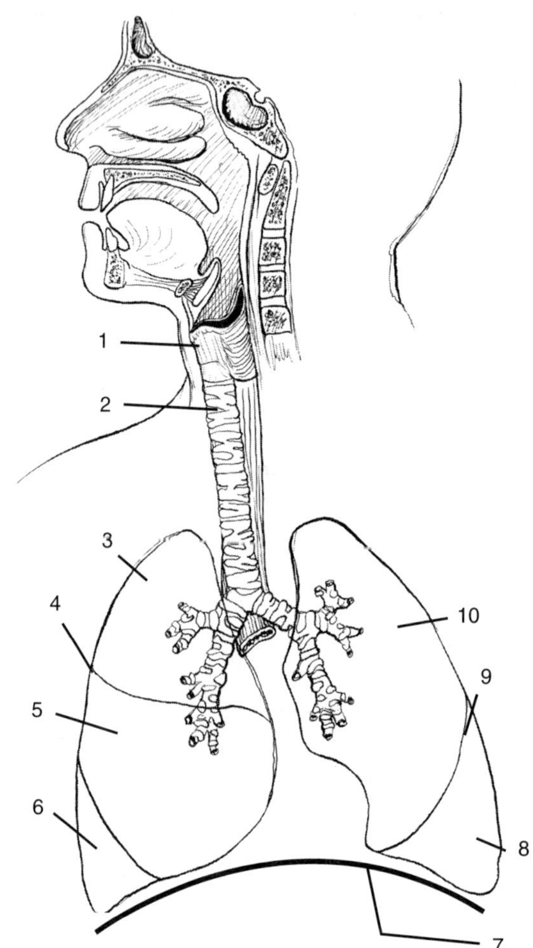

FIGURE 2.1 Lungs and associated structures, anterior view.

1.______________________ 6. ______________________

2.______________________ 7. ______________________

3.______________________ 8. ______________________

4.______________________ 9. ______________________

5.______________________ 10. ______________________

For questions 11-18, identify the anatomy of the bronchial tree in Figure 2.2.

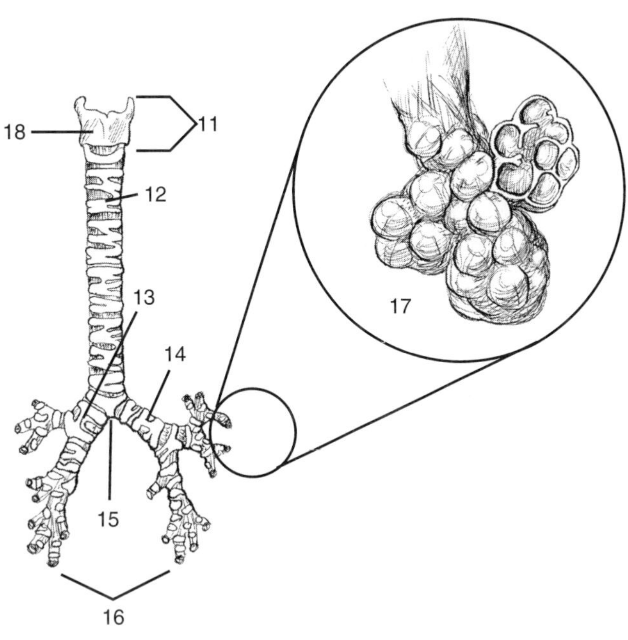

FIGURE 2.2 Bronchial tree, anterior view.

11. ____________________

12. ____________________

13. ____________________

14. ____________________

15. ____________________

16. ____________________

17. ____________________

18. ____________________

19. That portion of the chest that contains the heart, trachea, and esophagus is called the

_______________________________________.

20. The three parts of the upper airway are the larynx, trachea, and

_______________________________________.

21. The ______________ is responsible for voice production.

22. The right lung has ______________ lobes.

23. Gas exchange occurs in the

_______________________________________.

24. Both food and air pass through the nasopharynx.

a. true

b. false

25. The left primary bronchus is shorter, wider, and more vertical than the right primary bronchus.

a. true

b. false

26. The trachea serves as a passageway for both food and air.

a. true

b. false

27. The lobes of the left lung are separated by the:

a. mediastinum

b. oblique fissure

c. horizontal and oblique fissures

d. pleural cavity

28. Which structure is *not* located in the mediastinum?

a. trachea

b. esophagus

c. epiglottis

d. heart

29. The trachea bifurcates into the primary bronchi at the level of:

a. T1

b. T5

c. T8

d. T10

30. The part of the upper airway extending from the soft palate to the epiglottis is called the:

a. oropharynx

b. laryngopharynx

c. larynx

d. nasopharynx

31. Which structure consists of three paired and three unpaired cartilages?

a. larynx

b. laryngopharynx

c. trachea

d. oropharynx

32. The dilated, sac-like, terminal portion of the respiratory tree is called the:

a. primary bronchus

b. secondary bronchus

c. alveolus

d. trachea

33. A patient with pulmonary emphysema:

a. has smaller lungs than normal

b. has enlarged lungs with destruction of lung tissue

c. is more likely to develop lung cancer

d. has an increased ability to exchange oxygen in the lungs

34. The carina is:

a. the location of the vocal cords

b. one of the cartilages in the larynx

c. the area of bifurcation of the trachea

d. the structure preventing food from entering the upper airway

35. Food is directed to the esophagus by a cartilaginous fold called the:

a. larynx

b. alveolus

c. epiglottis

d. hilus

36. Place the following in the correct order that inspired air will travel.

1. nasopharynx

2. primary bronchus

3. nasal cavity

4. alveolus

5. terminal bronchiole

a. 3, 1, 5, 2, 4

b. 1, 3, 2, 4, 5

c. 3, 1, 2, 4, 5

d. 3, 1, 2, 5, 4

37. On deep inspiration, the diaphragm is:

a. relaxed

b. lowered

c. raised

d. does not move

38. Which hemidiaphragm is normally located higher?

a. left, because the stomach pushes it up

b. right, because the liver pushes it up

c. right, because the right lung is larger

d. both right and left hemidiaphragms should be equal height

Radiographic Procedures, Analysis, and Critical Thinking

For questions 39–46, identify the radiographic anatomy on the lateral chest projection in Figure 2.3A.

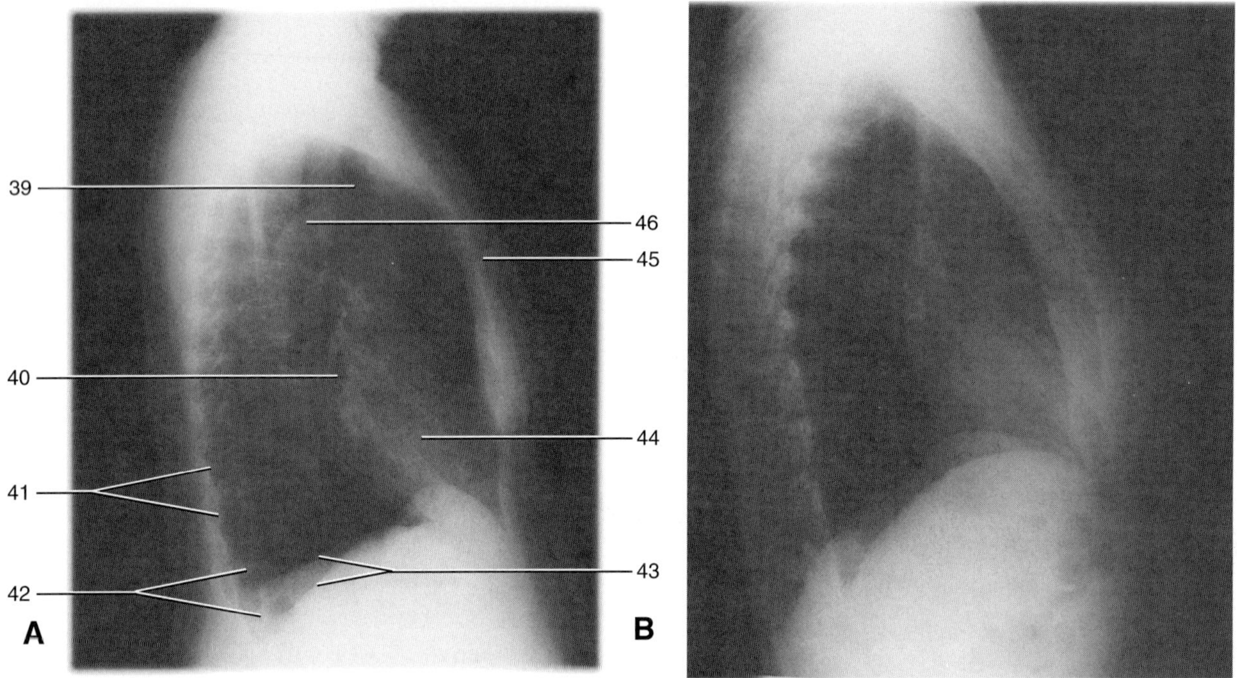

FIGURE 2.3 Radiograph of chest, lateral projection: (A) correct positioning, (B) incorrect positioning.

39. ______________________

40. ______________________

41. ______________________

42. ______________________

43. ______________________

44. ______________________

45. ______________________

46. ______________________

47. Compare the positioning quality of the correctly positioned radiograph in Figure 2.3A with that in Figure 2.3B. Describe the positioning error, explain what caused it, and give the step(s) necessary to correct the problem.

48. The film size used for most adult chest radiography is _______________ inches.

49. When positioning for a lateral chest, the _______________ plane is placed parallel to the film.

50. The lordotic projection of the chest demonstrates the _______________ portion of the lung.

51. The kVp for a routine lateral projection of the chest is the same as for a routine PA chest.

a. true

b. false

52. For the lateral decubitus positions of the chest, the arms are placed by the patient's sides with the shoulders rolled forward.

a. true

b. false

53. An oblique chest radiograph taken with the patient in an RAO position will demonstrate detail of the right lung.

a. true

b. false

54. Upper airway examinations are normally done on inspiration so that the trachea is filled with air.

a. true

b. false

For questions 55–59, identify the radiographic anatomy on the PA chest projection in Figure 2.4A.

55. Apex

a. 1

b. 2

c. 5

d. 10

56. Costophrenic angle

a. 4

b. 5

c. 6

d. 7

57. Aortic arch

a. 3

b. 5

c. 9

d. 10

58. Hilum

a. 1

b. 3

c. 7

d. 8

59. Diaphragm

a. 4

b. 5

c. 6

d. 7

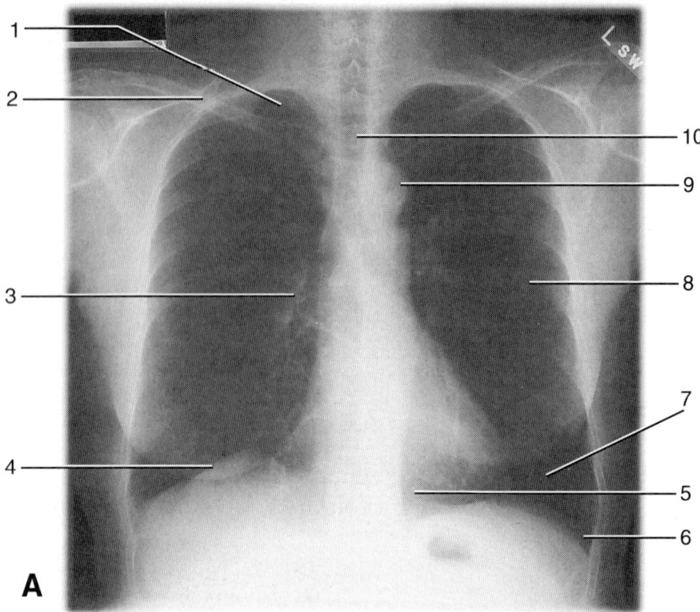

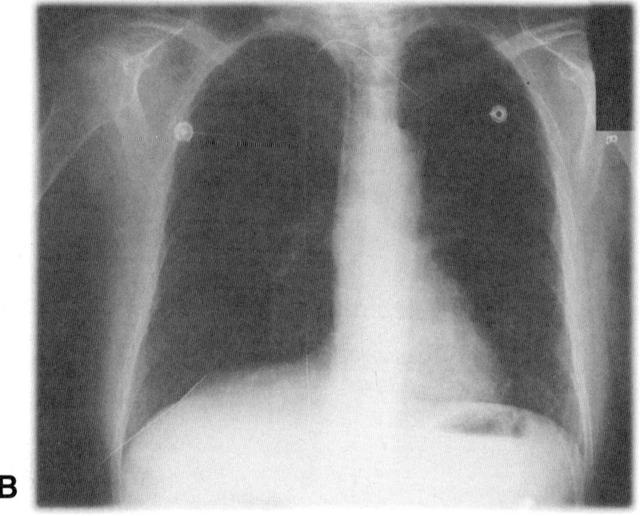

FIGURE 2.4: Radiograph of chest, PA projection: (A) correct positioning, (B) incorrect positioning.

60. Compare the positioning quality of the correctly positioned radiograph in Figure 2.4A with that in Figure 2.4B. Describe the positioning error, explain what caused it, and give the step(s) necessary to correct the problem.

61. Which of the following is true regarding visualization of the lower thoracic spine on a PA chest radiograph?

a. If the film has proper penetration, the vertebrae should not be seen.

b. Bony detail of the vertebrae should be clearly seen.

c. Visualization of the vertebrae is a sign of underexposure.

d. The vertebrae should be faintly visualized.

62. For an upright PA chest examination, the top of the film is placed:

a. 1.5 inches below the top of the shoulders

b. 2.5 inches below the top of the shoulders

c. 1.5 inches above the top of the shoulders

d. 2.5 inches above the top of the shoulders

63. On a PA chest radiograph, how many posterior ribs should be visualized above the diaphragm?

a. 4

b. 8

c. 10

d. 12

64. The shoulders are rolled forward for PA chest projections to:

a. remove the clavicles from the lung fields

b. move the diaphragm to its lowest position

c. remove the scapulae from the lung fields

d. minimize distortion

65. Why are chest x-rays ideally performed in the upright position?

1. to demonstrate possible air/fluid levels

2. to move the diaphragm to its lowest possible position

3. to minimize distortion/magnification of the heart and great vessels

a. 1 and 2

b. 1 and 3

c. 2 and 3

d. 1, 2, and 3

66. What is the best area on the radiograph to examine to detect rotation on a PA chest?

a. sternoclavicular joints

b. costophrenic angles

c. acromioclavicular joints

d. hilum

67. On a PA chest radiograph a radiographer observes that the SC joints are equidistant from the vertebral column. Which of the following conclusions may be reached?

a. The film needs to be repeated using deeper inspiration.

b. The lung apices were likely not included in their entirety on the film.

c. The patient was rotated.

d. The patient was correctly positioned.

68. What is the optimum kVp range for a PA projection of the chest taken with a grid?

a. 60–70

b. 70–80

c. 90–100

d. 100–120

69. On a supine AP projection of the chest, the central ray enters:

a. 3–4 inches below the sternal angle

b. 3–4 inches below the suprasternal notch

c. at the level of the xiphoid process

d. at the level of the suprasternal notch

70. The central ray for a lateral projection of the chest should be at the level of:

a. T3–T4

b. T6–T7

c. T9–T10

d. T11–T12

71. What is the best criterion to use to determine whether or not rotation exists on a lateral chest radiograph?

a. Sternum is in a true lateral.

b. Posterior ribs and lungs are mostly superimposed.

c. SC joints are equidistant from the vertebra.

d. The hila are superimposed.

72. To demonstrate a fluid level in the right thorax of a patient who is unable to stand, which of the following positions/projections should be used?

a. supine

b. Trendelenburg

c. left lateral decubitus

d. right lateral decubitus

73. In which projection are the pulmonary apices visualized below the clavicular shadows?

a. PA

b. AP supine

c. decubitus

d. lordotic

74. If a patient is too ill to be placed upright, the lordotic projection may be obtained by placing the patient supine and directing the central ray:

a. 15–20° cephalic

b. 15–20° caudal

c. 30–35° cephalic

d. 30–35° caudal

75. Which projection of the chest is performed to demonstrate the mediastinal structures removed from superimposition of the vertebral column?

a. lordotic

b. lateral decubitus

c. oblique

d. dorsal decubitus

76. Obliques of the chest require a patient rotation of:

a. 15°

b. 30°

c. 45°

d. 60°

77. A patient is prone and the beam is placed horizontally. This projection is called a:

a. right lateral decubitus

b. left lateral decubitus

c. ventral decubitus

d. dorsal decubitus

78. The central ray for an AP projection of the upper airway should be at the level of:

a. the mandible

b. C2–C3

c. the manubrium

d. the sternal angle

79. For a lateral projection of the upper trachea, the top of the film should be placed:

a. at the level of the gonion

b. at the level of the manubrial notch

c. at the level of the external auditory meatus

d. 1.5–2 inches below the level of the external auditory meatus

80. Children require a number of procedural modifications to obtain satisfactory PA chest films. Describe these modifications from the adult examination.

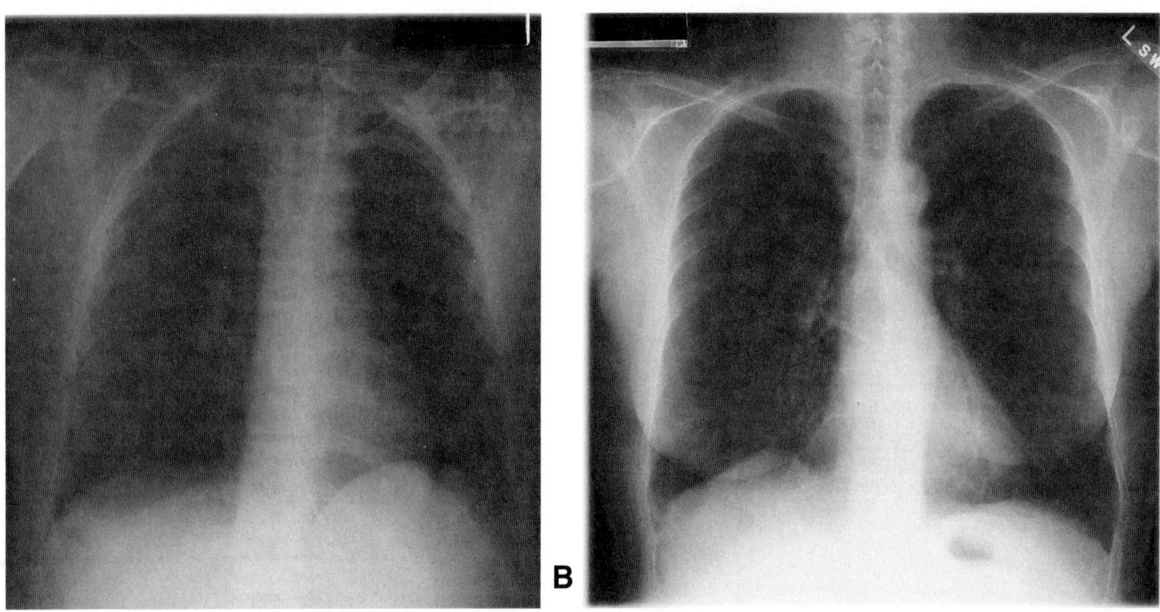

FIGURE 2.5 Radiograph of chest, frontal projections (A) and (B).

81. A patient arrives through the emergency room and is sent to the radiology department in a wheelchair for a chest x-ray. You have to decide whether to perform the examination with the patient standing, sitting, or lying down. Give at least three critical pieces of information that you would use to make your decision.

82. A radiographer is examining the two radiographs in Figure 2.5, a routine PA upright chest taken today and an AP supine chest taken last week. How can the radiographer determine which film is which, by comparing the anatomy demonstrated on the radiographs?

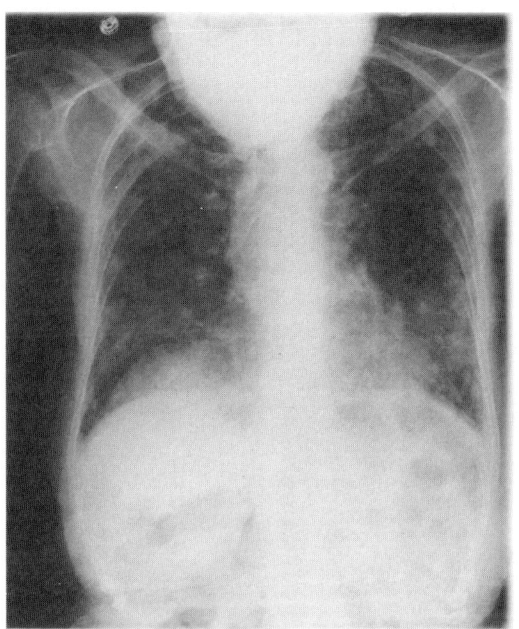

FIGURE 2.6 Radiograph of chest, PA projection with artifact.

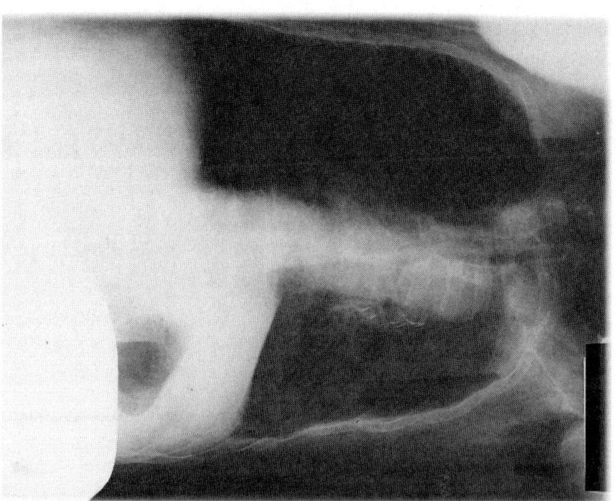

FIGURE 2.7 Radiograph of chest, fluid level.

83. A radiographer examines the PA chest radiograph in Figure 2.6 and is attempting to identify the radiopaque shadow covering the upper thoracic vertebrae. Describe the positioning error that likely caused this shadow and how it can be corrected.

84. Can you name the projection used to obtain the radiograph in Figure 2.7, given the fluid level demonstrated in the lung? If this film had been taken with the patient supine using a vertical beam, would this fluid level appear differently? What would the appearance of the fluid level have been if the patient were upright using a horizontal beam (PA chest)?

Do You Remember?

85. Which term refers to the longitudinal or long portion of a structure?

a. tangential

b. lordotic

c. decubitus

d. axial

86. Which term means lying down in any position?

a. decubitus

b. prone

c. supine

d. recumbent

87. A supine patient is rotated 45° toward the left side. This position is referred to as:

a. LAO

b. LPO

c. RAO

d. RPO

88. Which plane divides the body into front and back sections?

a. sagittal

b. midsagittal

c. transverse

d. coronal

89. The average body type that comprises approximately half of the population is called:

a. hyposthenic

b. sthenic

c. asthenic

d. hypersthenic

STUDY TIP: STUDY TIME

Trisha: "I can't believe I failed that test, I studied at least 30 hours."

Instructor Bob: "No kidding, 30 hours seems like a long time. That should have been enough to do well."

Trisha: "I did better on the previous test and I hardly studied. Maybe I should just study less from now on."

Conversations such as this occur daily in instructor offices. Study time is one of the most important factors affecting success on tests. It is well documented that, other factors being equal, the amount of study time is directly related to test scores. Simply stated, the more students study, the better their performance. How then can we explain Trisha's situation?

Instructor Bob: "Tell me about how and when you studied for last Monday's test."

Trisha: "Well, I studied from noon to 10:00 PM on Saturday and noon to 2:00 AM on Sunday/Monday."

Instructor Bob: "That's not 30 hours."

Trisha: "Oh, I just rounded off."

Trisha's problem is a common one—waiting until the last 2 days before a test to begin preparing. She studied 24 hours, which for Trisha was probably plenty of preparation time to do well on the test. Learning, however, takes time.

- Always prepare for a test at least a week in advance. The more material to be included on the test and the more important the test, the longer should be the preparation time.
- Try not to study more than 50 minutes without a 5- to 10-minute break and never study when tired. More than 2 hours in a single session is usually not productive. Trisha would have benefited much more by studying 2 hours per day for the 12 days preceding the test than by studying 24 hours 2 days before the test. The same amount of study time would likely have resulted in a very different test score.

> There is no such thing as too much studying. It is impossible for studying to lower your grade. If your grade becomes lower after studying, chances are it is because of *how* you studied (too much at one time) or *what* you studied (perhaps your notes were awful)!

CHAPTER 3

Abdomen

LEARNING OBJECTIVES

At the completion of this chapter, the student should be able to:

1. List and describe the soft tissue and bony anatomy of the abdomen.
2. Identify the quadrant in which abdominal organs are located.
3. Given drawings and radiographs, locate anatomic structures and landmarks.
4. Explain the rationale for each projection.
5. Explain the patient preparation required for each examination.
6. Describe the positioning used to visualize anatomic structures of the abdomen.
7. List or identify the central ray location and the extent of the field necessary for each projection.
8. Differentiate between the positioning and centering factors for an acute abdomen series and a routine supine and upright abdomen.
9. Explain the protective measures that should be taken for each examination.
10. Recommend the technical factors for producing an acceptable radiograph for each projection.
11. State the patient instructions for each projection.
12. Given radiographs, evaluate positioning and technical factors.
13. Describe modifications of procedures for atypical or impaired patients to better demonstrate the anatomic area of interest.

Routine and Alternative Positions/Projections

Part	Routine	Alternative
Abdomen	Supine/KUB	
	AP upright	Lateral decubitus
	Acute abdomen series	
		Lateral

QUESTIONS

Anatomy and Physiology

For questions 1–20, identify the anatomy of the abdominal viscera in Figure 3.1.

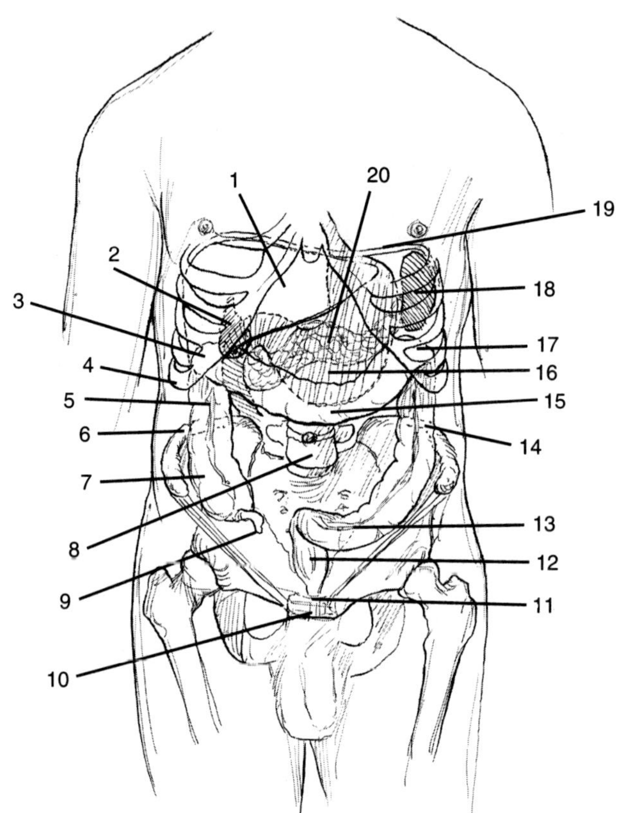

FIGURE 3.1 Diagram of abdominal viscera, anterior view.

1. ____________________
2. ____________________
3. ____________________
4. ____________________
5. ____________________
6. ____________________
7. ____________________
8. ____________________
9. ____________________
10. ____________________
11. ____________________
12. ____________________
13. ____________________
14. ____________________
15. ____________________
16. ____________________
17. ____________________
18. ____________________
19. ____________________
20. ____________________

For questions 21–29, identify the regions of the abdomen in Figure 3.2.

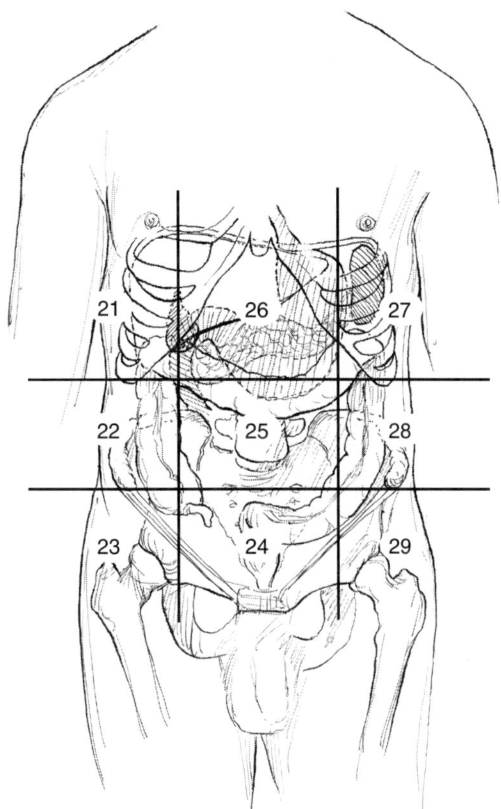

FIGURE 3.2 Diagram of abdominal regions.

21. ______________________

22. ______________________

23. ______________________

24. ______________________

25. ______________________

26. ______________________

27. ______________________

28. ______________________

29. ______________________

For questions 30–35, identify the abdominal muscles and urinary system anatomy in Figure 3.3.

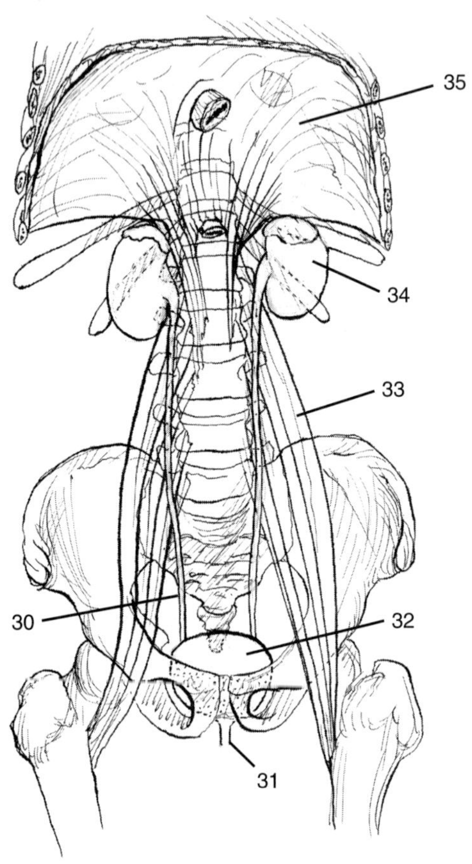

FIGURE 3.3 Diagram of abdominal muscles and urinary system, anterior view.

30. ____________________

31. ____________________

32. ____________________

33. ____________________

34. ____________________

35. ____________________

For questions 36–45, identify the anatomy of the accessory digestive organs in Figure 3.4.

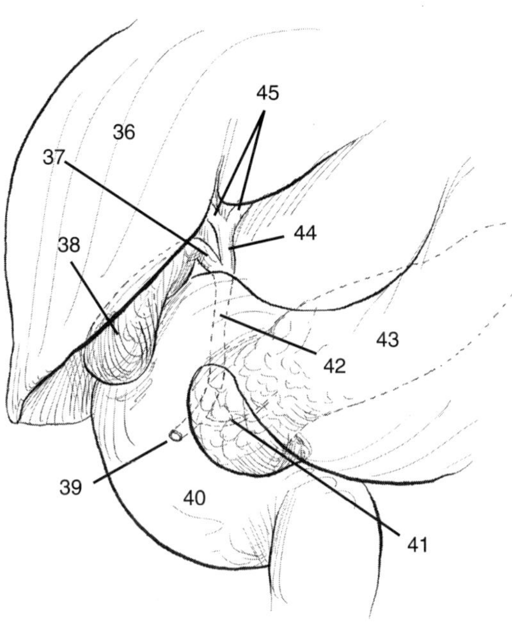

FIGURE 3.4 Diagram of the accessory digestive organs, anterior view.

36. ______________________

37. ______________________

38. ______________________

39. ______________________

40. ______________________

41. ______________________

42. ______________________

43. ______________________

44. ______________________

45. ______________________

46. The ______________ attaches most of the small intestine to the posterior abdominal wall.

47. Compared to the sthenic patient, the stomach on an asthenic patient is located

______________________________________.

48. The appendix is normally found in the ______________ ______________ region.

For questions 49–56, match the organ with the quadrant in which the majority of the organ lies.

	Organ	Quadrant
49._____	spleen	**a.** right upper
50._____	liver	**b.** right lower
51._____	cecum	**c.** left upper
52._____	sigmoid colon	**d.** left lower
53._____	stomach	
54._____	appendix	
55._____	hepatic flexure	
56._____	gallbladder	

57. The ASIS is inferior to the iliac crest.

a. true

b. false

58. The greater trochanter lies at the approximate level of the pubic symphysis.

a. true

b. false

59. Free air in the peritoneum will normally sink to the lowest point in the abdominopelvic cavity.

a. true

b. false

60. Which of the following is *not* one of the nine regions of the abdomen?

a. lumbar

b. hypochondrium

c. gastric

d. iliac

61. The position of the diaphragm will _____ during expiration.

a. lower

b. raise

c. remain unchanged

d. first lower then raise

62. The portion of the peritoneum that adheres to the abdominopelvic cavity is called the:

a. parietal peritoneum

b. visceral peritoneum

c. peritoneal cavity

d. serous peritoneum

63. The term retroperitoneal refers to _____ the peritoneum.

a. around

b. inside

c. in front of

d. behind

64. Which of the following is an organ that contains glands with both endocrine and exocrine functions?

a. gallbladder

b. liver

c. spleen

d. pancreas

65. Which organ is divided into head, body, and tail portions?

a. gallbladder

b. liver

c. stomach

d. pancreas

66. The iliac crest lies at the approximate level of:

a. T12

b. L1–L2

c. L3–L4

d. the sacrum

67. Which term refers to a bowel obstruction?

a. ileus

b. pneumoperitoneum

c. calculus

d. hernia

Radiographic Procedures, Analysis, and Critical Thinking

For questions 68–77, identify the radiographic anatomy of the abdomen in Figure 3.5A.

68. ______________________

69. ______________________

70. ______________________

71. ______________________

72. ______________________

73. ______________________

74. ______________________

75. ______________________

76. ______________________

77. ______________________

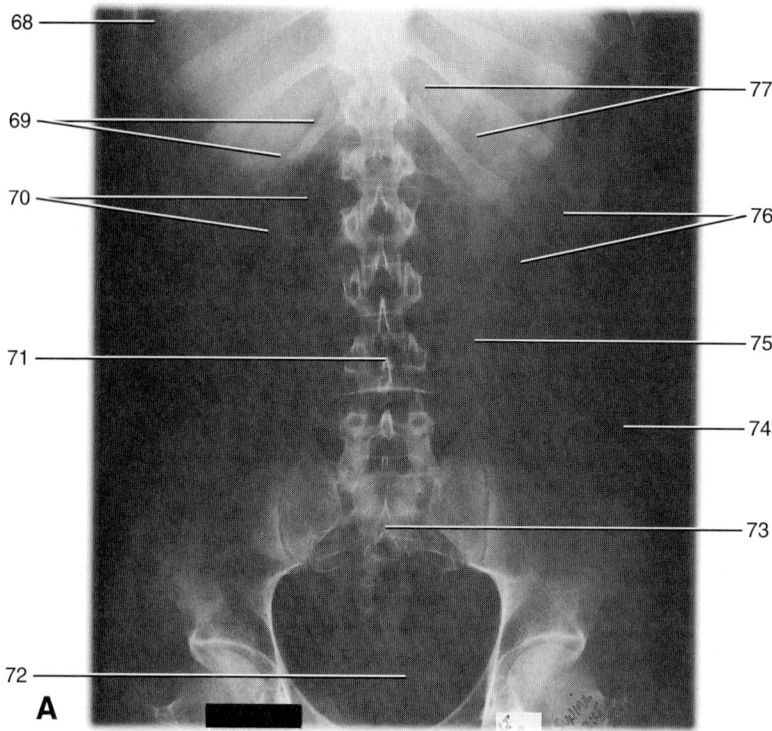

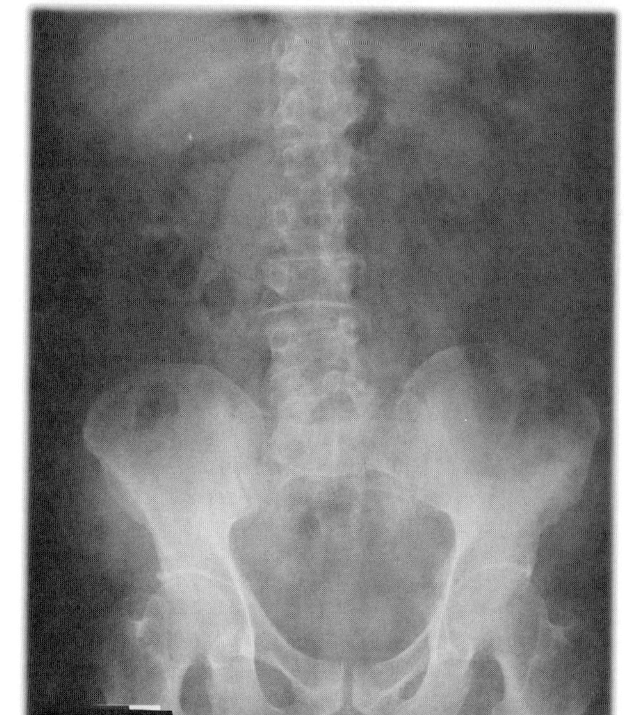

FIGURE 3.5 Abdomen, supine AP projection: (A) correct positioning, (B) incorrect positioning.

78. Compare the positioning quality of the correctly positioned radiograph in Figure 3.5A with that in Figure 3.5B. Describe the positioning error, explain what caused it, and give the step(s) necessary to correct the problem.

79. Although few muscles can be visualized radiographically, the psoas muscles are demonstrated on abdomen films because

______________________________.

80. Most abdominal radiographs require a kVp range of

______________________________.

81. What are the correct breathing instructions for abdominal radiography?

a. hold breath on full expiration

b. hold breath on full inspiration

c. shallow breathing during the exposure

d. no breathing instructions need to be given

82. Where is the central ray location for a KUB examination?

a. iliac crest

b. ASIS

c. 1.5 inches above the iliac crest

d. 1.5 inches below the iliac crest

83. Which of the following are *not* clearly demonstrated on a KUB?

1. gallbladder

2. pancreas

3. ilium

a. 1 and 2

b. 1 and 3

c. 2 and 3

d. 1, 2, and 3

84. Where is the central ray location for an upright AP projection of the abdomen?

a. iliac crest

b. ASIS

c. 2 inches above the iliac crest

d. 2 inches below the iliac crest

85. Where is the central ray location for a lateral projection of the abdomen?

a. at the midaxillary line

b. 2 inches anterior to the midaxillary line

c. 2 inches posterior to the midaxillary line

d. 4 inches anterior to the midaxillary line

86. Which projection of the abdomen best demonstrates calcifications of the aorta?

a. AP

b. upright AP

c. lateral

d. lateral decubitus

87. Where is the central ray location for an AP lateral decubitus projection of the abdomen?

a. iliac crest

b. ASIS

c. 2 inches above the iliac crest

d. 2 inches below the iliac crest

88. In the left lateral decubitus projection of the abdomen, free air will form shadows under the:

a. spleen

b. stomach

c. liver

d. right hemidiaphragm

89. Which of the following *must* be true to demonstrate air/fluid levels in the abdomen?

a. Patient must be upright.

b. Beam must be horizontal.

c. 40 inch SID must be used.

d. None of the above must be true.

90. If a patient is too ill to stand for an upright abdomen, which of the following should be substituted?

a. right lateral decubitus

b. left lateral decubitus

c. 45° semi-upright

d. supine KUB

91. Rupture of which of the following would be the *most* likely cause of free air on an upright abdomen radiograph?

a. colon

b. spleen

c. kidney

d. liver

92. In cases of suspected bowel obstructions, a lateral decubitus projection of the abdomen would be taken to demonstrate:

a. the location of the obstructive material

b. the mobility of the colon

c. the presence of gas or fluid levels

d. torn mesentery

93. An acute abdomen series includes:

1. supine AP projection of the abdomen/KUB

2. supine AP projection of the chest

3. upright AP projection of the abdomen

a. 1 and 2

b. 1 and 3

c. 2 and 3

d. 1, 2, and 3

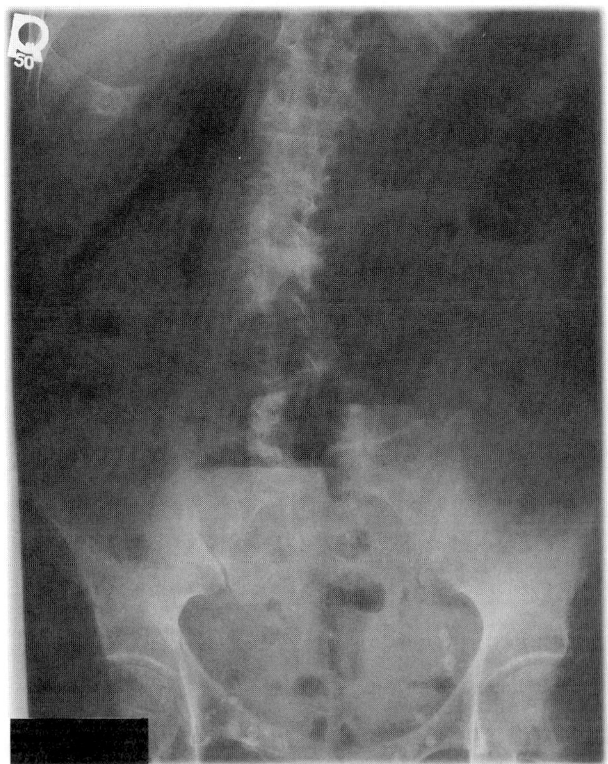

FIGURE 3.6 Radiograph of abdomen, upright AP projection.

94. The radiograph in Figure 3.6 was taken of a patient with a bowel obstruction. Describe structures on the radiograph that would lead you to conclude that this was taken with the patient upright rather than supine.

95. A radiographer takes an upright AP projection of the abdomen and notices that only the left hemidiaphragm is included on the radiograph. Should the film be repeated? Why or why not?

96. Explain why it is necessary to keep the patient upright for at least 5 minutes before taking an upright AP projection of the abdomen.

97. A radiographer is performing a left lateral decubitus abdomen on a hypersthenic patient who is too large to fit on a 14 x 17 inch film. Explain what positioning modifications should be taken to accommodate this patient.

98. Why are most abdominal organs difficult to visualize radiographically without the use of contrast media?

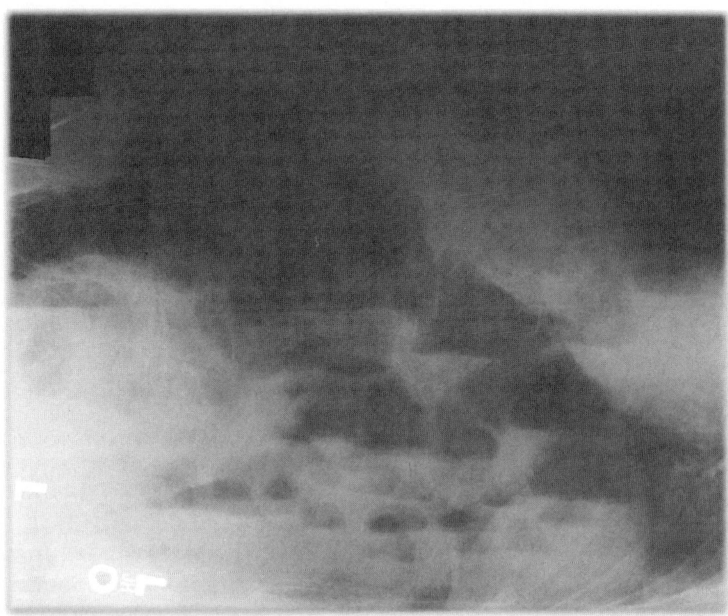

FIGURE 3.7 Radiograph of abdomen, left lateral decubitus with air-fluid levels.

99. Examine the radiograph in Figure 3.7. What cues indicate that this was a left lateral decubitus projection? If this film had been taken with the patient supine using a vertical beam, would this fluid level appear differently? What would the appearance of the fluid level have been if the patient were supine using a horizontal beam?

Do You Remember?

100. On a lateral chest the intervertebral joint spaces of the thoracic vertebrae should be clearly visible.

a. true

b. false

101. Bending a joint to decrease the angle of the two bones is known as:

a. extension

b. flexion

c. dorsiflexion

d. adduction

102. Which of the following is *not* a primary exposure factor?

a. source-image distance

b. milliamperage

c. time

d. kilovoltage

103. How many ribs should be demonstrated on a properly positioned PA projection of the chest?

a. 7

b. 8

c. 10

d. 12

104. The primary bronchi enter the lungs at the:

a. hilum

b. apex

c. base

d. carina

105. Which of the following must occur to demonstrate fluid in the pleural space?

a. Patient must be upright.

b. Patient must be supine.

c. Patient must be upright and the beam must be horizontal.

d. The beam must be horizontal.

106. Which term means the *opposite* of medial?

a. posterior

b. anterior

c. contralateral

d. lateral

STUDY TIP: OVERCOMING "BAD" TEACHERS

Pat: "I failed this test miserably and it's all the teacher's fault!"

Instructor Bob: "How could the teacher cause you to fail a test?"

Pat: "Ms. Collins is a terrible teacher. She talks too fast and skips around during the lecture. By the time I have written down the important things, she has moved on to something else."

Instructor Bob: "That's hard to believe. Ms. Collins has been teaching successfully here for many years, and her students always perform well on the Registry exam."

In fact, Ms. Collins does move quickly through the material. She is a global teacher who discusses the major concept or idea first and returns to the details later. Pat, on the other hand, is a linear learner who prefers that information be discussed in a sequential order. Pat is having trouble following this style of instruction and is blaming his teacher for his failure.

An experienced teacher is not likely to change teaching techniques for a single student in the class. It is not practical. Each student must learn "survival techniques" for dealing with the various types of instructors.

- In a private conference, politely ask the teacher if he or she can slow the pace. Be aware that most instructors have a set amount of material that they must cover to prepare students for the next class.
- Audiotape the lecture and listen to it later. Keep each lecture tape until after the course is completed so that you can use it to study for a comprehensive final examination.
- Find out what material is going to be covered ahead of time. Reading ahead will give you knowledge of the subject so you can more easily follow and understand the lecture.
- Borrow other students' notes after class to see if you missed any important points during the lecture.

In an ideal world, the instructor modifies his or her teaching to the learning styles of each student. In the real world, the student must develop strategies to cope with each instructor's teaching style. If you do poorly on a test, do not blame the teacher for your performance but instead focus on modifying your learning to match the teacher.

SECTION III

LIMBS and THORAX

CHAPTER 4

Upper Limb and Shoulder Girdle

LEARNING OBJECTIVES

At the completion of this chapter, the student should be able to:

1. List and describe the anatomy of the upper limb and shoulder girdle.
2. Given drawings and radiographs, locate anatomic structures and landmarks.
3. Explain the rationale for each projection.
4. Explain the patient preparation required for each examination.
5. Describe the positioning used to visualize anatomic structures in the upper limb and shoulder girdle.
6. List or identify the central ray location and the extent of the field necessary for each projection.
7. Explain the protective measures that should be taken for each examination.
8. Recommend the technical factors for producing an acceptable radiograph for each projection.
9. State the patient instructions for each projection.
10. Given radiographs, evaluate positioning and technical factors.
11. Describe modifications of procedures for atypical or impaired patients to better demonstrate the anatomic area of interest.

Routine and Alternative Positions/Projections

Part	Routine	Alternative
Finger	PA (tip: AP)	
	Oblique	
	Lateral	
Thumb	AP (tip: PA)	AP axial/First metacarpophalangeal joint
	Oblique	
	Lateral	
Hand	PA (tip: PA)	Ball-catcher's (Norgaard)
		AP axial (Brewerton)
	Oblique	
	Lateral	
Wrist	PA	Ulnar flexion
		Radial flexion
		Scaphoid (Stecher)
		Axial oblique (Clements-Nakayama)
		Tangential: carpal bridge
		Tangential: carpal canal (Gaynor-Hart)
	Oblique	
	Lateral	
		PA and lateral casted variations
Forearm	AP	
	Lateral	
Elbow	AP	Partial flexion (trauma AP)
		Acute flexion
	Obliques (medial/lateral)	Radial head/coronoid process (Coyle)
	Lateral	
		Radial head/lateromedial rotation
Humerus	AP	Transthoracic lateral
	Lateral	
Shoulder	AP internal rotation	
	AP external rotation	
	AP neutral rotation	

		Inferosuperior axial projection (Lawrence)
		Inferosuperior axial projection (West Point) (tip: Clements modification)
		AP axial/coracoid process
		Glenoid cavity (Grashey)
		Scapular Y
		Intertubercular groove
Scapula	AP	
	Lateral	
Clavicle	PA (tip: PA axial)	AP axial
		Tangential (Tarrant)
Acromioclavicular joints	AP with and without weight	

QUESTIONS

Anatomy and Physiology

For questions 1–10, identify the anatomy of the hand in Figure 4.1.

1. ______________________

2. ______________________

3. ______________________

4. ______________________

5. ______________________

6. ______________________

7. ______________________

8. ______________________

9. ______________________

10. ______________________

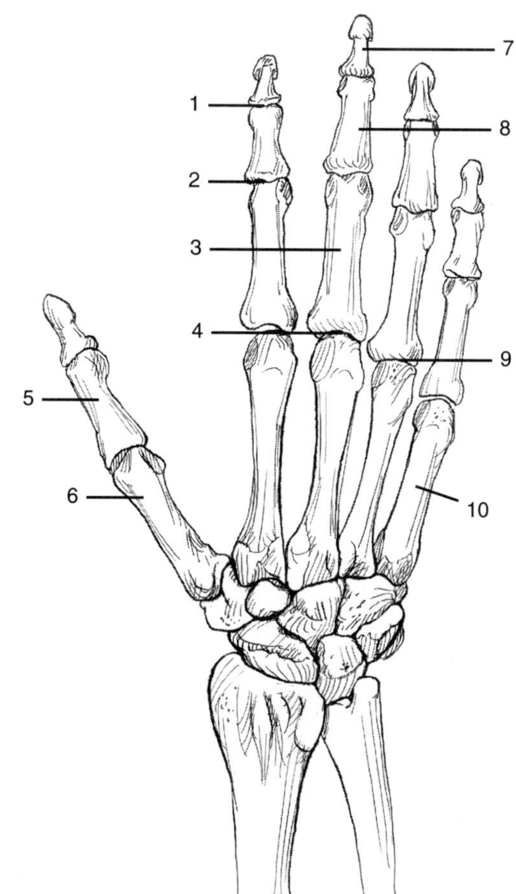

FIGURE 4.1 Diagram of hand, posterior view.

For questions 11–22, identify the anatomy of the wrist in Figure 4.2.

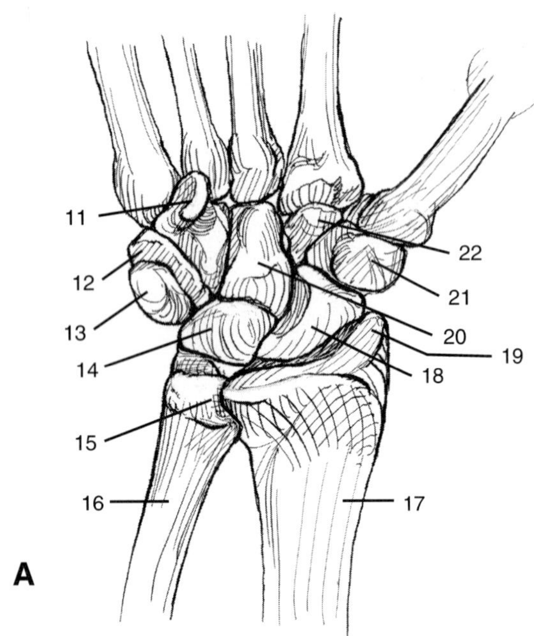

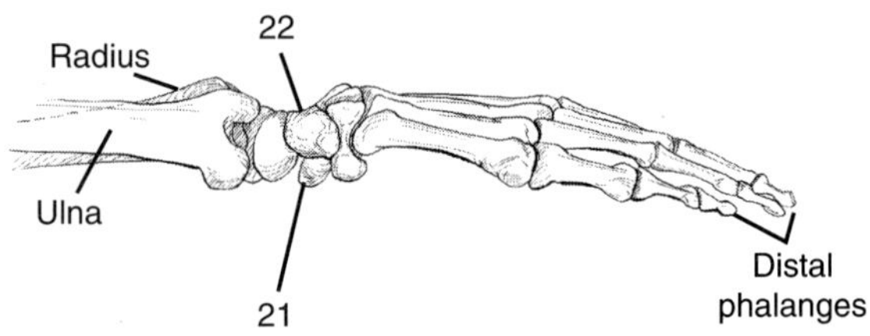

FIGURE 4.2 Diagram of wrist, (A) anterior and (B) lateral views.

11. ____________________

12. ____________________

13. ____________________

14. ____________________

15. ____________________

16. ____________________

17. ____________________

18. ____________________

19. ____________________

20. ____________________

21. ____________________

22. ____________________

For questions 23–34, identify the anatomy of the elbow in Figure 4.3.

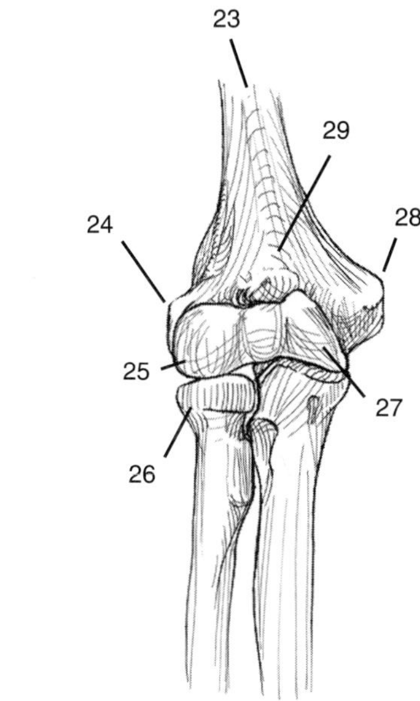

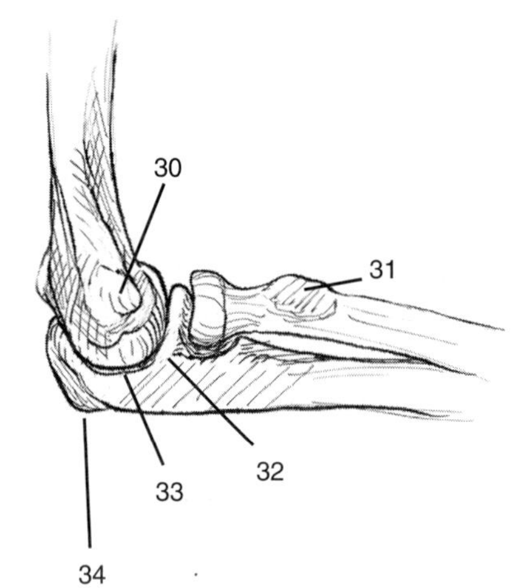

FIGURE 4.3 Diagram of elbow, (A) anterior and (B) lateral views.

23. ______________________

24. ______________________

25. ______________________

26. ______________________

27. ______________________

28. ______________________

29. ______________________

30. ______________________

31. ______________________

32. ______________________

33. ______________________

34. ______________________

For questions 35–44, identify the anatomy of the humerus in Figure 4.4.

35. ____________________

36. ____________________

37. ____________________

38. ____________________

39. ____________________

40. ____________________

41. ____________________

42. ____________________

43. ____________________

44. ____________________

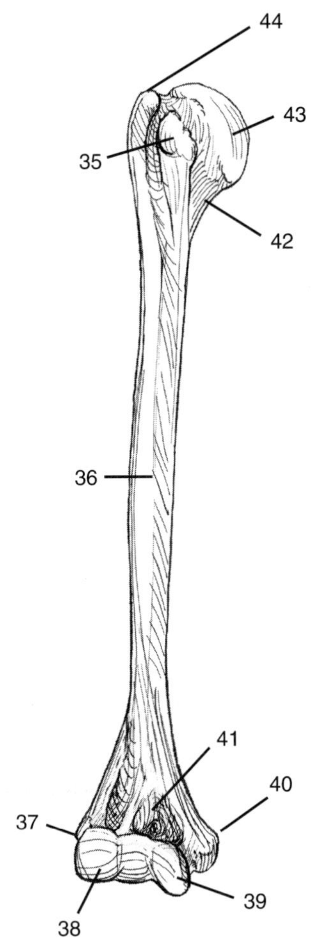

FIGURE 4.4 Diagram of humerus, anterior view.

For questions 45–52, identify the anatomy of the shoulder in Figure 4.5.

45. ____________________

46. ____________________

47. ____________________

48. ____________________

49. ____________________

50. ____________________

51. ____________________

52. ____________________

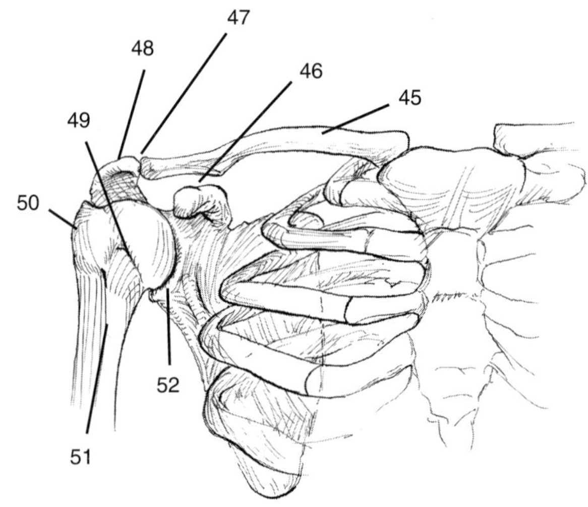

FIGURE 4.5 Diagram of shoulder, anterior view.

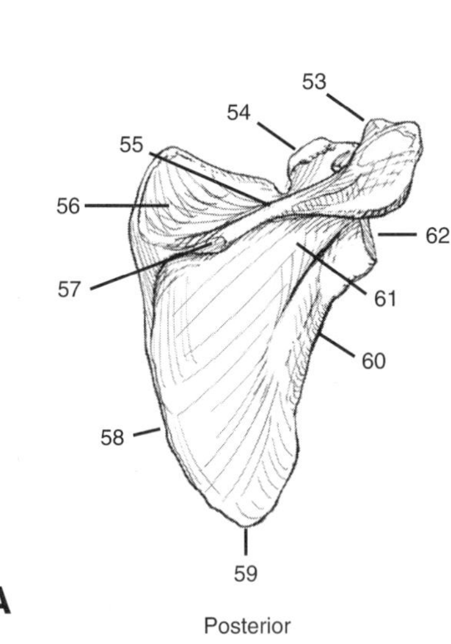

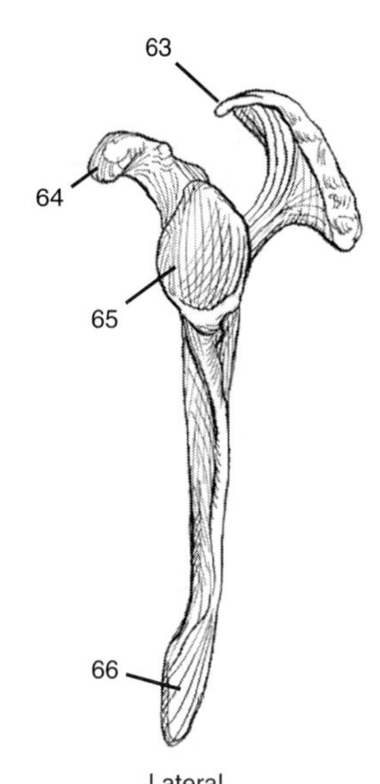

FIGURE 4.6 Diagram of scapula, (A) posterior and (B) lateral views.

For questions 53–66, identify the anatomy of the scapula in Figure 4.6.

53. ____________________	**60.** ____________________
54. ____________________	**61.** ____________________
55. ____________________	**62.** ____________________
56. ____________________	**63.** ____________________
57. ____________________	**64.** ____________________
58. ____________________	**65.** ____________________
59. ____________________	**66.** ____________________

For questions 67–74, match the preferred carpal name with its older name.

	Preferred Name	Older Name
67. _____	pisiform	**a.** os magnum
68. _____	triquetrum	**b.** unciform
69. _____	hamate	**c.** semilunar
70. _____	capitate	**d.** navicular
71. _____	lunate	**e.** greater multangular
72. _____	trapezoid	**f.** lesser multangular
73. _____	trapezium	**g.** triangular
74. _____	scaphoid	**h.** None of the above

75. The right hand normally possesses _____ phalanges.

a. 11

b. 12

c. 13

d. 14

76. The head of the radius articulates with the:

a. ulna

b. semilunar notch

c. trochlea

d. capitellum

77. The olecranon fossa is located on the:

a. anterior surface of the humerus

b. anterior surface of the ulna

c. posterior surface of the humerus

d. posterior surface of the ulna

78. Which of the following are in the *proximal* row of carpal bones?

a. capitate, hamate, and multangular

b. hamate, lunate, and navicular

c. capitate, lunate, and pisiform

d. lunate, scaphoid, and triquetrum

79. With the arm in the anatomic position, the radius is on the _____ side.

a. lateral

b. ventral

c. medial

d. posterior

80. Which process in the elbow is the most easily palpable?

a. radial tuberosity

b. lateral epicondyle

c. coracoid process

d. medial epicondyle

81. Which process of the scapula projects anteriorly?

a. coracoid

b. acromion

c. coronoid

d. glenoid

Radiographic Procedures, Analysis, and Critical Thinking

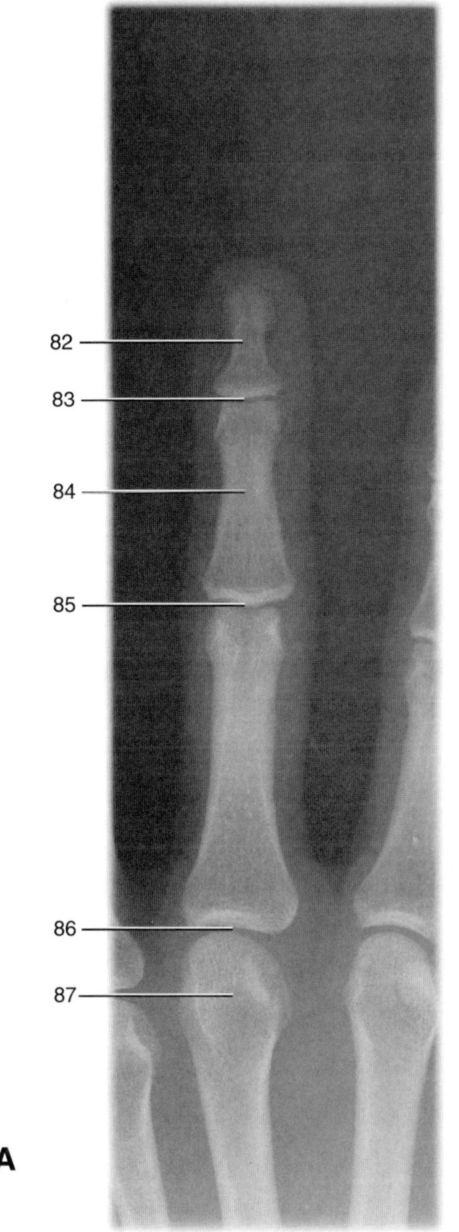

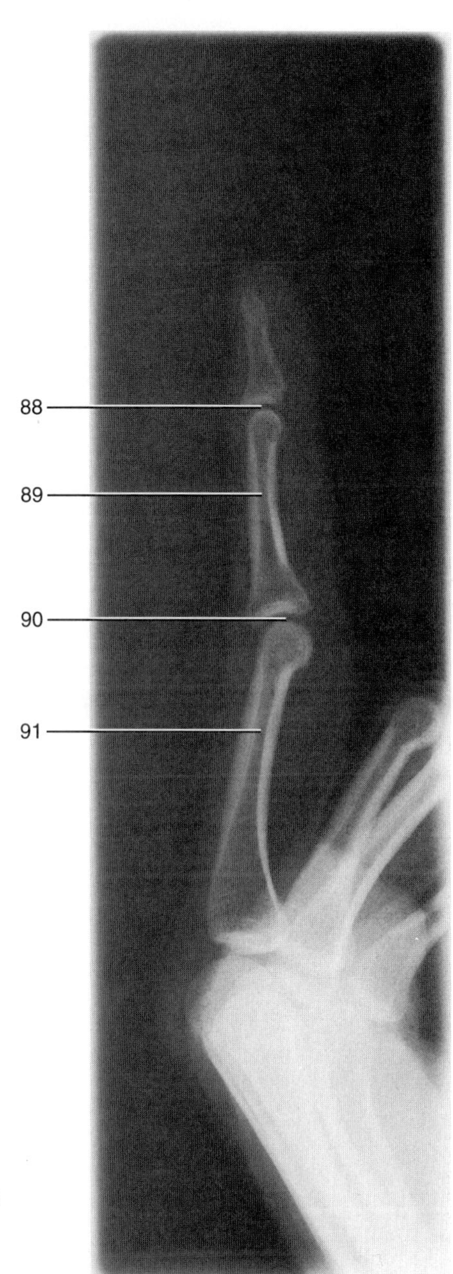

FIGURE 4.7 Radiograph of finger, (A) PA and (B) lateral projection.

For questions 82–91, identify the radiographic anatomy of the finger in Figure 4.7.

82. ______________________

83. ______________________

84. ______________________

85. ______________________

86. ______________________

87. ______________________

88. ______________________

89. ______________________

90. ______________________

91. ______________________

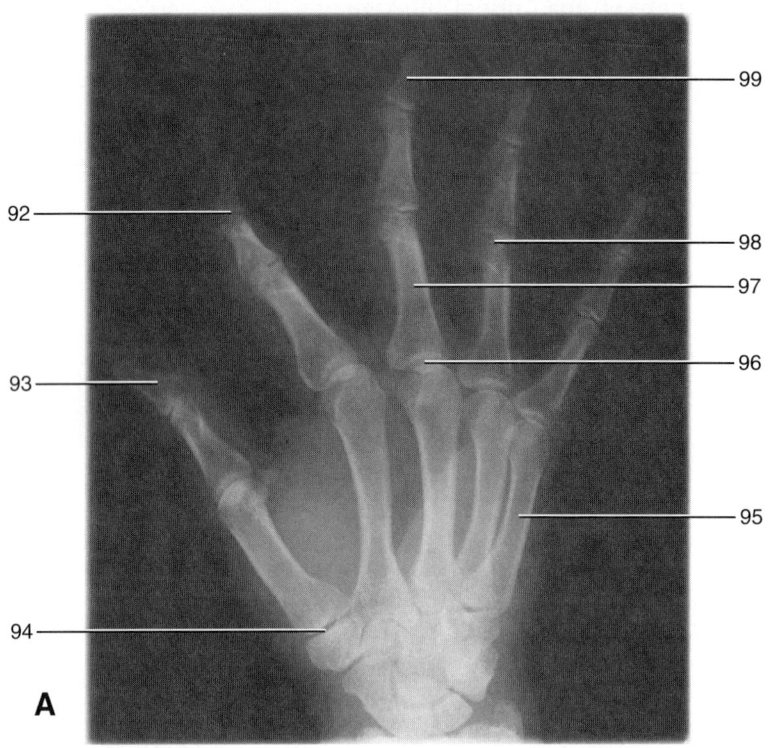

FIGURE 4.8A Radiograph of hand, oblique projection, correct positioning.

For questions 92–99, identify the anatomy on the oblique hand projection in Figure 4.8A.

92. ____________________

93. ____________________

94. ____________________

95. ____________________

96. ____________________

97. ____________________

98. ____________________

99. ____________________

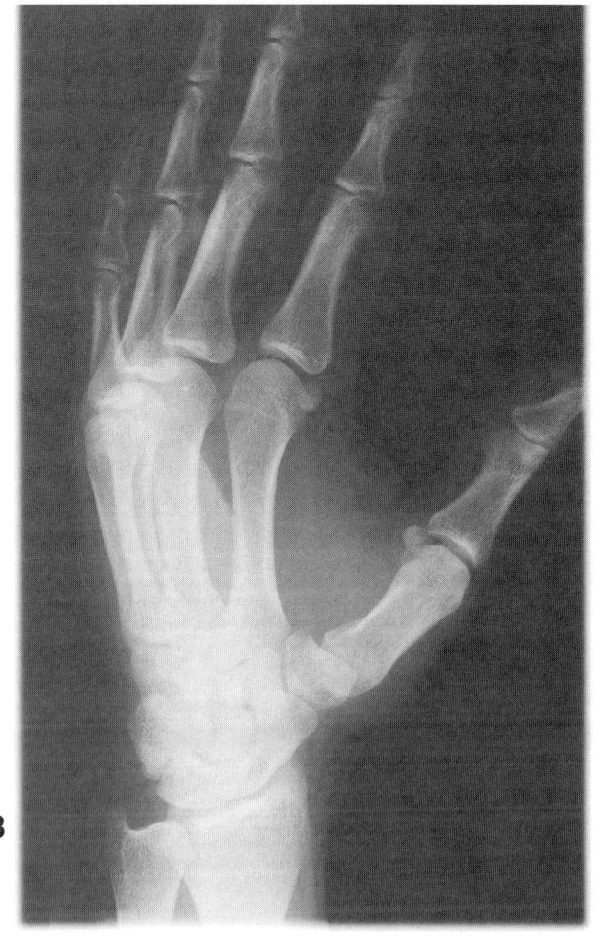

FIGURE 4.8B Radiograph of hand, oblique projection, incorrect positioning.

100. Compare the positioning quality of the correctly positioned radiograph in Figure 4.8A with that in Figure 4.8B. Describe the positioning error, explain what caused it, and give the step(s) necessary to correct the problem.

For questions 101–110, identify the radiographic anatomy of the wrist in Figure 4.9.

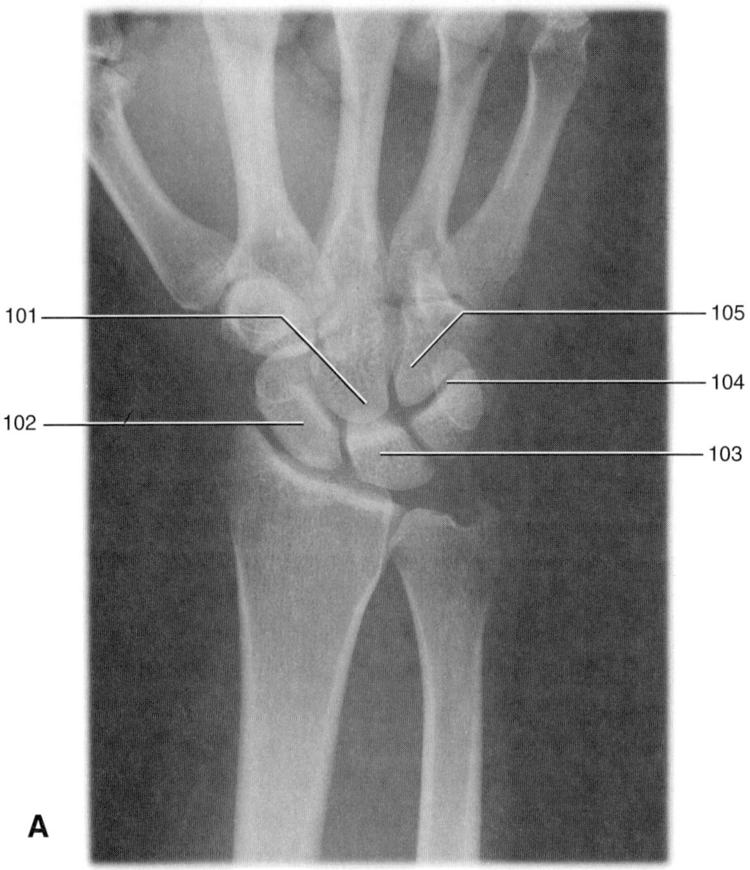

FIGURE 4.9A Radiograph of wrist, PA projection.

101. ______________________

102. ______________________

103. ______________________

104. ______________________

105. ______________________

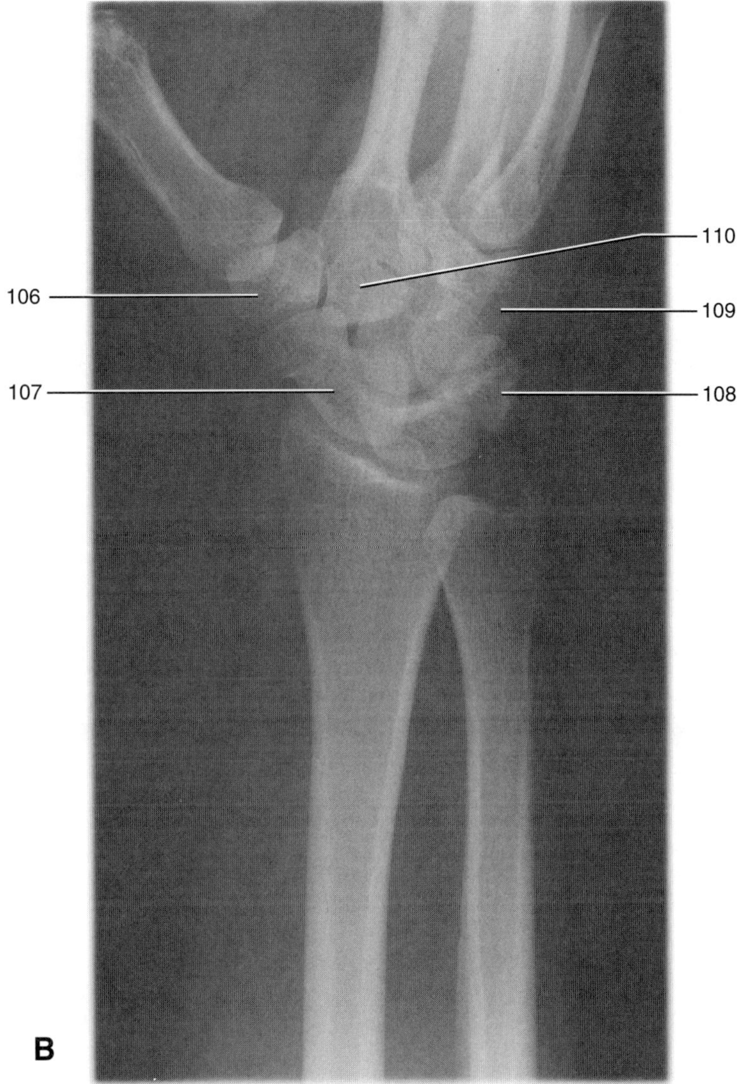

FIGURE 4.9B Radiograph of wrist, oblique projection.

106. ____________________

107. ____________________

108. ____________________

109. ____________________

110. ____________________

For questions 111–118, identify the radiographic anatomy on the lateral forearm projection in Figure 4.10A.

111. ______________________

112. ______________________

113. ______________________

114. ______________________

115. ______________________

116. ______________________

117. ______________________

118. ______________________

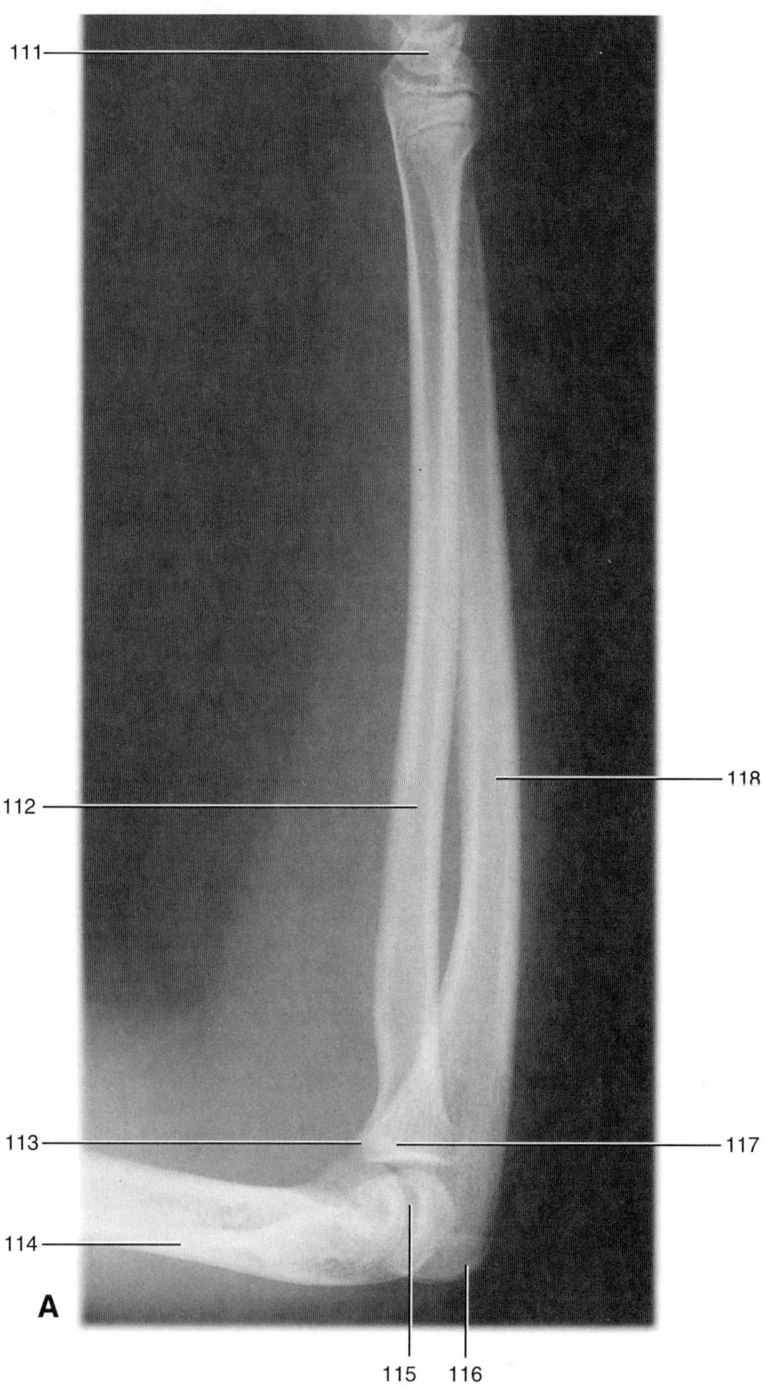

FIGURE 4.10A Radiograph of forearm, lateral projection, correct positioning.

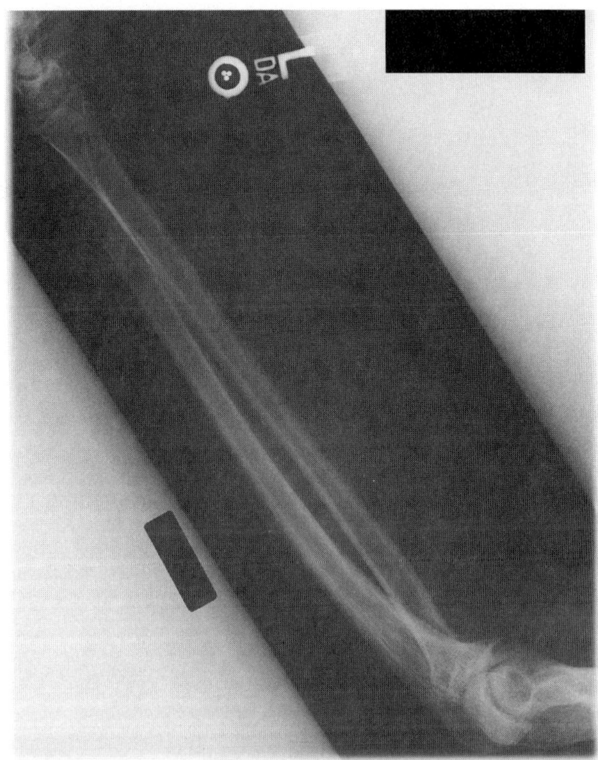

FIGURE 4.10B Radiograph of forearm, lateral projection,incorrect positioning.

119. Compare the positioning quality of the correctly positioned radiograph in Figure 4.10A with that in Figure 4.10B. Describe the positioning error, explain what caused it, and give the step(s) necessary to correct the problem.

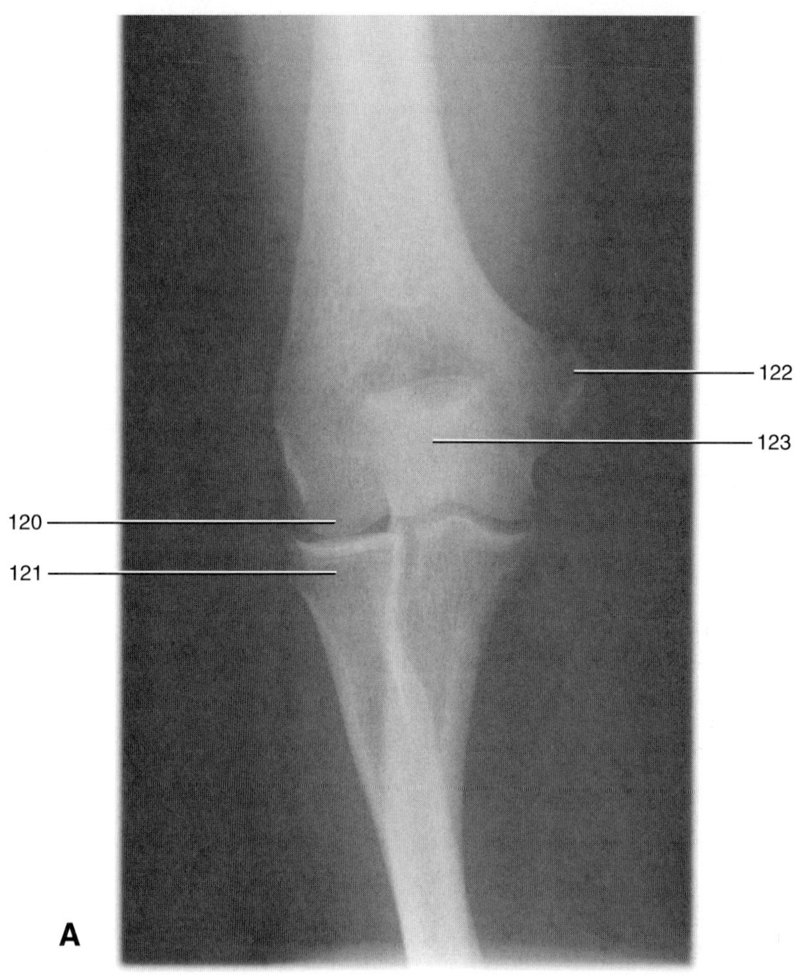

FIGURE 4.11A Radiograph of elbow, oblique projection, internal.

For questions 120–130, identify the radiographic anatomy on the oblique elbow in Figure 4.11.

120. ____________________

121. ____________________

122. ____________________

123. ____________________

124. ____________________

125. ____________________

126. ____________________

127. ____________________

128. ____________________

129. ____________________

130. ____________________

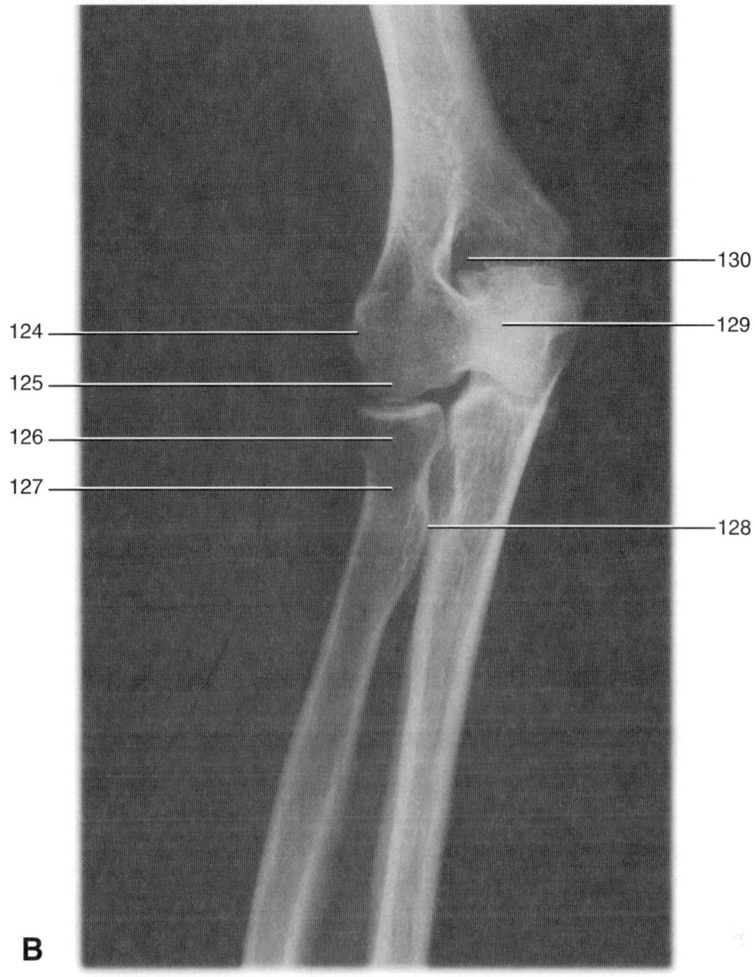

FIGURE 4.11B Radiograph of elbow, oblique projection external.

131. Compare the two elbow radiographs in Figures 4.11 (A) and (B), describing observed differences in the anatomic appearance of the two projections, and determine which is the internal oblique.

For questions 132–137, identify the radiographic anatomy on the lateral elbow projection in Figure 4.12A.

132. ______________________

133. ______________________

134. ______________________

135. ______________________

136. ______________________

137. ______________________

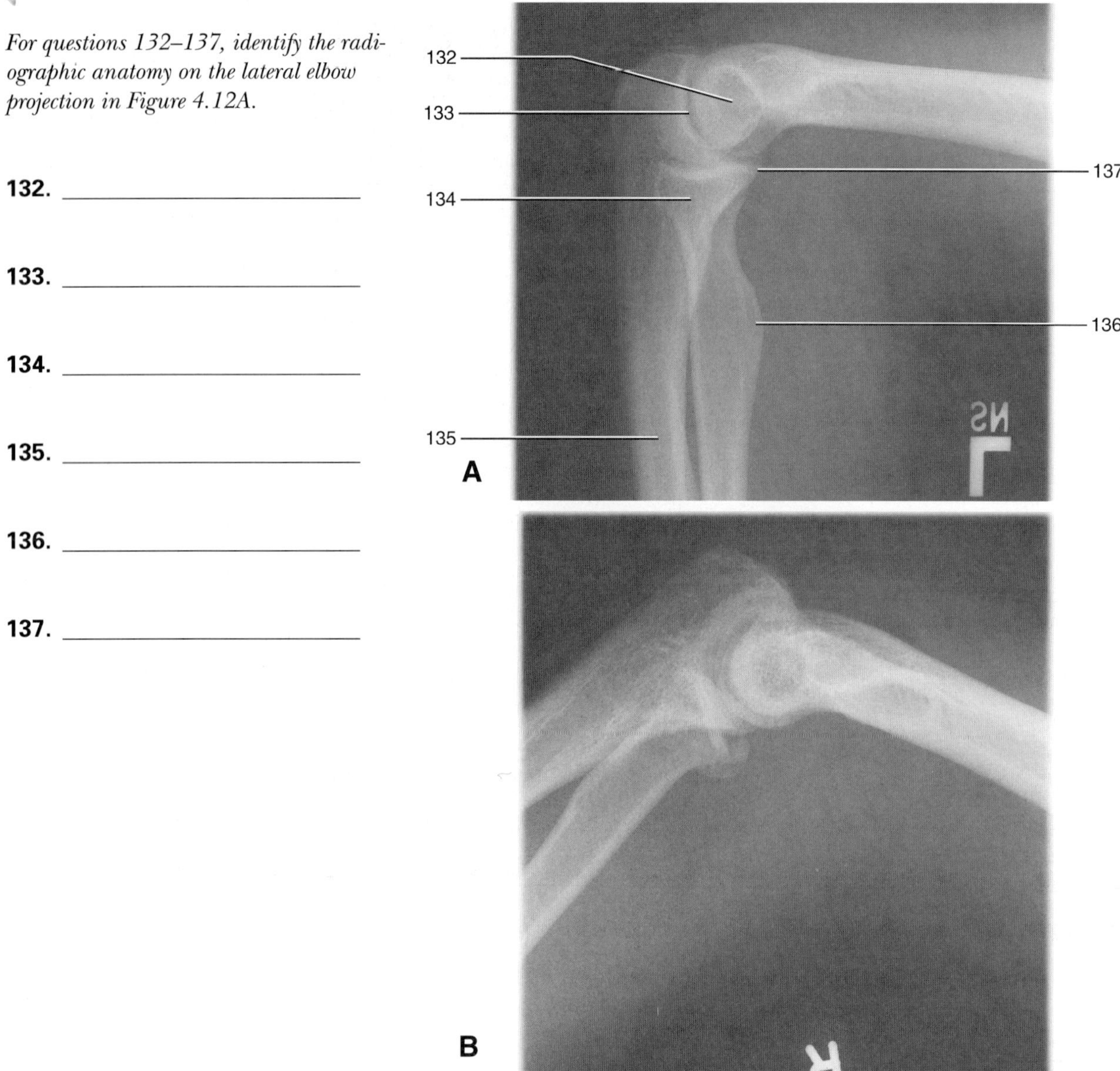

FIGURE 4.12 Radiograph of elbow, lateral projection, (A) correct positioning and (B) incorrect positioning.

138. Compare the positioning quality of the correctly positioned radiograph in Figure 4.12A with that in Figure 4.12B. Describe the positioning error, explain what caused it, and give the step(s) necessary to correct the problem.

For questions 139–148, identify the radiographic anatomy of the shoulder in Figure 4.13.

139. ____________________

140. ____________________

141. ____________________

142. ____________________

143. ____________________

144. ____________________

145. ____________________

146. ____________________

147. ____________________

148. ____________________

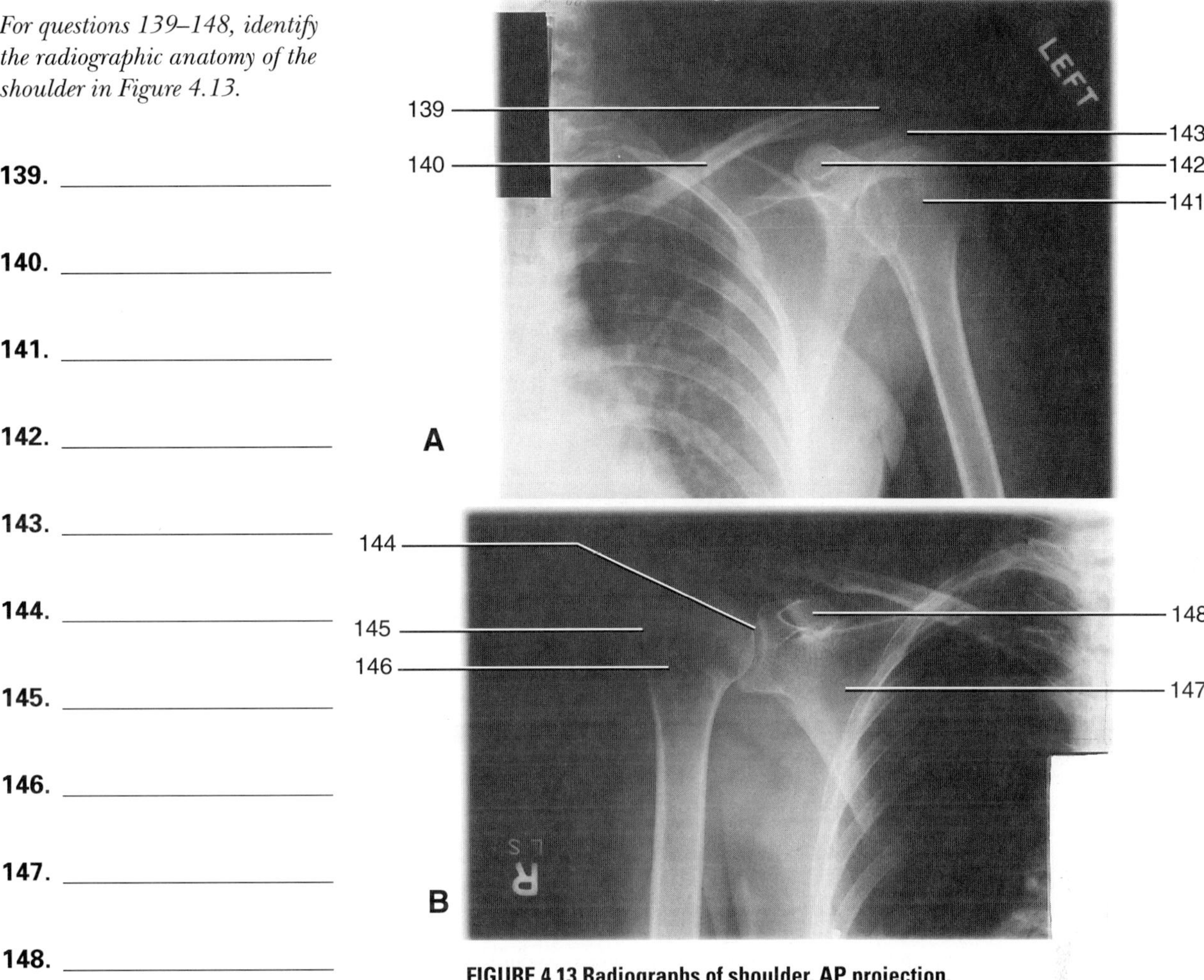

FIGURE 4.13 Radiographs of shoulder, AP projection.

149. Compare the two shoulder radiographs in Figure 4.13, describing observed differences in the anatomic appearance of the two projections, and determine which is the internal rotation.

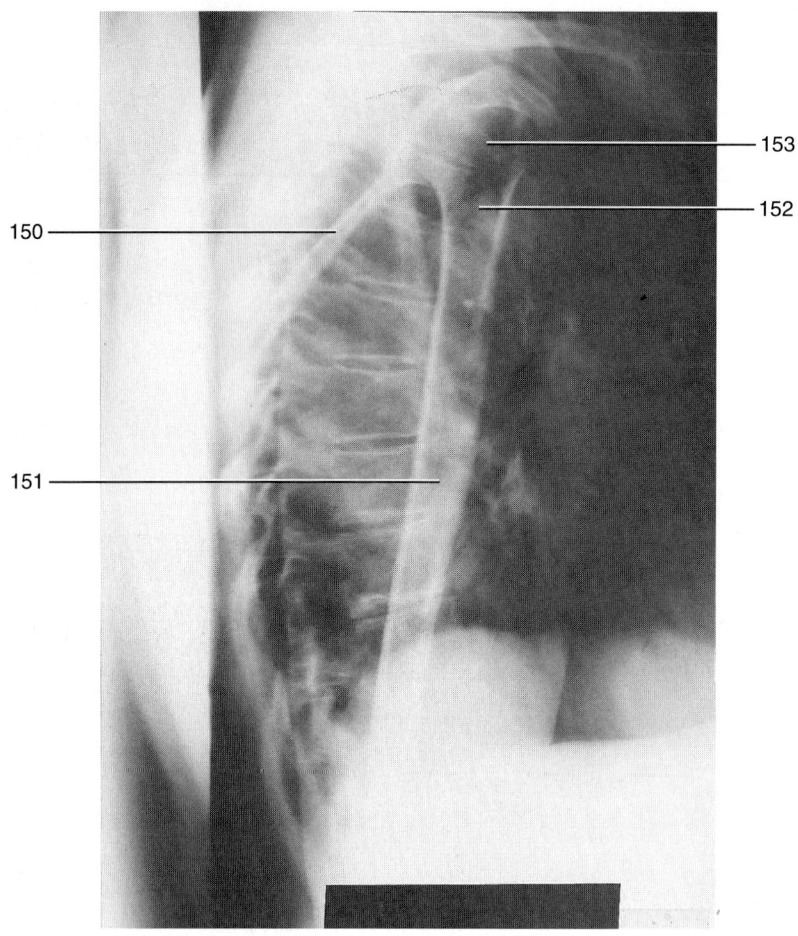

FIGURE 4.14 Radiograph of shoulder, transthoracic projection.

For questions 150–153, identify the radiographic anatomy on the transthoracic shoulder projection in Figure 4.14.

150. ________________________

151. ________________________

152. ________________________

153. ________________________

For questions 154–159, identify the radiographic anatomy of the clavicle in Figure 4.15.

154. ____________________

155. ____________________

156. ____________________

157. ____________________

158. ____________________

159. ____________________

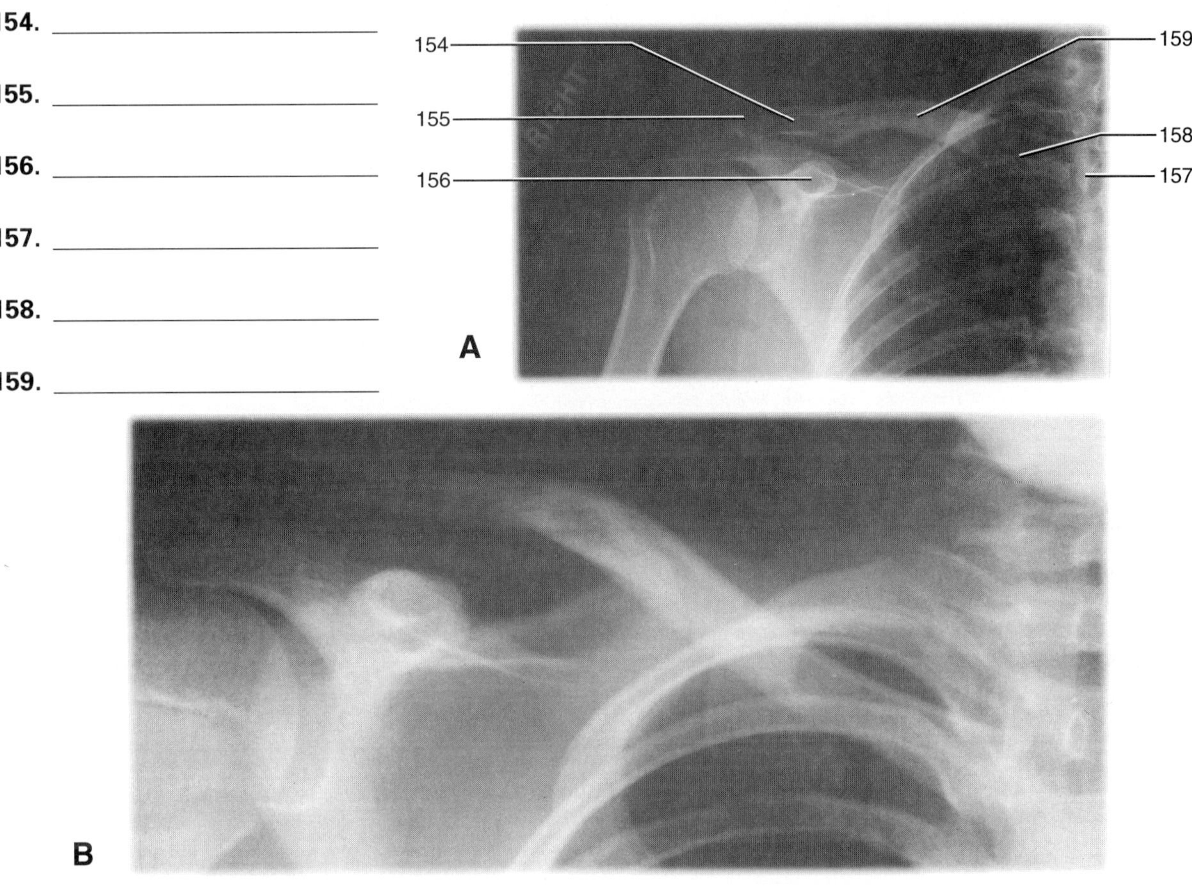

FIGURE 4.15 Radiograph of clavicle, AP axial projection, (A) shallow and (B) steep angle tube angulation.

160. Compare the two clavicle radiographs in Figure 4.15, describing observed differences in the anatomic appearance of the two projections, and determine which used more tube angle.

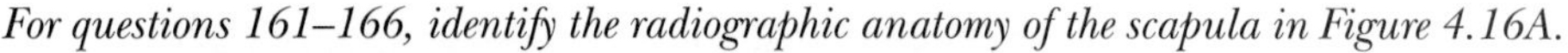

For questions 161–166, identify the radiographic anatomy of the scapula in Figure 4.16A.

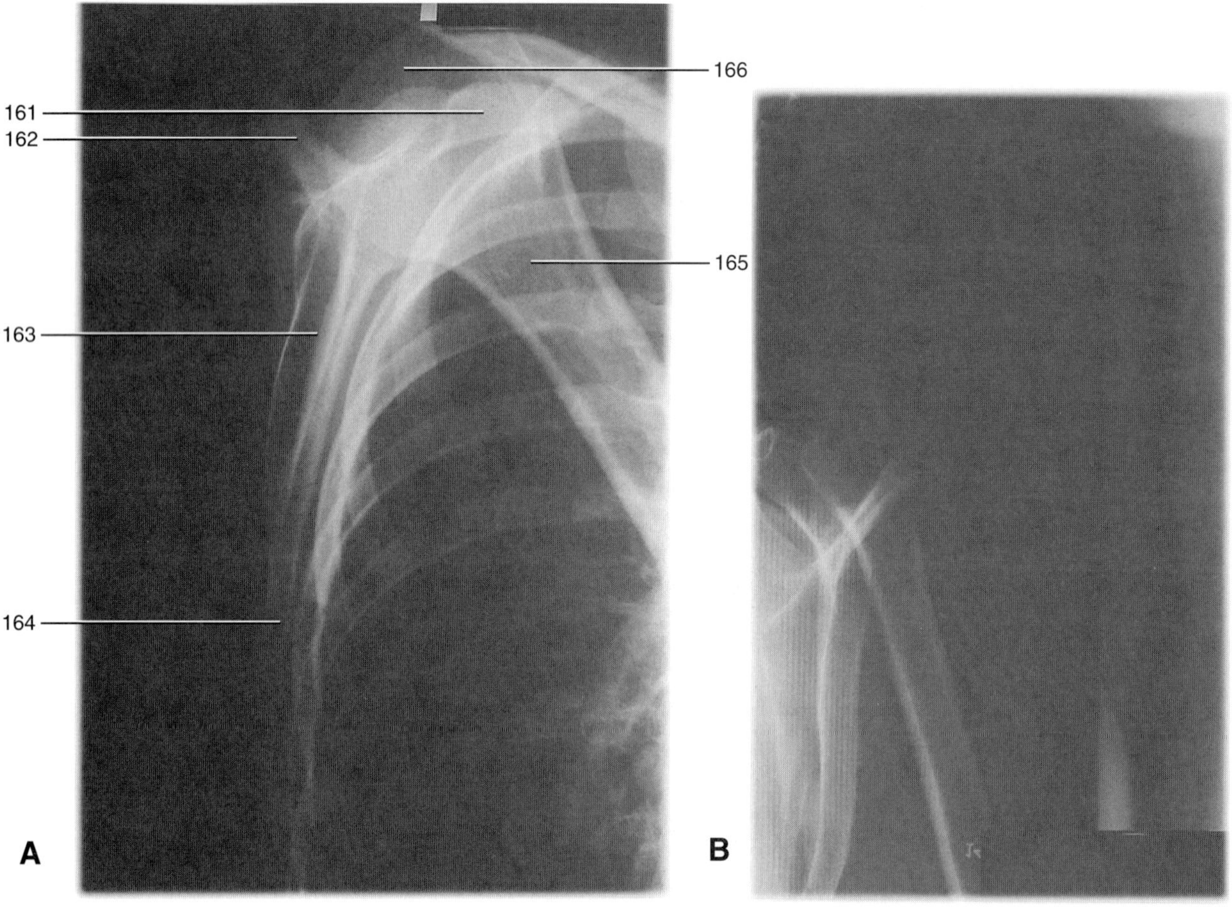

FIGURE 4.16 Radiograph of scapula, lateral projection, (A) correct positioning and (B) incorrect positioning.

161. ____________________

162. ____________________

163. ____________________

164. ____________________

165. ____________________

166. ____________________

167. Compare the positioning quality of the correctly positioned radiograph in Figure 4.16A with that in Figure 4.16B. Describe the positioning error, explain what caused it, and give the step(s) necessary to correct the problem.

168. Compared to PA and oblique projections of the hand, the lateral requires a technical factor change of approximately

____________________________________.

169. The PA axial (Clements-Nakayama) projection of the wrist is primarily taken to demonstrate fractures of the

____________________________________.

170. The radial head and neck are best demonstrated on the ___________ projection of the ___________.

171. The inferosuperior axial (West Point) projection of the shoulder requires a tube angle of __________ degrees medially and __________ degrees anteriorly.

172. To place the part parallel to the film for an AP scapula, the arm is

____________________________________.

173. Gonadal shielding is not necessary for radiography of the upper limb because the x-ray beam is far away from the gonad area.

a. true

b. false

174. The purpose of the fan lateral of the hand is to separate the metacarpals so that each is individually demonstrated.

a. true

b. false

175. For tangential projections demonstrating the carpal bridge, the wrist is hyperextended.

a. true

b. false

176. For postreduction films of the wrist in a cast, it is essential to take two films at 90° to each other.

a. true

b. false

177. When evaluating a radiograph of a lateral forearm, the humeral epicondyles should be mostly superimposed.

a. true

b. false

178. To prevent superimposition on a transthoracic lateral humerus (Lawrence), a 15° caudal angle can be used.

a. true

b. false

179. A scapular Y projection will have to be repeated if the shaft of the humerus is superimposed on the body of the scapula.

a. true

b. false

For questions 180–184, identify the radiographic anatomy of the hand in Figure 4.17.

180. Number 1

a. second metacarpal

b. fourth metacarpal

c. second proximal phalanx

d. fourth proximal phalanx

181. Number 2

a. proximal phalangeal joint

b. interphalangeal joint

c. distal phalangeal joint

d. metacarpophalangeal joint

182. Number 3

a. proximal interphalangeal joint

b. interphalangeal joint

c. distal interphalangeal joint

d. phalangeal joint

183. Number 4

a. head of fourth metacarpal

b. head of second metacarpal

c. base of fourth metacarpal

d. base of second metacarpal

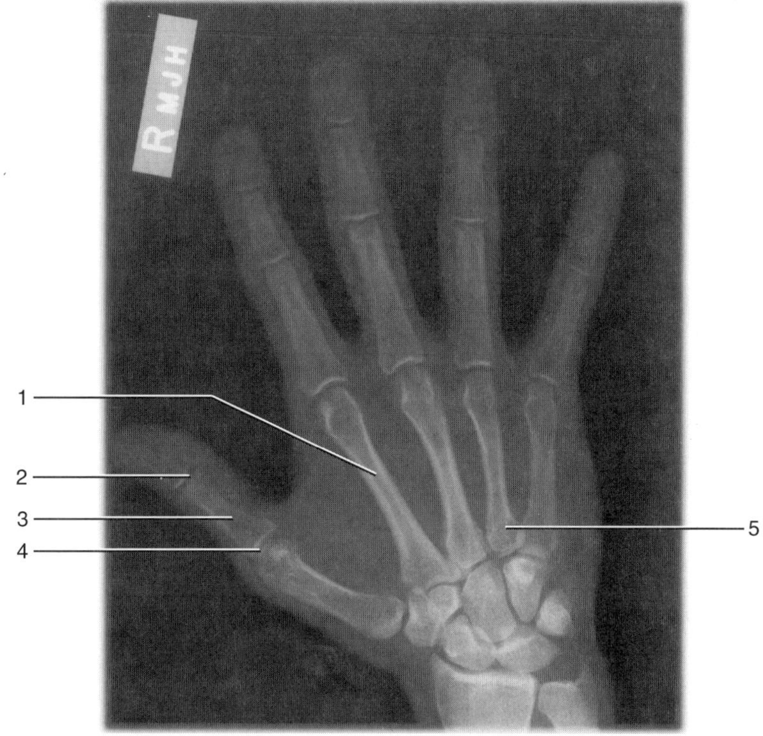

FIGURE 4.17 Radiograph of hand, PA projection.

184. Number 5

a. proximal phalanx

b. distal phalanx

c. middle phalanx

d. metacarpal

185. The optimum kVp for upper limb examinations performed on the table top with an extremity cassette is:

a. 50

b. 60

c. 70

d. 80

186. Which of the following is *not* clearly demonstrated on a lateral projection of the fourth finger?

a. fourth metacarpal

b. proximal phalanx of the fourth digit

c. fourth metacarpophalangeal joint

d. proximal interphalangeal joint of the fourth digit

187. For all projections of the thumb, the central ray is directed to the:

a. interphalangeal joint

b. proximal interphalangeal joint

c. distal interphalangeal joint

d. metacarpophalangeal joint

188. A PA projection of the hand demonstrates a(an) _____ projection of the first finger.

a. PA

b. AP

c. oblique

d. lateral

189. The central ray for a PA projection of the hand is directed through the:

a. third metacarpophalangeal joint

b. midportion of the middle phalanx

c. third interphalangeal joint

d. midshaft of the third metacarpal

190. For the ball-catcher's projection, which of the following best describes the position of the hands?

a. semisupinated at a 45° angle to the cassette

b. posterior surface of the hands flat on the cassette

c. semipronated at a 45° angle to the cassette

d. anterior surface of the hands flat on the cassette

191. For the AP axial projection of the first carpometacarpal joint, the central ray is placed at a _____ angle toward the forearm.

a. 15°

b. 25°

c. 35°

d. 45°

192. For the ulnar flexion projection of the wrist, the central ray is angled _____ toward the forearm.

a. 5–10°

b. 15–20°

c. 25–35°

d. 45°

193. The acute flexion projection of the elbow should clearly demonstrate the:

a. semilunar notch

b. radial head

c. olecranon process

d. coronoid process

194. Which of the following is sometimes done to place the carpals more parallel to the cassette for a PA wrist projection?

a. spread the fingers

b. flex the wrist

c. flex the radius

d. clench the fist

195. Although the PA oblique is more common when examining the wrist, the AP oblique is sometimes performed to better demonstrate the _____.

a. scaphoid

b. capitate

c. trapezium

d. pisiform

196. For the lateral projection of the wrist, it is most important to:

a. extend the fingers

b. extend the wrist

c. flex the wrist

d. flex the fingers

197. Why is the tube angled for the ulnar flexion projection of the wrist?

a. to give better sharpness of detail

b. to reduce radiation exposure to the patient

c. to elongate the navicular and separate it from the others

d. to superimpose the navicular on the distal radius

198. Which of the following are done to project the navicular free from superimposition?

1. Hand is placed in ulnar flexion.

2. Tube is angled 20° toward the forearm/elbow.

3. Thumb is placed in true lateral.

a. 1 and 2

b. 1 and 3

c. 2 and 3

d. 1, 2, and 3

199. A patient pronates the hand and bends the fingers backward as far as possible. The central ray is angled 25–30° toward the forearm. What is the name of this radiographic projection?

a. tangential/carpal bridge

b. tangential/carpal canal (Gaynor-Hart)

c. scaphoid projection (Stecher)

d. PA axial (Clements-Nakayama)

200. If the radius and ulna are crossed over each other on an AP forearm radiograph, the hand was likely:

a. obliqued

b. lateral

c. pronated

d. supinated

201. Which of the following criteria are used to evaluate a radiograph of a medial (internal) oblique projection of the elbow?

1. Coronoid process is seen in profile.
2. Radius and ulna are mostly superimposed.
3. Radial head, neck, and tuberosity are projected free of the ulna.

a. 1 and 2

b. 1 and 3

c. 2 and 3

d. 1, 2, and 3

202. In the lateral projection of the elbow, the arm should be flexed so that the forearm and humerus form an angle of ____.

a. 30°

b. 45°

c. 90°

d. 180°

203. Which elbow position/projection best demonstrates the olecranon process in profile?

a. AP

b. lateral

c. medial (internal) oblique

d. lateral (external) oblique

204. Which of the following are true for an AP projection of the elbow?

1. Epicondylar plane is parallel to the cassette.
2. Arm is fully extended.
3. Hand is pronated.

a. 1 and 2

b. 1 and 3

c. 2 and 3

d. 1, 2, and 3

205. For the lateral projection of the elbow, it is important to place the:

a. epicondylar plane perpendicular to the plane of the film

b. epicondylar plane parallel to the plane of the film

c. hand pronated

d. hand supinated

206. The lateral (external) oblique projection of the elbow clearly demonstrates the:

a. lateral epicondyle of the humerus

b. olecranon process

c. radial head and neck

d. coronoid process

207. What is the position of the arm for trauma projections of the elbow (Coyle method)?

a. elbow fully extended

b. elbow extended and obliqued medially 45°

c. elbow extended and obliqued laterally 45°

d. elbow flexed approximately 80–90°

208. For trauma AP projections of the elbow (partial flexion), two films are taken:

a. with two different tube angles

b. one with the forearm parallel to the cassette, the other with the humerus parallel to the cassette

c. at right angles to one another

d. one with the forearm parallel to the cassette, the other with the forearm perpendicular to the cassette

209. The transthoracic lateral projection is a useful projection for demonstration of the:

1. humerus

2. shoulder

3. elbow

a. 1 and 2

b. 1 and 3

c. 2 and 3

d. 1, 2, and 3

210. The AP projection of the shoulder with external rotation best demonstrates the:

a. lesser tubercle in profile

b. greater tubercle in profile

c. coracoid process in profile

d. scapula in a lateral perspective

211. For which projection of the shoulder is the posterior surface of the hand placed on the lateral surface of the thigh?

a. internal rotation

b. external rotation

c. neutral rotation

d. transthoracic

212. For all routine AP shoulder projections, the central ray enters at the:

a. coracoid process

b. acromion process

c. coronoid process

d. glenoid fossa

213. Which of the following would likely be included in a shoulder routine for patients with acute trauma to the proximal humerus?

1. AP neutral rotation

2. inferosuperior axial (Lawrence)

3. scapular Y

a. 1 and 2

b. 1 and 3

c. 2 and 3

d. 1, 2, and 3

214. For the glenoid cavity projection of the shoulder (Grashey), the patient is rotated _____ the affected side.

a. 15–20° toward

b. 15–20° away from

c. 35–40° toward

d. 35–40° away from

215. The affected arm is abducted 90° from the body with the central ray horizontal and entering through the axilla. Which shoulder projection has been described?

a. transthoracic

b. scapular Y

c. glenoid cavity (Grashey)

d. inferosuperior axial (Lawrence)

216. For the AP projection of the scapula, which of the following are true?

1. The arm is abducted.

2. The central ray is at the coracoid process.

3. A grid is required.

a. 1 and 2

b. 1 and 3

c. 2 and 3

d. 1, 2, and 3

217. In the lateral scapula projection, the scapula forms the letter Y. What two structures make up the top portion of the Y?

a. glenoid fossa and humeral head

b. scapular spine and vertebral border

c. acromion and coracoid processes

d. vertebral border and acromion process

218. Which patient position/projection can be used to demonstrate the left scapula in a lateral perspective?

a. RAO

b. LPO

c. LAO

d. transthoracic

219. Which of the following will project the clavicle free from superimposition and result in the least amount of magnification of the clavicle?

a. PA, 20° cephalad tube angle

b. AP, 20° cephalad tube angle

c. PA, 20° caudal tube angle

d. AP, 20° cephalad tube angle

220. Which of the following are true for AP projections of the acromioclavicular joints?

1. The patient should be upright, if possible.

2. The central ray is angled 15–20° cephalad.

3. Weights should be used bilaterally.

a. 1 and 2

b. 1 and 3

c. 2 and 3

d. 1, 2, and 3

Questions 221–223: A patient arrives in the emergency room with obvious severe trauma to the right arm. A complete right arm x-ray is ordered. The patient is in severe pain and still bleeding.

221. For the humerus examination on this patient, it is acceptable to include only the joint closest to the affected region.

a. true

b. false

222. The correct humerus routine for this patient should be:

a. AP and lateral

b. AP only

c. AP and transthoracic

d. AP and inferosuperior

223. Describe all the films that should be taken, specifying the film sizes.

224. Compare the radiographic appearance of a lateral scapula to that produced by a scapular Y projection of the shoulder.

225. Although angling the tube can increase radiographic distortion, it can also be used to demonstrate certain structures more clearly. Explain the role of the tube angle in clavicle radiography.

226. Motion is almost always detrimental to film quality. Explain why and how motion may actually improve film quality on transthoracic humerus radiographs.

Do You Remember?

227. Formation of bile is the major function of the gallbladder.

a. true

b. false

228. Gonadal shielding is usually not used when performing AP abdomen or KUB radiographs on females.

a. true

b. false

229. Which projection is performed to demonstrate pleural effusions in the left lung?

a. lordotic

b. left lateral decubitus

c. right lateral decubitus

d. ventral decubitus

230. Which region lies directly superior to the umbilical region?

a. epigastric

b. hypochondriac

c. hyperchondriac

d. hypergastric

231. The ____ is attached to the surface of all abdominal viscera.

a. omentum

b. mesentery

c. parietal peritoneum

d. visceral peritoneum

232. For optimum contrast, a kVp range of _____ should be used for routine abdominal radiography.

a. 50–59

b. 60–69

c. 70–79

d. 80–89

233. A patient is lying on his left side with a horizontal beam entering at the umbilicus. What is the name of this projection?

a. AP right lateral decubitus

b. PA right lateral decubitus

c. AP left lateral decubitus

d. PA left lateral decubitus

234. Which of the following is the best criterion for evaluating a PA chest radiograph for rotation.

a. symmetry of the breast shadows

b. superimposition of the posterior ribs

c. distance of the sternoclavicular joints from the vertebral column

d. equal radiographic density in both lungs

STUDY TIP: QUALITY STUDY TIME

When we last saw Briana and Dean, they were talking in the hallway about how insulted they were that instructor Bob was teaching them study skills. Six weeks have now passed.

Dean: After failing that first quiz, I took your advice about studying; now I study more frequently but in shorter sessions. No more marathon cramming sessions for me!

Instructor Bob: Hey that's great but I haven't noticed your grades rising very rapidly. Where exactly do you study?

Dean: I study either with Briana or at home.

Instructor Bob: Studying with a classmate is a great idea as long as you spend your time studying and not socializing. What about home; in what room do you study?

Dean: I have to study in the family room, because my twin girls will tear up the house if I don't keep a close eye on them.

Instructor Bob: Are you sure you can study effectively while watching children and TV?

Dean: Oh yeah, I've been doing that for years.

The amount of study time is directly related to class performance, but so is the quality of study time. Some students put in huge amounts of study time but the quality is poor and the result is nonoptimal class performance.

- Minimize as many distractions as possible in your study environment. The study room should be well lit. Televisions should be turned off. Although soft music can stimulate studying, loud music and talk radio are definitely out.

- Small children are always time intensive and it is difficult for working parents to juggle studying and family time. If at all possible, try to find someone to watch the children while you study in a different room or study when the children are sleeping or at a sitter's home.

- If you study with classmates, you must carefully limit socialization time. Build some social time into the session. Set a timer for 40–50 minutes of intensive group studying where only class material is discussed. When the timer goes off, reset it for 10–20 minutes of social time, then start over with an additional 40–50 minutes of intensive study. If you use this method, socialization will not "creep" into your study time to break your concentration and momentum.

> One hour of quiet, high quality study time is worth several hours of studying with distractions. Plan your study time to minimize as many distractions as possible.

CHAPTER 5

Lower Limb and Pelvis

LEARNING OBJECTIVES

At the completion of this chapter, the student should be able to:

1. List and describe the bony anatomy of the lower limb and pelvis.
2. Given drawings and radiographs, locate anatomic structures and landmarks.
3. Explain the rationale for each projection.
4. Explain the patient preparation required for each examination.
5. Describe the positioning used to visualize anatomic structures in the lower limb and pelvis.
6. List or identify the central ray location and the extent of the field necessary for each projection.
7. Explain the protective measures that should be taken for each projection.
8. Recommend the technical factors for producing an acceptable radiograph for each projection.
9. State the patient instructions for each projection.
10. Given radiographs, evaluate positioning and technical factors for radiographs of the lower limb and pelvis.
11. Describe modifications of procedures for atypical or impaired patients to better demonstrate the anatomic area of interest.

Routine and Alternative Positions/Projections

Part	Routine	Alternative
Toes	AP	
	Oblique	
	Lateral	
		Tangential sesamoids (Lewis)
Foot	AP (dorsoplantar)	Ap weight-bearing
	Oblique	
	Lateral	Lateral weight-bearing
Calcaneus	Axial (plantodorsal)	
	Lateral	
		Lateral subtalar joint (Broden)
Ankle	AP	AP mortise
		AP stress
	Oblique	
	Lateral	
Lower leg	AP	
	Lateral	
		Oblique
Knee	AP	AP weight-bearing
	Internal oblique	External oblique
	Lateral	
Patella	PA	
	Lateral	
		Tangential (Settegast)
		Tangential (Hughston)
		Tangential (Merchant)
Intercondyloid fossa	Axial (Holmblad)	Axial (Camp-Coventry)
		Axial (Beclere)
Femur	AP	
	Lateral	Translateral
Pelvis	AP	Axial AP (Taylor)

Hip	AP	
	Lateral (frog)	Bilateral (Modified Cleaves)
		Superoinferior (Danelius-Miller)
		Superoinferior (Clements-Nakayama)
Sacroiliac joints	Axial AP	
	Oblique	

QUESTIONS

Anatomy and Physiology

For questions 1–15, identify the anatomy of the foot in Figure 5.1.

1. ____________________
2. ____________________
3. ____________________
4. ____________________
5. ____________________
6. ____________________
7. ____________________
8. ____________________
9. ____________________
10. ____________________
11. ____________________
12. ____________________
13. ____________________
14. ____________________
15. ____________________

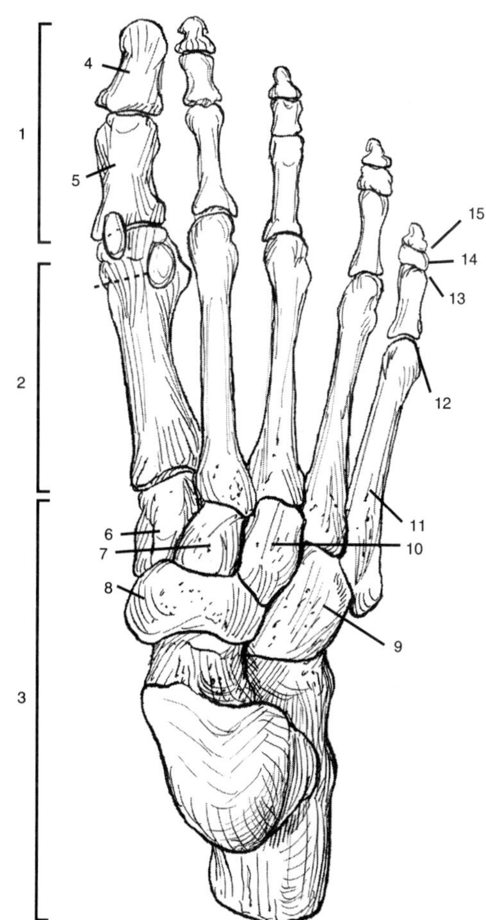

FIGURE 5.1 Diagram of foot, anterior view.

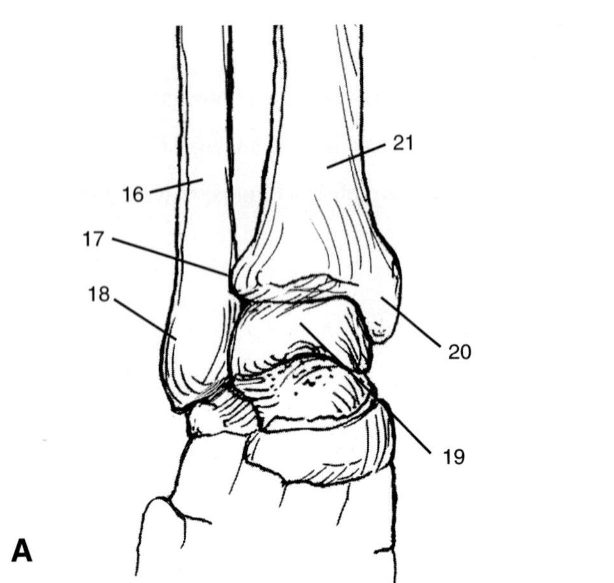

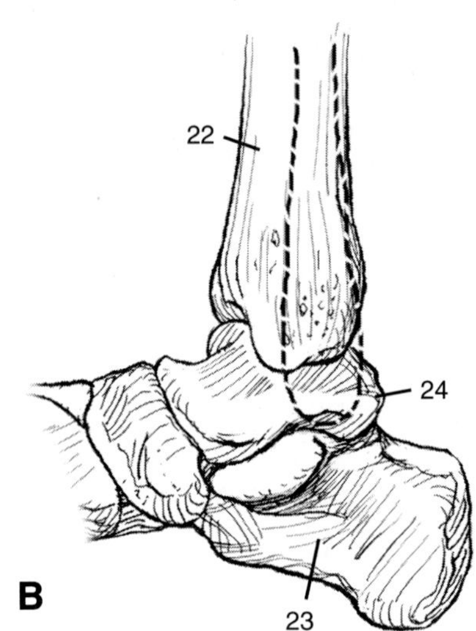

FIGURE 5.2 Diagram of ankle, (A) anterior and (B) lateral views.

For questions 16–24, identify the anatomy of the ankle in Figure 5.2.

16. ______________________

17. ______________________

18. ______________________

19. ______________________

20. ______________________

21. ______________________

22. ______________________

23. ______________________

24. ______________________

For questions 25–37, identify the anatomy of the knee in Figure 5.3.

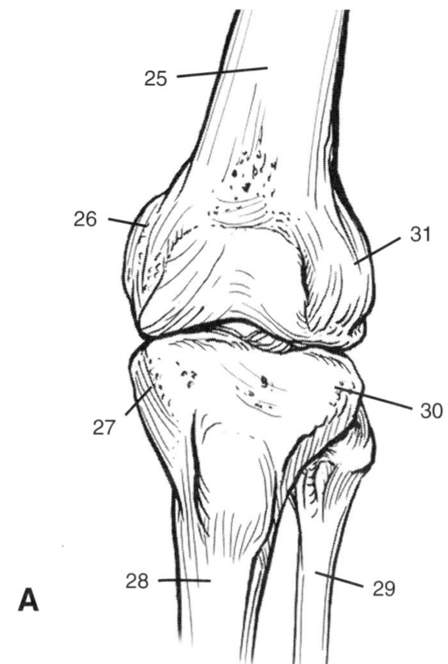

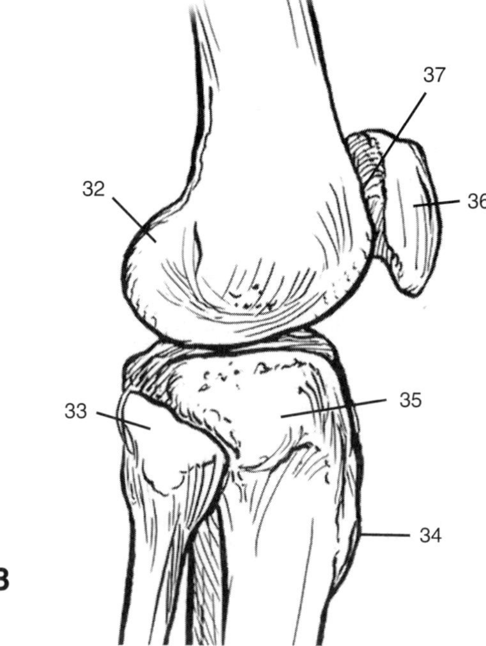

FIGURE 5.3 Diagram of knee, (A) anterior and (B) lateral views.

25. ______________________

26. ______________________

27. ______________________

28. ______________________

29. ______________________

30. ______________________

31. ______________________

32. ______________________

33. ______________________

34. ______________________

35. ______________________

36. ______________________

37. ______________________

For questions 38–51, identify the anatomy of the pelvis in Figure 5.4.

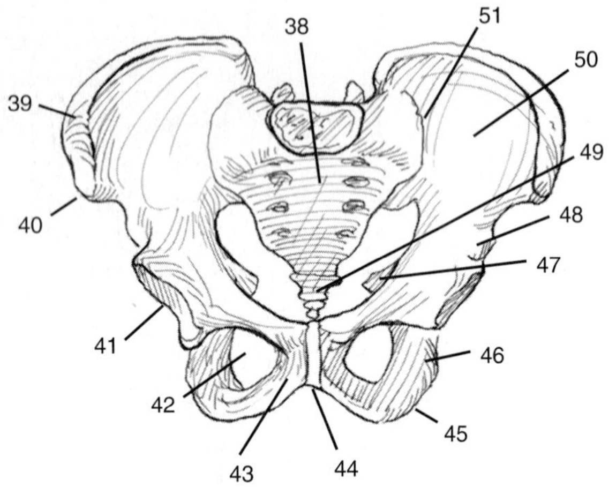

FIGURE 5.4 Diagram of pelvis, anterior view.

38. ______________________

39. ______________________

40. ______________________

41. ______________________

42. ______________________

43. ______________________

44. ______________________

45. ______________________

46. ______________________

47. ______________________

48. ______________________

49. ______________________

50. ______________________

51. ______________________

For questions 52–67, identify the anatomy of the pelvis in Figure 5.5.

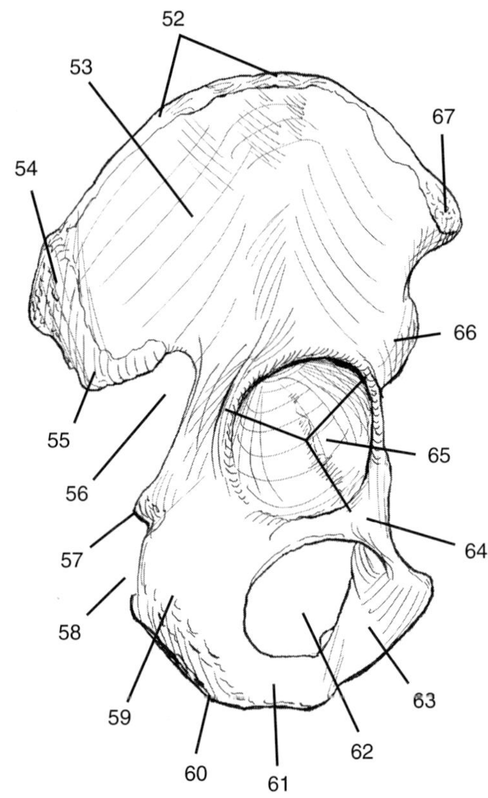

FIGURE 5.5 Diagram of pelvis, lateral view.

52. ______________________

53. ______________________

54. ______________________

55. ______________________

56. ______________________

57. ______________________

58. ______________________

59. ______________________

60. ______________________

61. ______________________

62. ______________________

63. ______________________

64. ______________________

65. ______________________

66. ______________________

67. ______________________

68. The three bones comprising the ankle joint are the tibia, fibula, and the

______________________________.

69. The cartilage pads located on the tibial plateau are called

______________________________.

70. The lesser trochanter is located on the ______________, ______________ aspect of the femur.

71. The ischium joins the inferior pubic ramus to form the lower boundary of the

______________________________.

72. In the left foot there are ______________ phalanges.

73. The symphysis pubis is classified as an immovable, synarthrosis type joint.

a. true

b. false

74. The lesser pelvis is also known as the true pelvis.

a. true

b. false

75. Gonadal shielding should be applied for all lower extremity examinations, unless it would obstruct necessary anatomy.

a. true

b. false

76. Compared to men, women generally have a narrower pelvis with a smaller angle to the subpubic arch.

a. true

b. false

77. Which bone lies on the lateral side of the foot?

a. first cuneiform

b. navicular

c. cuboid

d. talus

78. How many tarsals are in a foot?

a. 3

b. 5

c. 4

d. 7

79. The sustentaculum tali is a bony projection on which bone?

a. talus

b. calcaneus

c. navicular

d. cuboid

80. The calcaneus is also called the:

a. talus

b. astragalus

c. os calcis

d. os magnum

81. The cruciate and collateral ligaments stabilize which joint?

a. patellofemoral

b. fibiotibial

c. tibiofemoral

d. ankle

82. The knee is considered what type of joint?

1. hinge

2. synovial

3. diarthroidal

a. 1 and 2

b. 1 and 3

c. 2 and 3

d. 1, 2, and 3

83. The joint space of the knee is located:

a. 1 cm superior to the tibial tuberosity

b. 1 cm inferior to the patellar base

c. 1 cm inferior to the patellar apex

d. at the midpoint of the patella

84. The intercondylar fossa is on the:

a. femur

b. tibia

c. patella

d. ilium

85. When seated, most of the body rests on the:

a. ischial tuberosity

b. greater trochanter

c. pubic symphysis

d. ilium

86. Which structure articulates with the head of the femur?

a. glenoid fossa

b. tibial plateau

c. tibial condyle

d. acetabulum

87. The obturator foramen is formed by the fusion of which bones?

1. pubic

2. ilium

3. ischium

a. 1 and 2

b. 1 and 3

c. 2 and 3

d. 1, 2, and 3

For questions 88–91, match the process to the bone on which it is located.

	Process	Bone
88.	_____ sciatic notch	a. tibia
89.	_____ intercondylar eminence	b. fibula
90.	_____ anterior superior iliac spine	c. femur
91.	_____ medial malleolus	d. ilium
		e. ischium

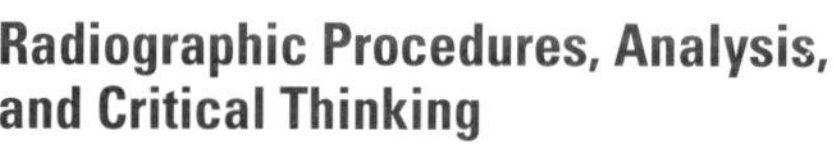

Radiographic Procedures, Analysis, and Critical Thinking

For questions 92–98, identify the radiographic anatomy of the toes in Figure 5.6.

92. ____________________

93. ____________________

94. ____________________

95. ____________________

96. ____________________

97. ____________________

98. ____________________

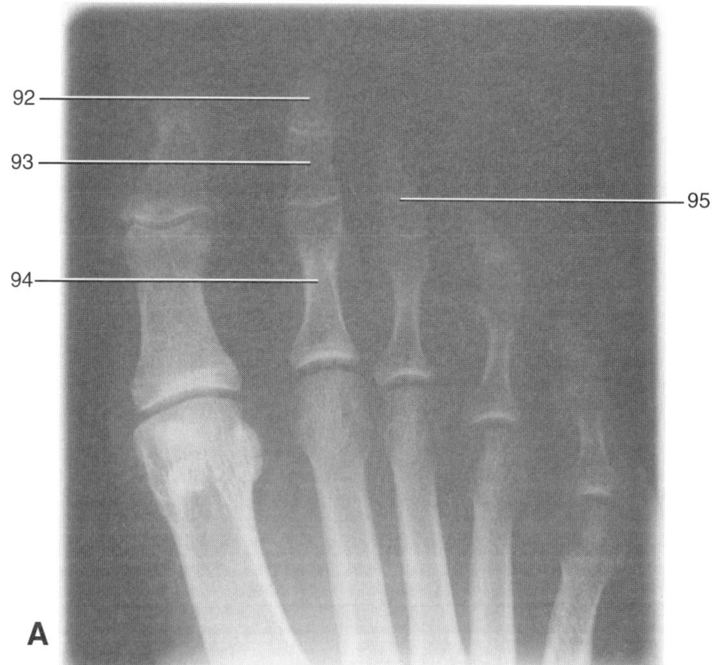

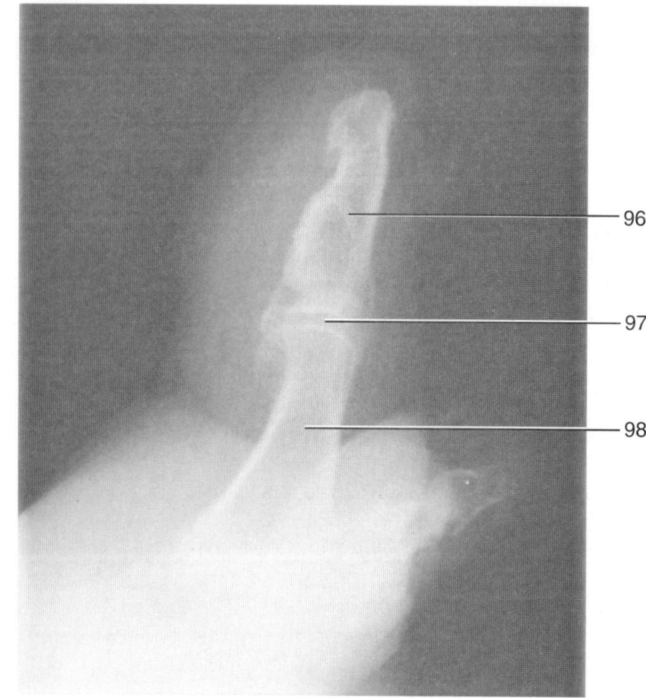

FIGURE 5.6 Radiograph of toes, (A) AP and (B) lateral projections.

For questions 99–105, identify the radiographic anatomy of the calcaneus in Figure 5.7.

99. ______________________________

100. ______________________________

101. ______________________________

102. ______________________________

103. ______________________________

104. ______________________________

105. ______________________________

99

101

100

A

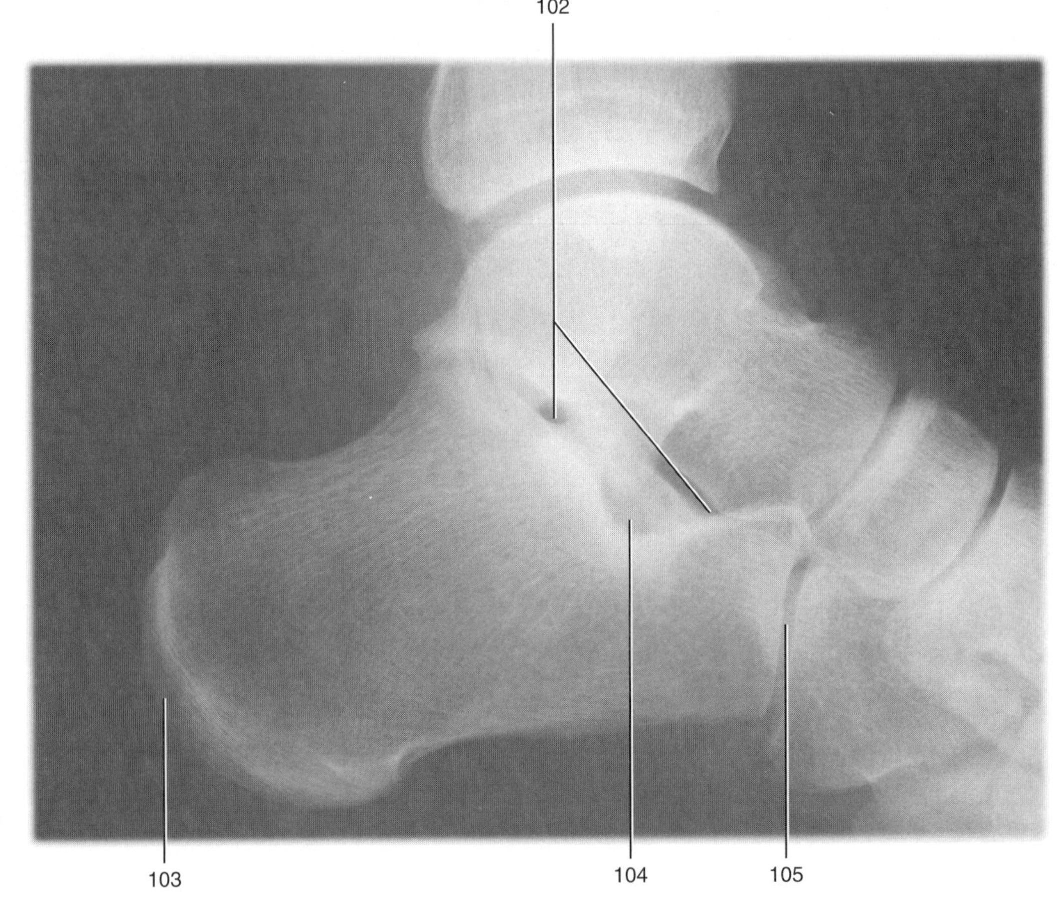

FIGURE 5.7 Radiograph of calcaneus, (A) axial and (B) lateral projections.

For questions 106–111, identify the radiographic anatomy of the foot in Figure 5.8A.

106. ______________________

107. ______________________

108. ______________________

109. ______________________

110. ______________________

111. ______________________

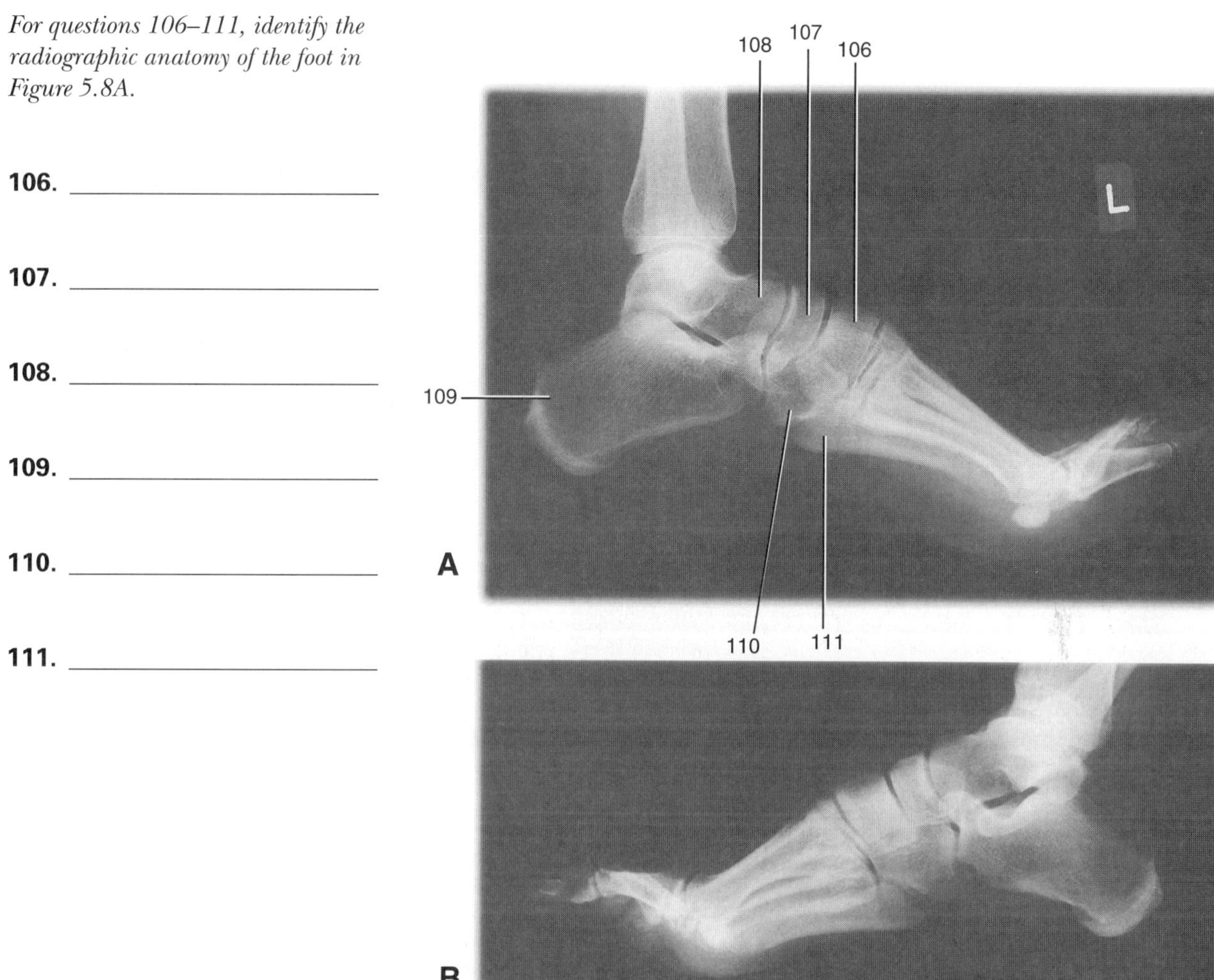

FIGURE 5.8 Radiograph of foot, lateral projection, (A) correct positioning and (B) incorrect positioning.

112. Compare the positioning quality of the correctly positioned radiograph in Figure 5.8A with that in Figure 5.8B. Describe the positioning error, explain what caused it, and give the step(s) necessary to correct the problem.

For questions 113–118, identify the radiographic anatomy of the ankle in Figure 5.9A.

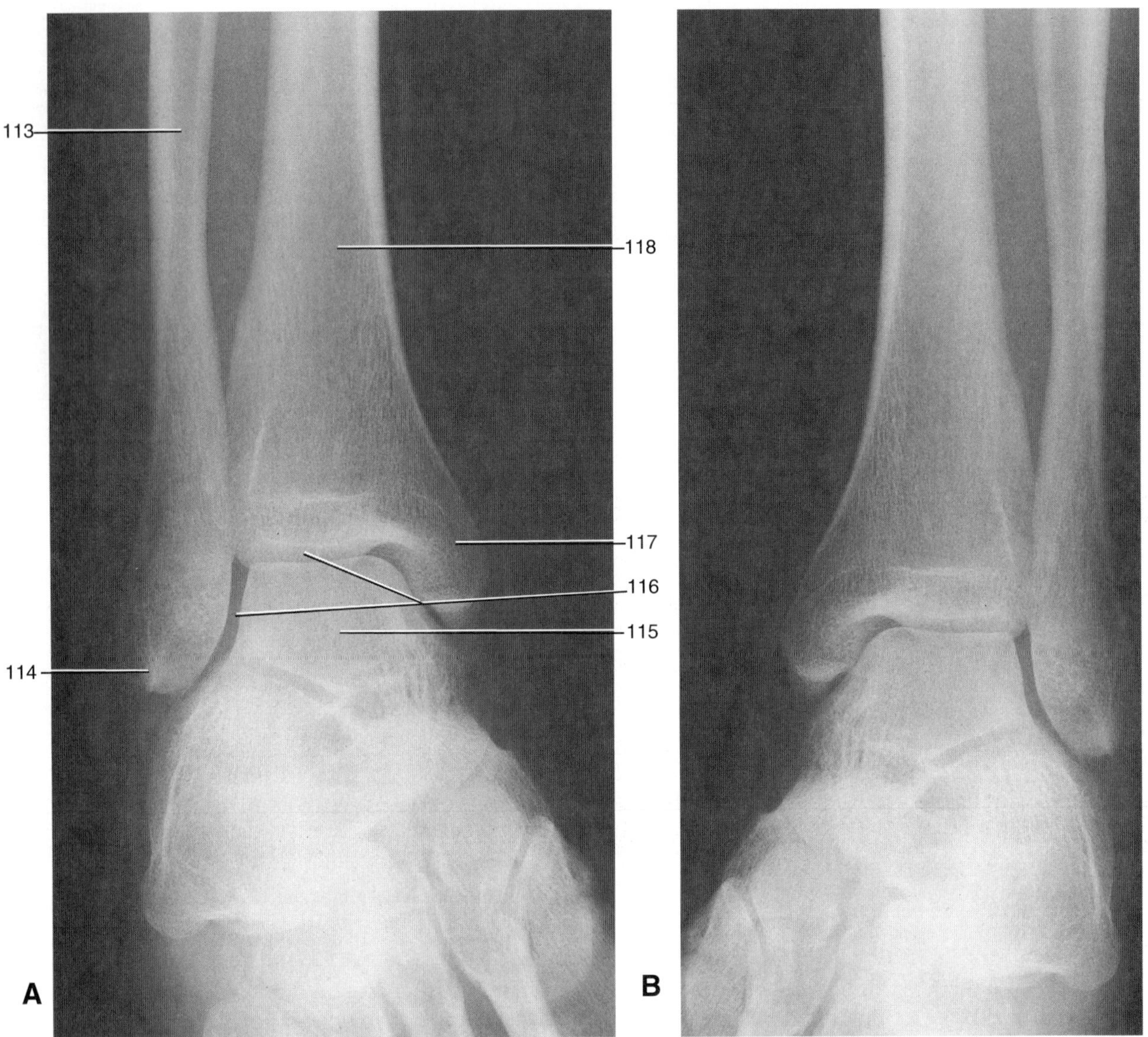

FIGURE 5.9 Radiograph of ankle, oblique projection, (A) correct positioning and (B) incorrect positioning.

113. ____________________

114. ____________________

115. ____________________

116. ____________________

117. ____________________

118. ____________________

119. Compare the positioning quality of the correctly positioned radiograph in Figure 5.9A with that in Figure 5.9B. Describe the positioning error, explain what caused it, and give the step(s) necessary to correct the problem.

For questions 120–129, identify the radiographic anatomy of the knee in Figure 5.10.

120. ____________________

121. ____________________

122. ____________________

123. ____________________

124. ____________________

125. ____________________

126. ____________________

127. ____________________

128. ____________________

129. ____________________

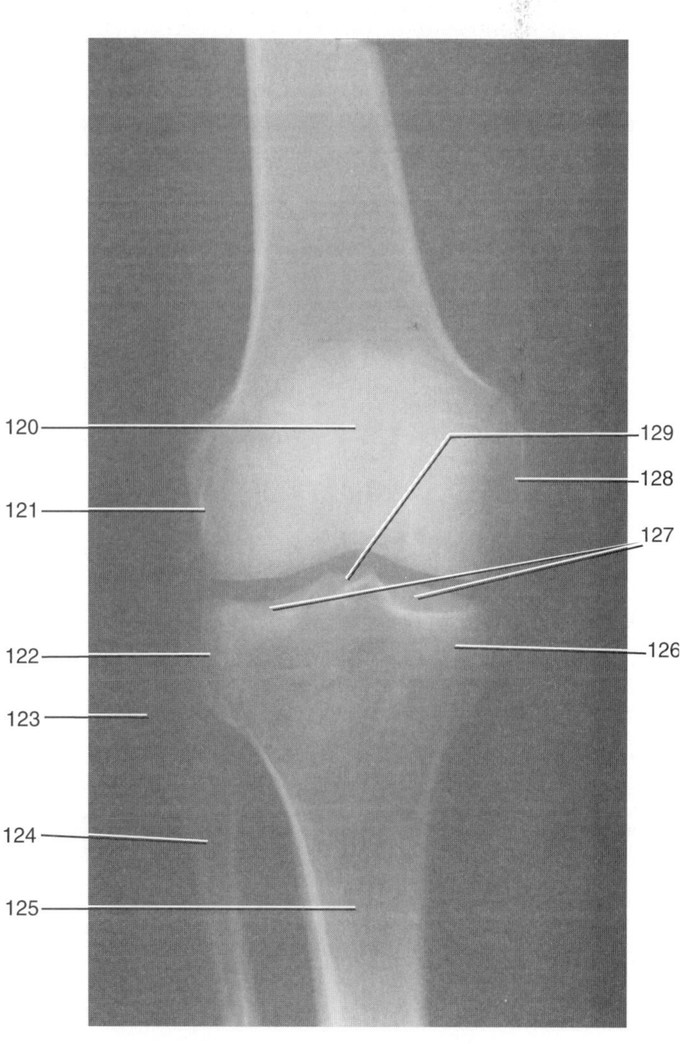

FIGURE 5.10 Radiograph of knee, AP projection.

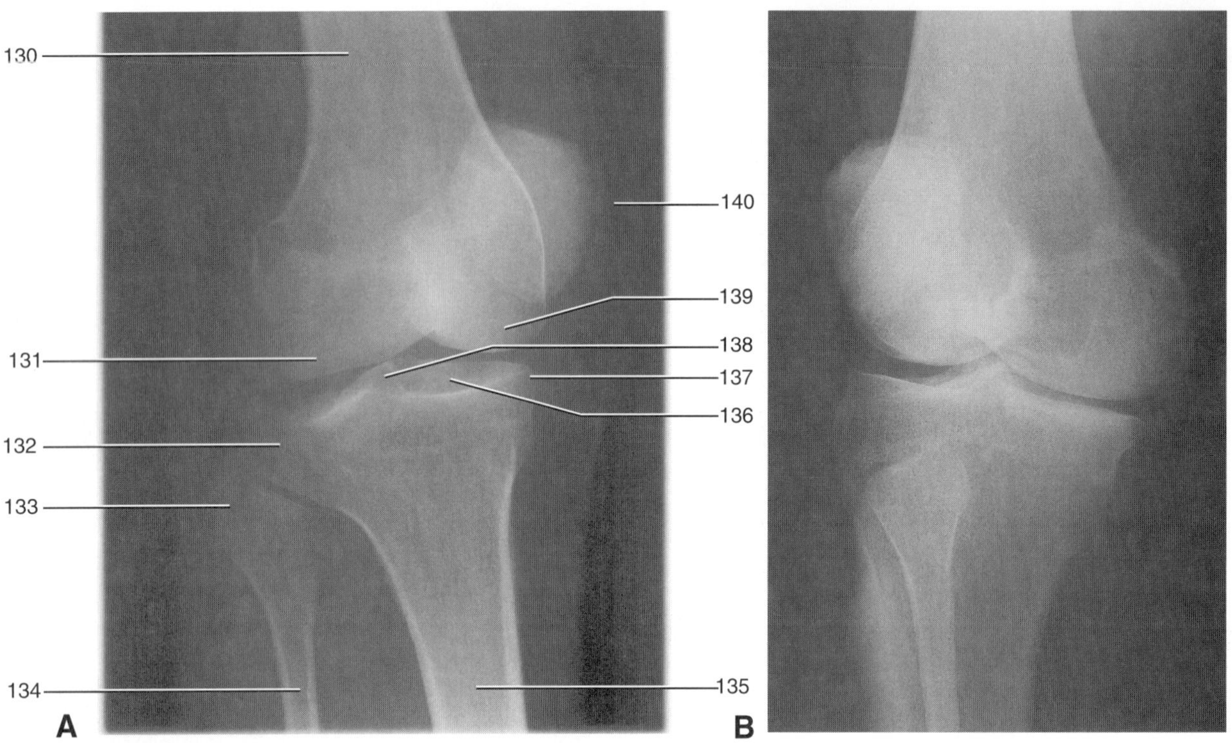

FIGURE 5.11 (A) and (B) Radiographs of knee, oblique projection.

For questions 130–140, identify the radiographic anatomy of the knee in Figure 5.11.

130. ______________________

131. ______________________

132. ______________________

133. ______________________

134. ______________________

135. ______________________

136. ______________________

137. ______________________

138. ______________________

139. ______________________

140. ______________________

141. Compare the two knee radiographs in Figure 5.11. Describe observed differences in the anatomic appearance of the two projections and determine which is the internal oblique.

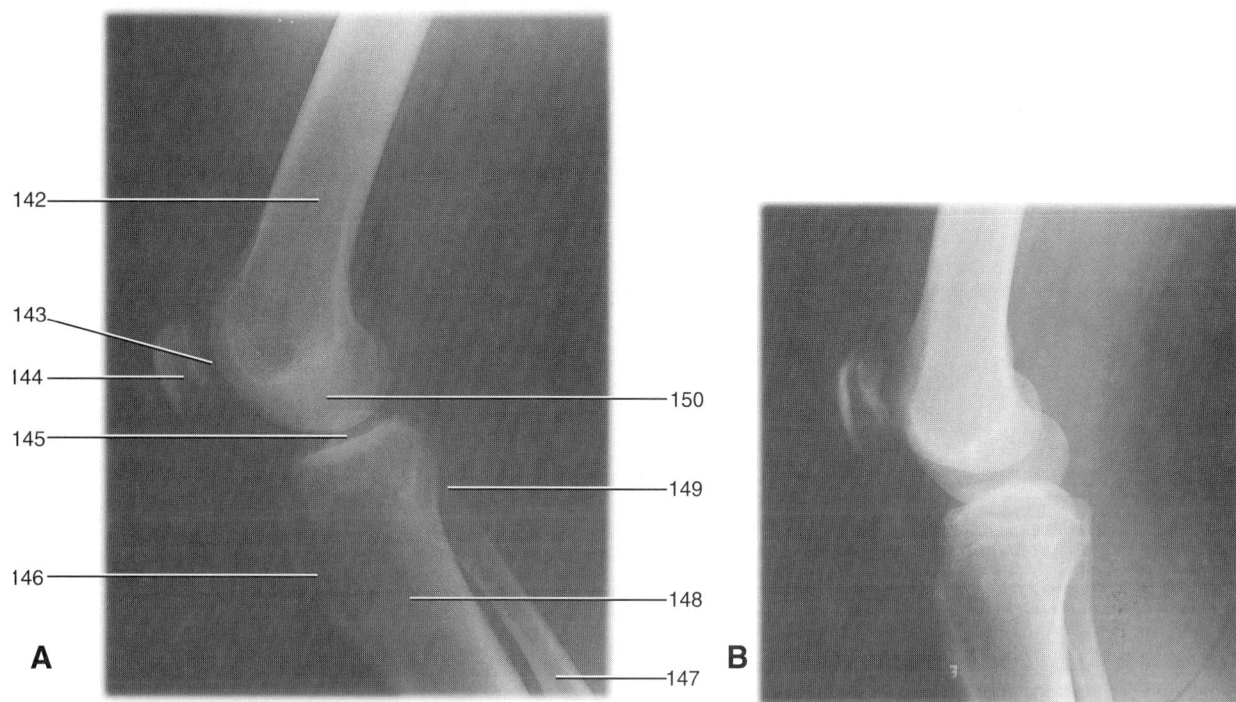

FIGURE 5.12 Radiograph of knee, lateral projection, (A) correct positioning and (B) incorrect positioning.

For questions 142–150, identify the radiographic anatomy of the knee in Figure 5.12A.

142. ____________________

143. ____________________

144. ____________________

145. ____________________

146. ____________________

147. ____________________

148. ____________________

149. ____________________

150. ____________________

151. Compare the positioning quality of the correctly positioned radiograph in Figure 5.12A with that in Figure 5.12B. Describe the positioning error, explain what caused it, and give the step(s) necessary to correct the problem.

For questions 152–157, identify the radiographic anatomy of the knee in Figure 5.13.

152. ______________________

153. ______________________

154. ______________________

155. ______________________

156. ______________________

157. ______________________

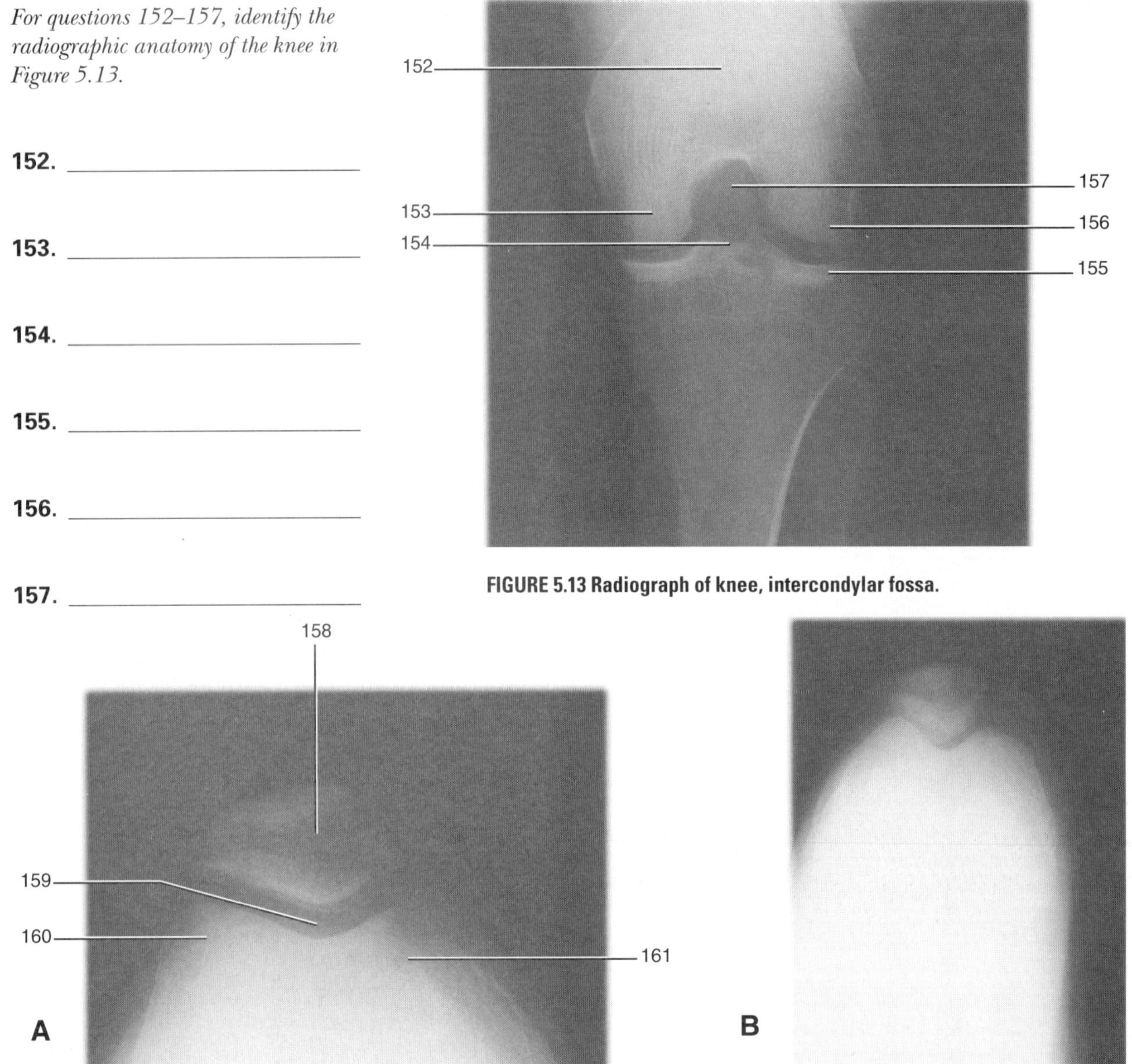

FIGURE 5.13 Radiograph of knee, intercondylar fossa.

FIGURE 5.14 Radiograph of patella, tangential projection, (A) correct positioning and (B) incorrect positioning.

For questions 158–161, identify the radiographic anatomy of the knee in Figure 5.14A.

158. ______________________

159. ______________________

160. ______________________

161. ______________________

162. Compare the positioning quality of the correctly positioned radiograph in Figure 5.14A with that in Figure 5.14B. Describe the positioning error, explain what caused it, and give the step(s) necessary to correct the problem.

For questions 163–169, identify the radiographic anatomy of the hip in Figure 5.15.

163. ______________________

164. ______________________

165. ______________________

166. ______________________

167. ______________________

168. ______________________

169. ______________________

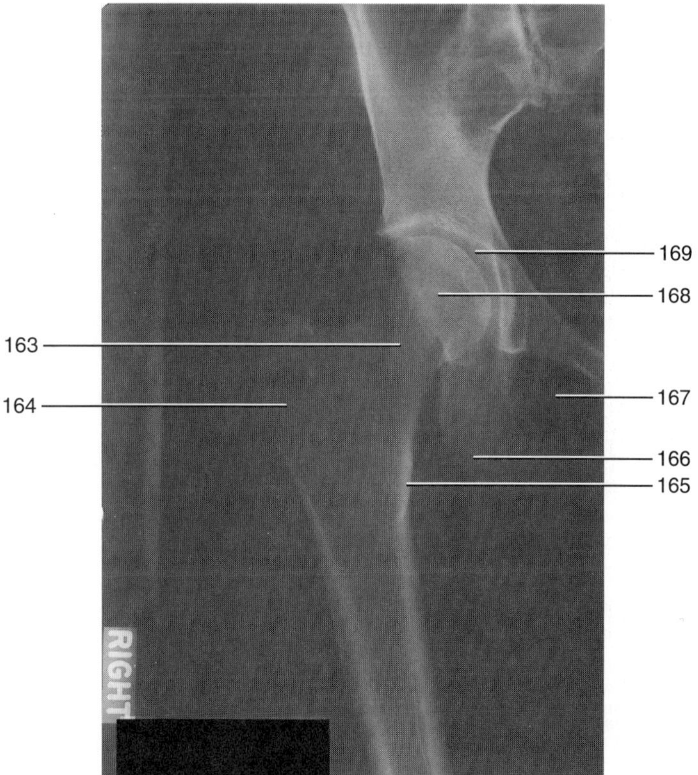

FIGURE 5.15 Radiograph of hip, AP projection.

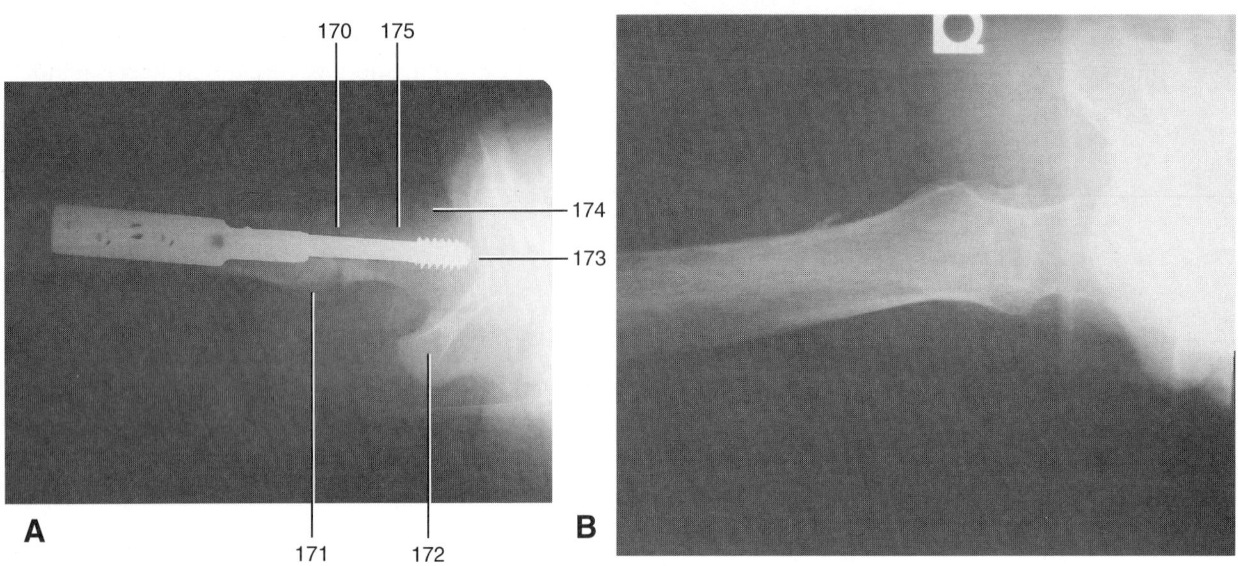

FIGURE 5.16 Radiograph of hip, lateral projection, (A) correct positioning and (B) incorrect positioning.

For questions 170–175, identify the radiographic anatomy of the hip in Figure 5.16A.

170. ______________________

171. ______________________

172. ______________________

173. ______________________

174. ______________________

175. ______________________

176. Compare the positioning quality of the correctly positioned radiograph in Figure 5.16A with that in Figure 5.16B. Describe the positioning error, explain what caused it, and give the step(s) necessary to correct the problem.

177. The AP projection of the foot is also called the _______________ projection.

178. The central ray is angled for an AP projection of the foot to

____.

179. For the axial calcaneus, the central ray is angled _______________ degrees in the _______________ direction.

180. For lateral projections of the ankle, the intermalleolar line is placed parallel to the cassette.

a. true

b. false

181. Tangential projections of the patella generally do not require a grid.

a. true

b. false

182. Weight-bearing projections of the knee are taken primarily to demonstrate small fractures of the tibial plateau.

a. true

b. false

183. For the AP projection of the female pelvis, it is not advisable to use gonadal shielding.

a. true

b. false

184. Gonadal shielding of male patients is not recommended for the superoinferior projection (Danelius-Miller) of the hip.

a. true

b. false

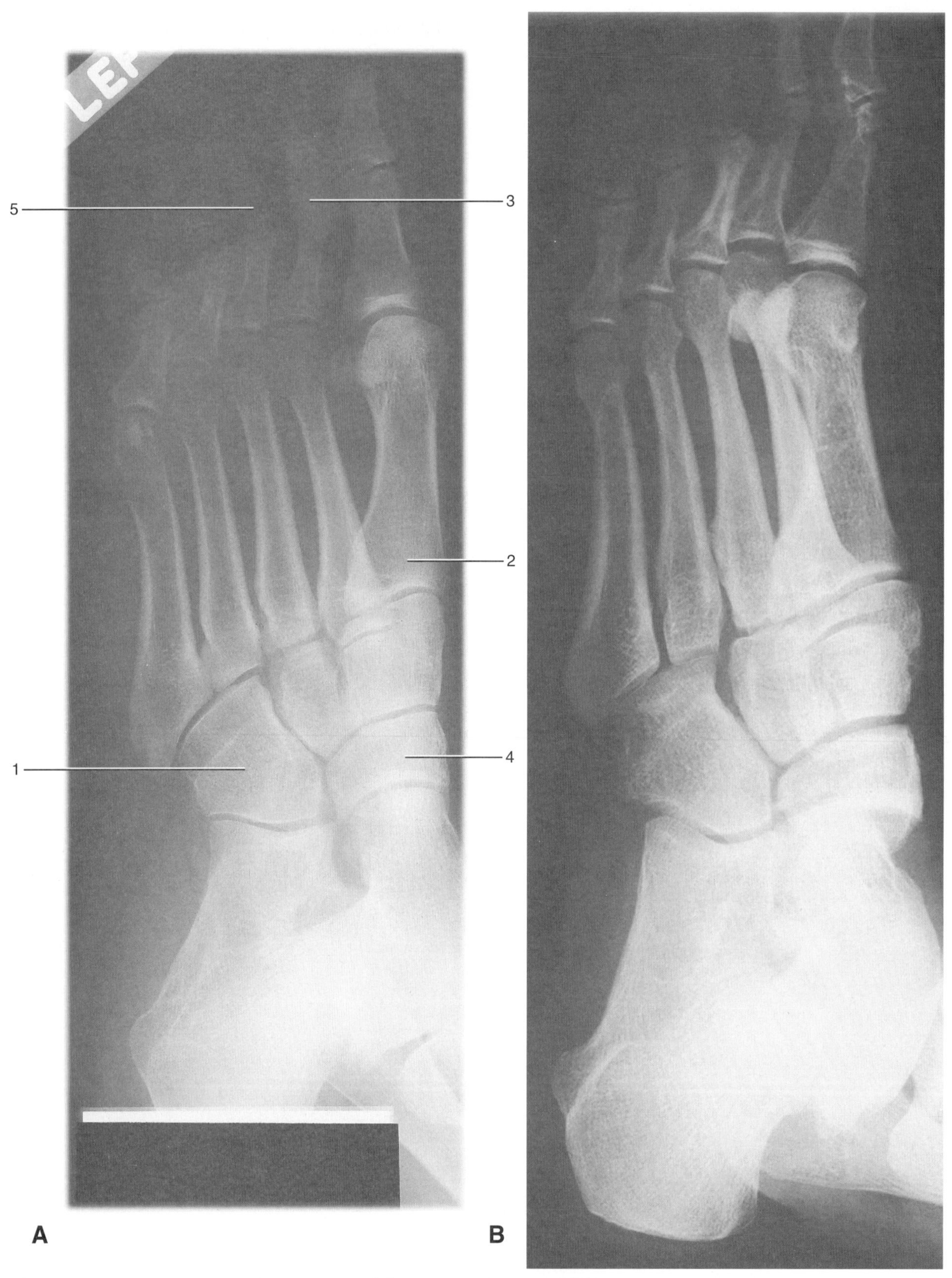

FIGURE 5.17 Radiograph of foot, oblique projection, (A) correct positioning and (B) incorrect positioning.

For questions 185–189, identify the radiographic anatomy of the foot in Figure 5.17A.

185. Number 1

a. cuboid

b. third cuneiform

c. first cuneiform

d. navicular

186. Number 2

a. head of first metatarsal

b. base of first metatarsal

c. sesamoid bone

d. first metacarpophalangeal joint

187. Number 3

a. proximal metatarsophalangeal joint

b. distal interphalangeal joint

c. proximal interphalangeal joint

d. interphalangeal joint

188. Number 4

a. talus

b. calcaneus

c. navicular

d. cuboid

189. Number 5

a. proximal phalanx

b. middle phalanx

c. distal phalanx

d. phalanx

190. Compare the positioning quality of the correctly positioned radiograph in Figure 5.17A with that in Figure 5.17B. Describe the positioning error, explain what caused it, and give the step(s) necessary to correct the problem.

For questions 191–197, identify the radiographic anatomy of the pelvis in Figure 5.18A.

191. Anterior superior iliac spine

a. 2

b. 3

c. 4

d. 15

192. Ischial tuberosity

a. 4

b. 7

c. 9

d. 13

193. Iliac crest

a. 1

b. 2

c. 3

d. 15

194. Superior pubic ramus

a. 7

b. 8

c. 10

d. 13

195. Greater trochanter

a. 5

b. 6

c. 12

d. 14

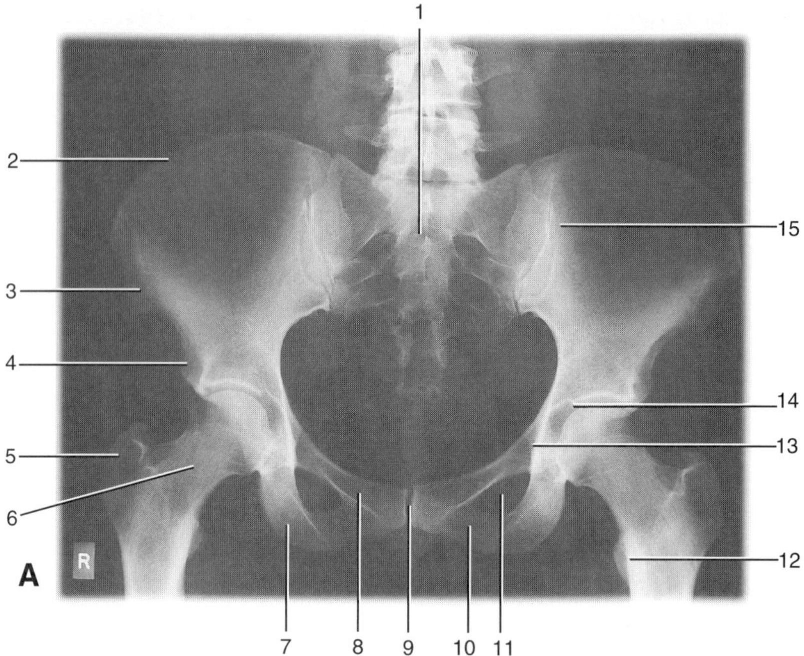

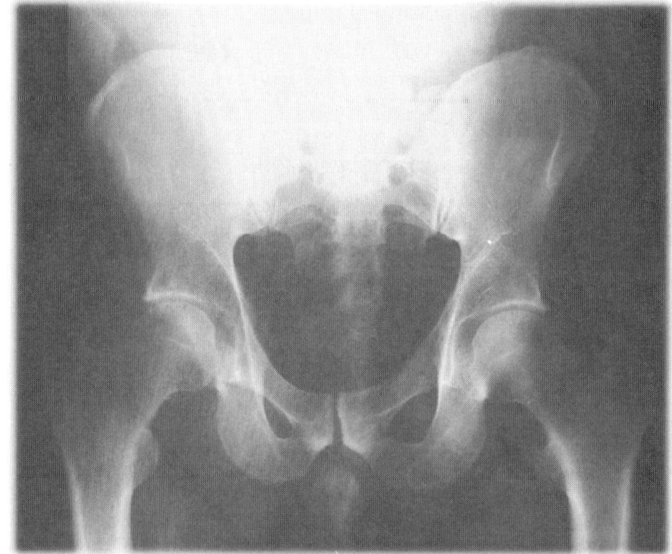

FIGURE 5.18 Radiograph of pelvis, AP projection, (A) correct positioning and (B) incorrect positioning.

196. Obturator foramen

a. 7

b. 8

c. 11

d. 13

197. Sacroiliac joint

a. 1

b. 9

c. 14

d. 15

198. Compare the positioning quality of the correctly positioned radiograph in Figure 5.18A with that in Figure 5.18B. Describe the positioning error, explain what caused it, and give the step(s) necessary to correct the problem.

199. For the AP and oblique projections of the toes, the central ray is directed perpendicular to the:

a. third metatarsophalangeal joint

b. second metatarsophalangeal joint

c. third proximal interphalangeal joint

d. second proximal interphalangeal joint

200. Which of the following is *not* well demonstrated on a lateral projection of the second toe?

a. distal phalanx

b. interphalangeal joints

c. metatarsophalangeal joint

d. head of metatarsal

201. For the routine lateral projection of the foot, the _____ surface of the foot is resting on the cassette.

a. plantar

b. dorsal

c. medial

d. lateral

202. Which of the following is *not* clearly demonstrated on an AP projection of the foot?

a. fifth metatarsal

b. calcaneus

c. cuboid

d. third cuneiform

203. Which projection of the foot best demonstrates the cuboid and bases of the metatarsals free from superimposition?

a. AP

b. internal oblique

c. external oblique

d. lateral

204. In the oblique projection of the foot, the part is rotated _____.

a. 5°

b. 15°

c. 30°

d. 60°

205. When radiographing the sesamoids, the position of the foot is:

a. plantoflexed

b. dorsiflexed

c. medial rotation

d. lateral rotation

206. Weight-bearing films of the longitudinal arch of the foot are taken as _____ projections.

a. plantodorsal

b. AP

c. lateral

d. medial oblique

207. When radiographing the calcaneus in an axial projection, the position of the foot is:

a. plantar flexed

b. dorsiflexed

c. lateral

d. medial oblique

208. A patient arrives in the emergency room for an axial calcaneus examination. Her foot is slightly extended and she is unable to place the plantar surface of the foot perpendicular to the cassette. The radiographer should:

a. use a 40° tube angle

b. use less than 40° tube angle

c. use more than 40° tube angle

d. ask the attending physician how to adjust positioning

209. Which projection best demonstrates the upper portion of the talus?

a. tangential calcaneus

b. AP ankle

c. plantodorsal foot

d. oblique foot

210. For an oblique projection of the ankle, the leg is rotated _____ .

a. internally, 45°

b. externally, 45°

c. internally, 30–35°

d. externally, 30–35°

211. For an AP projection of the ankle, the plantar surface of the foot should be placed _____ to the cassette.

a. parallel

b. perpendicular

c. at a 45° angle

d. at a 15° angle

212. The lateromedial projection of the subtalar joint requires that the foot be dorsiflexed and rotated medially _____ .

a. 0°

b. 15°

c. 45°

d. 60°

213. Which projection best demonstrates the ankle mortise?

a. AP

b. 45° oblique

c. 20° oblique

d. lateral

214. To demonstrate a ligamentous tear at the ankle joint, which of the following should be taken?

a. both internal and external oblique projections

b. routine ankle projections

c. stress views of the ankle

d. bilateral AP mortise projections

215. On a radiograph of an AP projection of the lower leg, the tibia and fibula should be free from superimposition at:

a. the proximal ends

b. the distal ends

c. both the proximal and distal ends

d. neither the proximal nor distal ends

216. For an internal oblique projection of the knee, the part should be rotated _____.

a. 15°

b. 30°

c. 45°

d. 60°

217. Which projection of the knee best demonstrates the tibia and fibula free of superimposition by each other?

a. AP

b. internal oblique

c. external oblique

d. lateral

218. Which projection of the knee opens the femoropatellar space?

a. AP

b. internal oblique

c. external oblique

d. lateral

219. How many degrees should the knee be flexed for a lateral projection of the knee?

a. 20–30°

b. 90°

c. 10–15°

d. 60–75°

220. To better visualize the joint space of the knee the tube may be angled:

a. 5° cephalad

b. 15° cephalad

c. 5° caudal

d. 15° caudal

221. The external oblique projection of the knee best demonstrates the:

a. patellofemoral joint space

b. medial femoral and tibial condyles

c. attachments for the cruciate ligaments

d. fibula free from superimposition of the tibia

222. Which projections are taken to demonstrate patellar fractures?

1. PA axial (Holmblad)

2. tangential (Hughston)

3. tangential (Settegast)

a. 1 and 2

b. 1 and 3

c. 2 and 3

d. 1, 2, and 3

223. Why is the PA projection preferred over the AP for radiography of the patella?

a. The PA opens the patellofemoral space.

b. The prone position is more comfortable for the patient.

c. The PA gives greater sharpness of detail.

d. All of the above

224. For the tangential patella (Settegast) projection, the patient is placed in the _____ position and the knee is flexed ____ .

a. prone, 15°

b. prone, 100°

c. supine, 15°

d. supine, 100°

225. A radiographer is attempting a tangential patella (Settegast) projection; however, the patient can only bend the leg so that it forms a 90° angle with the film. The correct tube angle should be approximately _____.

a. 15°

b. 40°

c. 30°

d. 50°

226. Which of the following is true for the PA axial (Camp-Coventry) projection of the intercondylar fossa?

a. Long axis of the tibia is placed at a 90° angle to the cassette.

b. Central ray is perpendicular to the long axis of the tibia.

c. Central ray is placed 30° to the long axis of the tibia.

d. Knee is flexed approximately 15°.

227. For the AP axial (Beclere) projection of the intercondylar fossa, the central ray should be perpendicular to the:

a. patella

b. long axis of femur

c. long axis of tibia

d. all of the above

228. Which projection demonstrates the intercondylar fossa with the patient in the supine position?

a. AP axial (Beclere)

b. tangential (Settegast)

c. PA axial (Camp-Coventry)

d. PA axial (Holmblad)

229. Which projection would benefit from the use of a curved knee cassette to reduce the part-film distance?

a. PA axial (Holmblad)

b. AP axial (Beclere)

c. PA axial (Camp-Coventry)

d. tangential (Settegast)

230. Which structures are well demonstrated on an intercondylar fossa projection?

1. patella

2. intercondylar fossa

3. tibial spine

a. 1 and 2

b. 1 and 3

c. 2 and 3

d. 1, 2, and 3

231. Which projection of the femur best demonstrates the lesser trochanter?

a. AP

b. internal oblique

c. lateral

d. external oblique

232. Which of the following is true for examinations of the femur?

a. AP and lateral films must include both the knee and hip joints.

b. AP and lateral films must include only the joint closest to the site of injury.

c. The joint closest to the pathology is included on the AP and the opposite joint on the lateral.

d. AP and lateral films must include only the joint requested by the physician.

233. For an AP projection of the femur on a non-trauma patient, the leg should:

a. have no rotation

b. be rotated 15° medially

c. be rotated 15° laterally

d. be rotated 25° medially

234. For an AP projection of the pelvis, the cassette should be placed so the upper border is:

a. 1.5 inches above the iliac crest

b. 1.5 inches below the iliac crest

c. 2.5 inches above the iliac crest

d. at the iliac crest

235. The patient is supine with the central ray perpendicular to the cassette at a point 2 inches medial to the ASIS at a level just above the greater trochanters. This projection is an AP:

a. pelvis

b. hip

c. femur

d. axial hip

236. A radiographer obtains an AP projection of the hip and observes that the lesser trochanter is not visualized on the film. This most likely indicates that the:

a. leg was not internally rotated

b. toes were not pointing straight up

c. patient probably has an intertrochanteric fracture

d. patient is correctly positioned

237. Which of the following should be considered when performing an axiolateral (Danelius-Miller) of the hip?

1. Use a grid.

2. Invert the foot of the affected side, if patient condition permits.

3. Use 70–80 kVp for adequate penetration.

a. 1 and 2

b. 1 and 3

c. 2 and 3

d. 1, 2, and 3

238. Which projections should be included for patients with severe bilateral hip trauma?

a. AP pelvis

b. both superoinferiors (Danelius-Miller)

c. both frog-leg laterals

d. both a and b

239. To locate the femoral neck using topographical landmarks, the radiographer should go down ____ inch(es) from the middle of an imaginary line between the ASIS and symphysis pubis.

a. 1/2

b. 1–1 1/2

c. 2–2 1/2

d. 3

240. For the axiolateral hip (Danelius-Miller), which of the following is placed perpendicular to the film?

a. central ray

b. femoral neck

c. femoral shaft

d. greater trochanter

241. The AP axial projection of the SI joints requires a tube angle of:

a. 10–15° cephalad

b. 30–35° caudal

c. 10–15° caudal

d. 30–35° cephalad

242. Which patient position can be used to demonstrate the right sacroiliac joint?

a. LAO

b. RAO

c. RPO

d. lateral

243. What is the correct central ray location for an AP oblique projection of the SI joints?

a. 1 inch medial to the elevated ASIS

b. at the elevated ASIS

c. 1 inch lateral to the elevated ASIS

d. 1 inch superior to and 1 inch medial to the elevated ASIS

244. The central ray angle for an AP axial of the pelvis (Taylor) for a male patient is:

a. 25° caudal

b. 25° cephalic

c. 40° caudal

d. 40° cephalic

245. The AP axial projection (modified Cleaves) is most useful for demonstrating:

a. small fractures of the acetabulum

b. anterior-posterior displacements of pubic bone fractures

c. subluxation of the pubic symphysis

d. congenital hip disease

246. A student measures a patient's lower leg to be 17 inches from joint to joint. Describe the projections that must be included for this nontrauma patient, specifying film sizes.

247. A radiographer obtains an axiolateral (Danelius-Miller) projection of the hip on a severely injured patient. The fracture is clearly shown but the entire acetabulum is not included on the radiograph. Would the film have to be repeated? Why or why not?

248. A patient arrives in the emergency room with severe trauma to the right leg, which is fully extended in a splint. The physician requests that the splint remain on the patient during the x-ray examination and orders knee and lower leg procedures. Describe the specific projections that should be done for this patient's knee and lower leg, specifying film sizes.

Do You Remember?

249. Why is the central ray placed 1–2 inches higher for an upright abdomen than for a supine abdomen?

a. The upright film is taken on full expiration.

b. The supine film must include the bladder.

c. The upright film must include the diaphragm.

d. The upright film must include both the bladder and the diaphragm.

250. The gallbladder is in the:

a. RUQ

b. RLQ

c. LLQ

d. LUQ

251. If a patient for an acute abdomen series is too ill to stand, which projection should be substituted for the upright abdomen?

a. ventral decubitus

b. dorsal decubitus

c. right lateral decubitus

d. left lateral decubitus

252. To move a limb *toward* the body is called:

a. flexion

b. extension

c. abduction

d. adduction

253. Both the femur and the _____ have epicondyles.

a. radius

b. ulna

c. humerus

d. tibia

254. There are 7 tarsals in each foot and _____ carpals in each hand.

a. 6

b. 7

c. 8

d. 10

255. The large rough process on the lateral surface of the proximal humerus is called the:

a. greater trochanter

b. lesser tuberosity

c. greater tuberosity

d. lesser trochanter

256. The navicular bone of the wrist is on the _____ side in the _____ row of carpals.

a. lateral, proximal

b. medial, distal

c. lateral, distal

d. medial, proximal

257. With the patient prone, the approximate tube angle for the axial clavicle is:

a. 15° cephalic

b. 30° caudal

c. 15° caudal

d. 30° cephalic

258. Which region lies bilaterally in the lowest part of the abdomen?

a. hypochondriac

b. lumbar

c. inguinal

d. hypogastric

STUDY TIP: CHALLENGING THE INSTRUCTOR

Instructor Bob tries to calm an angry student who is raising an emotional issue during procedures class.

Jean: I want two more points for this essay question.

Instructor Bob: Jean, I know you want an A on this test but I have reread your answer several times and I still don't agree. I feel you left out several important points that I covered in class and that also were included in your assigned readings.

Jean: You never covered this stuff in class and I have tapes to prove it. This isn't fair. You gave Jim full credit for this question and his answer was not as good as mine.

Instructor Bob: Jean, I have considered your points and I still do not think you should get full credit for your answer. There are plenty of quizzes and tests left this term for you to raise your grade.

Jean: Look at my notes—you never covered this in class and I'm going to prove it.

Grades are a strong motivator for some students and can produce strong emotions from both the student and the instructor. If you feel you have a legitimate complaint about a test or how it was graded, there are several important points to remember, if you want to avoid a situation like the one described above.

- Always discuss these types of problems in private. Never "gang up" on an instructor in class because this action tends to make the teacher very defensive. A teacher is more likely to be supportive and understanding on an individual basis than in a classroom full of angry students.

- Asking instructor Bob to reconsider his grading of the paper was acceptable and proper. Instructor Bob reread the answer, listened to Jean's issues, and made his decision. Teachers' decisions on test questions, however, should be considered as final.

- It is unlikely that further discussion such as the one above will lead to more points for Jean. In fact, it will probably cause instructor Bob to become defensive and stick more stubbornly to his original decision. These discussions lead only to negative emotions for both the teacher and the students and have the potential to interfere with future learning.

Review all tests for possible grading errors and bring any questions to the attention of the instructor privately. Once a decision is made, spend your time and energy preparing for the next examination, rather than pursuing a negative course of action that could lead to more anger and frustration.

CHAPTER 6

Ribs and Sternum

LEARNING OBJECTIVES

At the completion of this chapter, the student should be able to:

1. List and describe the anatomic structures of the ribs and sternum.
2. Given drawings and radiographs, locate anatomic structures and landmarks.
3. Explain the rationale for each projection.
4. Explain the patient preparation required for each examination.
5. Describe the positioning used to visualize anatomic structures of the bony thorax.
6. List or identify the central ray location and the extent of the field necessary for each projection.
7. Explain the protective measures that should be taken for each examination.
8. Recommend the technical factors for producing an acceptable radiograph for each projection.
9. State the patient instructions for each projection.
10. Given radiographs, evaluate positioning and technical factors.
11. Describe modifications of procedures for atypical or impaired patients to better demonstrate the anatomic area of interest.

Routine Positions/Projections

Part	Routine
Ribs	AP (above diaphragm)
	AP (below diaphragm)
	PA (above diaphragm)
	Oblique
Sternum	Right anterior oblique
	Lateral
Sternoclavicular joints	PA
	Oblique

QUESTIONS

Anatomy and Physiology

For questions 1–8, identify the anatomy of the rib in Figure 6.1.

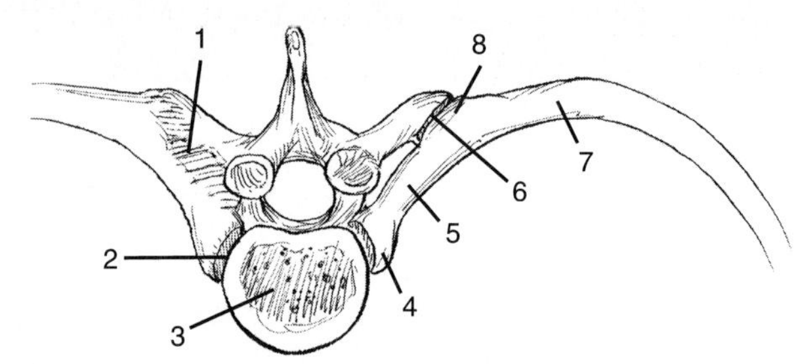

FIGURE 6.1 Diagram of rib with associated thoracic vertebra, oblique view.

1. ______________________

2. ______________________

3. ______________________

4. ______________________

5. ______________________

6. ______________________

7. ______________________

8. ______________________

For questions 9–16, identify the anatomy of the sternum in Figure 6.2.

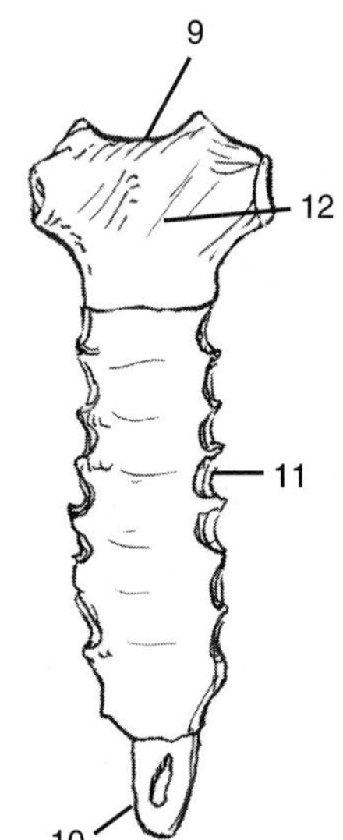

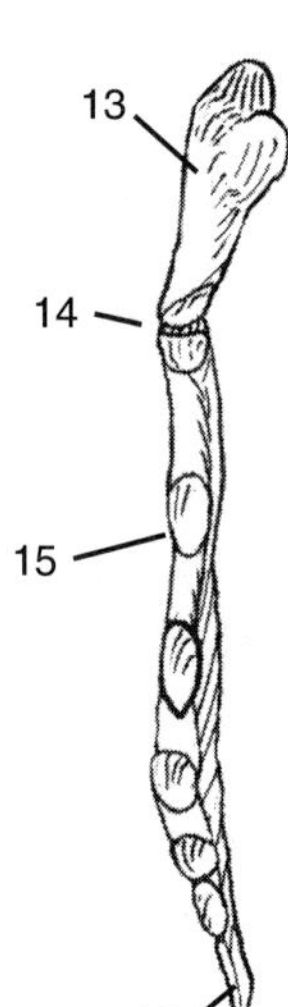

FIGURE 6.2 Diagram of sternum, (A) anterior and (B) lateral views.

9. ______________________

10. ______________________

11. ______________________

12. ______________________

13. ______________________

14. ______________________

15. ______________________

16. ______________________

17. The bony thorax consists of the ____________, ____________, and the ____________.

18. The articulations between the ribs and the vertebrae are called __________ joints and __________ joints.

19. The last ____________ pairs of ribs are called floating ribs because ____________.

20. The major divisions of the sternum are the ____________, ____________ and ____________.

21. The thorax is widest at the level of the 12th pair of ribs.

a. true

b. false

22. There are seven pairs of true ribs in the body.

a. true

b. false

23. The head of the rib articulates with the:

a. spinous process of the vertebrae

b. transverse process of the vertebrae

c. sternum

d. body of the vertebrae

24. The junction between the tubercle of a rib and the transverse process of a thoracic vertebra is known as a _____ joint.

a. costovertebral

b. zygapophyseal

c. costotransverse

d. intervertebral

25. Where are demifacets located?

a. ribs

b. thoracic vertebrae

c. sternum

d. between the sternum and the clavicles

26. Some pairs of ribs are called true ribs because they:

a. attach directly to vertebrae

b. attach to both vertebrae and the sternum

c. attach directly to the sternum via costal cartilage

d. do not attach to vertebrae or the sternum

27. Which portion of the sternum contains the suprasternal notch?

a. xiphoid

b. body

c. ensiform

d. manubrium

28. The suprasternal notch lies at the level of:

a. T1

b. T3

c. T6

d. T10

29. The sternal angle lies at the level of:

a. T2

b. T4

c. T8

d. T10

30. The tip of the xiphoid lies at the level of:

a. T6

b. T8

c. T10

d. T12

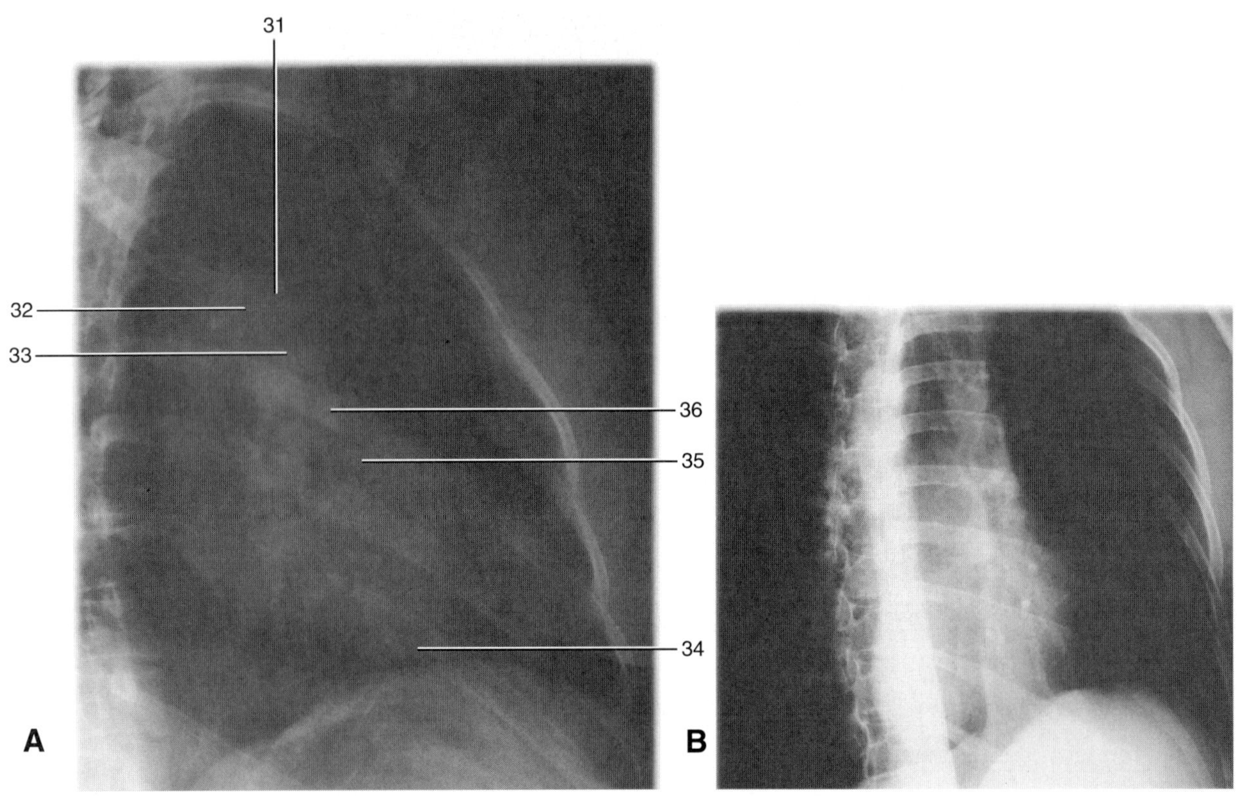

FIGURE 6.3 Radiograph of sternum, PA oblique projection, (A) correct positioning and (B) incorrect positioning.

Radiographic Procedures, Analysis, and Critical Thinking

For questions 31–36, identify the radiographic anatomy of the RAO sternum in Figure 6.3A.

31. ____________________

32. ____________________

33. ____________________

34. ____________________

35. ____________________

36. ____________________

37. Compare the positioning quality of the correctly positioned radiograph in Figure 6.3A with that in Figure 6.3B. Describe the positioning error, explain what caused it, and give the step(s) necessary to correct the problem.

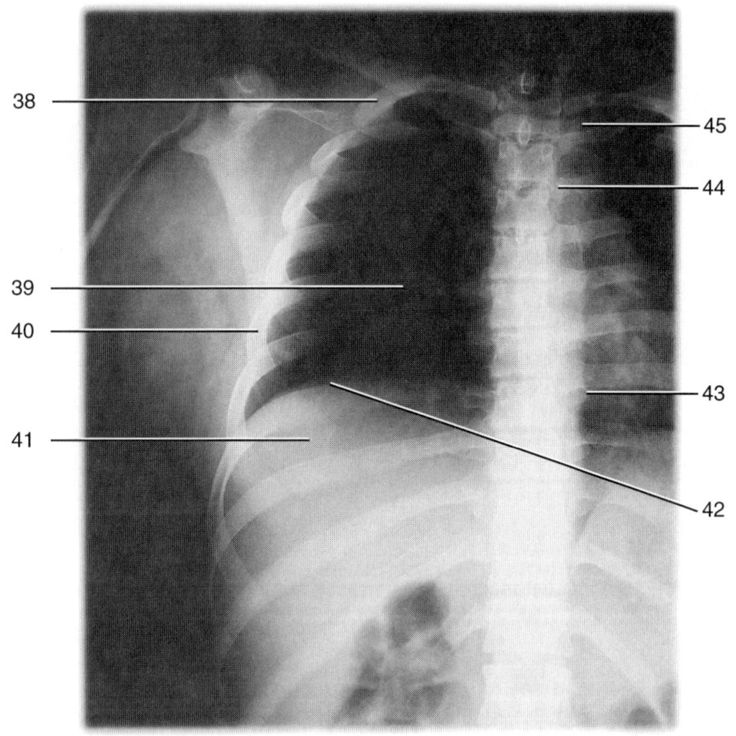

FIGURE 6.4 Radiograph of upper ribs, AP projection.

For questions 38–45, identify the radiographic anatomy of the AP ribs in Figure 6.4.

38. ______________________

39. ______________________

40. ______________________

41. ______________________

42. ______________________

43. ______________________

44. ______________________

45. ______________________

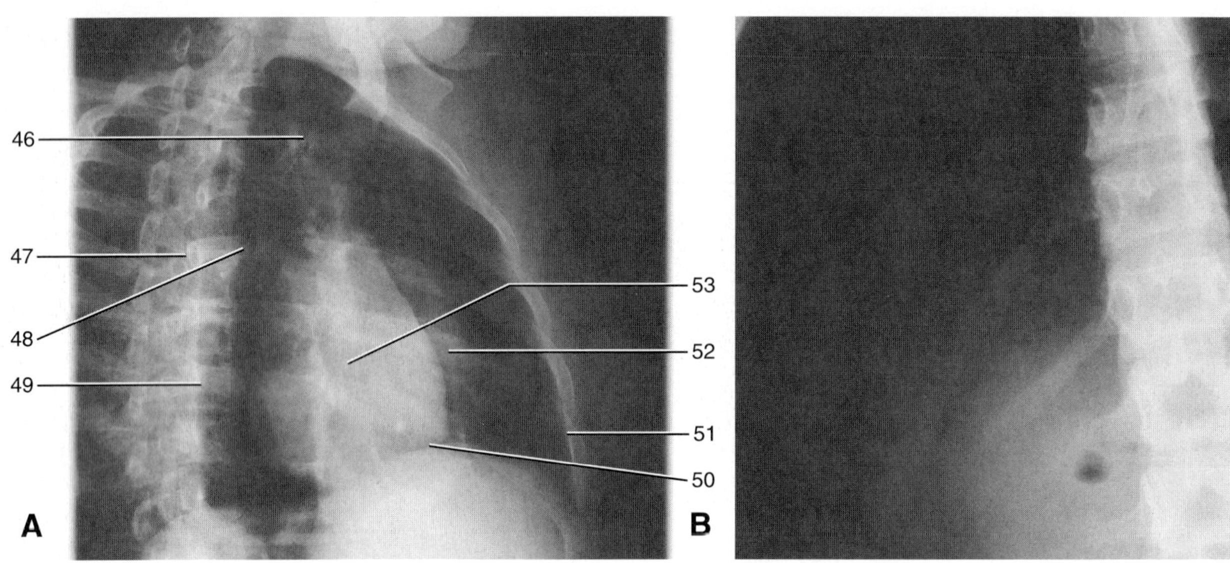

FIGURE 6.5 Radiograph of lower ribs, AP oblique projection, (A) correct positioning and (B) incorrect positioning.

For questions 46–53, identify the radiographic anatomy of the oblique ribs in Figure 6.5A.

46. ______________________

47. ______________________

48. ______________________

49. ______________________

50. ______________________

51. ______________________

52. ______________________

53. ______________________

54. Compare the positioning quality of the correctly positioned radiograph in Figure 6.5A with that in Figure 6.5B. Describe the positioning error, explain what caused it, and give the step(s) necessary to correct the problem.

55. The kVp range for upper ribs is

____________________________________.

56. The AP projection of the ribs below the diaphragm should be taken on full inspiration.

a. true

b. false

57. For injuries to the anterior portion of the upper right ribs, the correct oblique position is RAO.

a. true

b. false

For questions 58–62, identify the radiographic anatomy of the lateral sternum in Figure 6.6.

58. Suprasternal notch

a. 1

b. 2

c. 3

d. 4

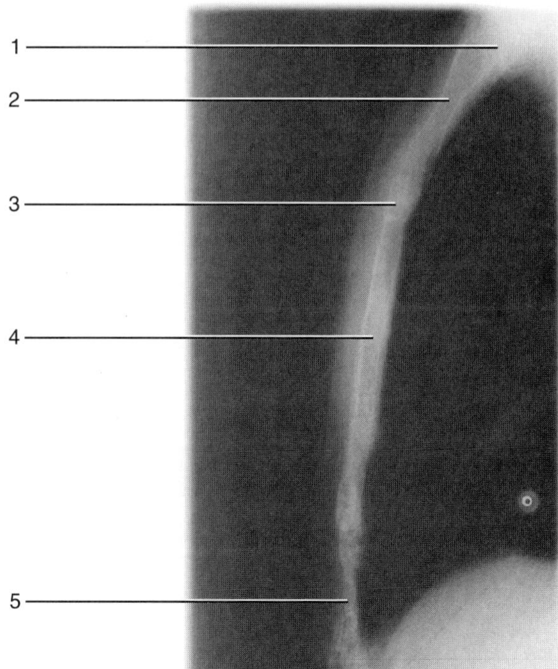

FIGURE 6.6 Radiograph of sternum, lateral projection.

59. Manubrium

a. 1

b. 2

c. 3

d. 4

60. Sternal angle

a. 2

b. 3

c. 4

d. 5

61. Xiphoid process

a. 2

b. 3

c. 4

d. 5

62. Body of sternum

a. 2

b. 3

c. 4

d. 5

63. Normal film size for sternum radiography is ____ inch.

a. 8 x 10

b. 10 x 12

c. 11 x 14

d. 7 x 17

64. For the oblique sternum projection, the patient should be rotated _____.

a. 15°

b. 30°

c. 45°

d. 60°

65. For the oblique sternum projection, the central ray should enter approximately:

a. 2 inches to the right of the spine

b. 4 inches to the right of the spine

c. 2 inches to the left of the spine

d. 4 inches to the left of the spine

66. For the lateral sternum projection, the top of the cassette should be placed approximately:

a. 2 inches above the level of the suprasternal notch

b. 2 inches above the level of the sternal angle

c. level with the uppermost border of the shoulders

d. at the level of the sternoclavicular joints

67. The RAO position of the sternum is preferred over the LAO because:

a. the RAO projects the sternum over the lung markings

b. the RAO projects the sternum over the heart shadow

c. the RAO projects the sternum over the vertebral shadows

d. the sternum is placed into a true frontal perspective

68. Which of the following are true concerning radiography of the sternum in the oblique position?

1. The patient should be instructed to breathe during the exposure.

2. A longer than normal SID is used.

3. A long exposure time is needed.

a. 1 and 2

b. 1 and 3

c. 2 and 3

d. 1, 2, and 3

69. For oblique projections of the sternoclavicular articulations, the patient should be rotated _____.

a. 15°

b. 30°

c. 45°

d. 60°

70. To demonstrate the left sternoclavicular articulation with minimum superimposition, the patient should be placed in the _____ position.

a. lateral

b. LPO

c. LAO

d. RAO

71. Rib examinations are performed upright if possible because:

a. there is less distortion and magnification on the radiograph

b. bony detail is improved on the radiograph

c. the diaphragm can move lower, thus demonstrating more ribs on the radiograph

d. it is more comfortable for patients with bony thorax injuries

72. For the AP projection of the upper ribs, the top of the cassette should be placed _____ the upper border of the shoulders.

a. 1 inch below

b. level with

c. 1 inch above

d. 2 inches above

73. The AP projection for upper ribs should demonstrate the first _____ pairs of ribs.

a. 5–6

b. 7–8

c. 9–10

d. 11–12

74. For the AP projection of the lower ribs, the lower border of the cassette is placed:

a. 1 inch below the iliac crest

b. level with the inferior rib margin

c. 1/2 inch below the inferior rib margin

d. 2 inches below the inferior rib margin

75. For lower ribs in the RPO position, the lower border of the cassette is placed:

a. 1 inch below the iliac crest

b. level with the inferior rib margin

c. 1 1/2–2 inches below the inferior rib margin

d. at the umbilicus

76. Which of the following best demonstrates fractures of the axillary portions of the left ribs?

a. AP

b. LPO

c. RPO

d. left lateral

77. For oblique projections of the ribs, the patient should be rotated _____.

a. 15°

b. 30°

c. 45°

d. 60°

78. Which of the following is *not* a routine projection for examinations of the ribs?

a. AP

b. lateral

c. PA oblique

d. AP oblique

79. Which ribs are best demonstrated with the patient in the LPO position?

a. left ribs

b. right ribs

c. all ribs

d. obliques do not demonstrate ribs well

80. Which of the following should be taken on full inspiration?

1. AP upper ribs
2. lateral sternum
3. RAO sternum

a. 1 and 2

b. 1 and 3

c. 2 and 3

d. 1, 2, and 3

81. Most rib examinations require that a routine PA chest be included, despite the fact that this film will not demonstrate satisfactory bony rib detail. Explain why this film is included.

82. The kVp range differs for upper and lower ribs. Furthermore the upper rib kVp range differs from the PA chest kVp range. Explain these apparent discrepancies.

Do You Remember?

83. Which region lies bilaterally in the most superior part of the abdomen?

a. hypochondriac

b. lumbar

c. inguinal

d. hypogastric

84. In asthenic patients the stomach lies horizontally and away from the midline.

a. true

b. false

85. The central ray for a PA projection of the chest enters at the level of:

a. T4–T5

b. T6–T7

c. T8–T9

d. T10–T11

86. Which of the following are true regarding the pancreas?

1. It lies in the retroperitoneal space.

2. It lies primarily in the right upper quadrant.

3. Its portions include three lobes and a fundus.

a. 1 and 2

b. 1 and 3

c. 2 and 3

d. 1, 2, and 3

87. The Grashey position of the shoulder primarily demonstrates the:

a. glenoid fossa

b. acromioclavicular joint

c. acromion process

d. greater tubercle

88. The triquetrum is also called the:

a. triangular

b. trapezium

c. greater multangular

d. unciform

89. Which of the following is not a position used to demonstrate the intercondylar fossa?

a. PA axial (Camp-Coventry)

b. PA axial (Holmblad)

c. AP axial (Taylor)

d. AP axial (Beclere)

90. The AP mortise projection demonstrates ligamentous tears of the:

a. elbow

b. shoulder

c. ankle

d. hip

91. The largest tarsal bone is the:

a. calcaneus

b. talus

c. navicular

d. cuboid

92. In which projection is the patella completely free of superimposition from the femur?

a. AP

b. internal oblique

c. PA axial (Camp-Coventry)

d. lateral

STUDY TIP: NOTE-TAKING

Instructor Bob: Ishmial, you don't seem to be doing well in this class. Are you studying enough?

Ishmial: I studied just like you said—at least 2 hours a night in a quiet place. I just don't seem to be studying the things you ask on the test. For example, look in my notes—do you see anywhere that you talked about pneumothorax? Yet there were two questions on the test I missed.

Instructor Bob: Let me take a look at those notes. Hey, Ishmial, these are pretty messy and look at this section, I can't even read it.

Ishmial: Yeah, I think I fell asleep right then; I worked all night the night before the lecture. But I always take good notes.

Instructor Bob: I think the problem is that your notes are not complete enough. Do you rewrite them or check the text or someone else's notes as a check on your accuracy?

Ishmial: I'll give it a try.

Instructors who lecture tend to use notes as a primary source for test questions. If a student takes incomplete notes (whether awake or asleep) this will create "holes" in the learning process. Notes must be taken carefully and completely.

- Borrow or photocopy someone else's notes to check yours for accuracy.
- If the instructor talks faster than you can write, consider audiotaping the lecture. Later, you can play it back at your own pace and fill in any missing gaps. Listening twice also adds to comprehension of the material.
- Rewrite and organize the notes, adding any extra material from the text.

> Note-taking is a skill that must be learned to succeed in college. If you find that the instructor is testing on material that you have not studied, incomplete notes may be the reason.

SECTION IV

VERTEBRAL COLUMN

CHAPTER 7

Cervical Spine

LEARNING OBJECTIVES

At the completion of this chapter, the student should be able to:

1. List and describe the bony anatomy of the cervical spine.
2. Given drawings and radiographs, locate anatomic structures and landmarks.
3. Explain the rationale for each projection.
4. Explain the patient preparation required for each examination.
5. Describe the positioning used to visualize anatomic structures of the cervical spine.
6. List or identify the central ray location and identify the extent of field necessary for each projection.
7. Explain the protective measures that should be taken for each projection.
8. Recommend the technical factors for producing an acceptable radiograph for each projection.
9. State the patient instructions for each projection.
10. Given radiographs, evaluate positioning and technical factors for radiographs of the cervical spine.
11. Describe modifications of procedures for atypical or impaired patients to better demonstrate the anatomic area of interest.

Routine and Alternative Positions/Projections

Part	Routine	Alternative
Cervical spine	AP	
	AP open mouth	AP wagging jaw (Otonello)
		AP odontoid process (Fuchs)
		PA odontoid process (Judd)
	Oblique	
	Lateral	Flexion/extension laterals
		AP vertebral arch

QUESTIONS

Anatomy and Physiology

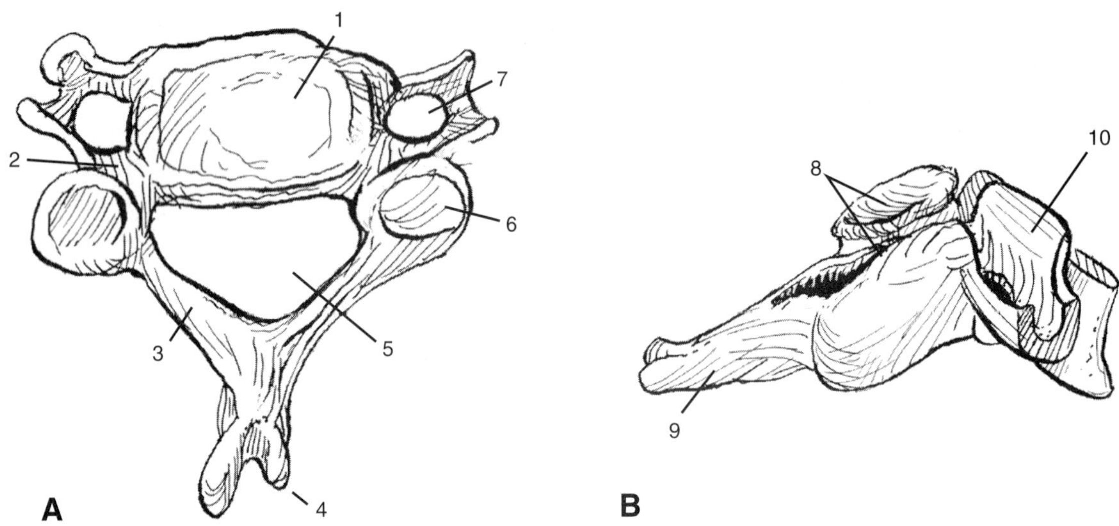

FIGURE 7.1 Diagram of typical cervical vertebra, (A) superior and (B) lateral views.

For questions 1–10, identify the anatomy of a typical cervical vertebra in Figure 7.1.

1. ______________________
2. ______________________
3. ______________________
4. ______________________
5. ______________________
6. ______________________
7. ______________________
8. ______________________
9. ______________________
10. ______________________

For questions 11–17, identify the anatomy of the first cervical vertebra in Figure 7.2.

11. ______________________
12. ______________________
13. ______________________
14. ______________________
15. ______________________
16. ______________________
17. ______________________

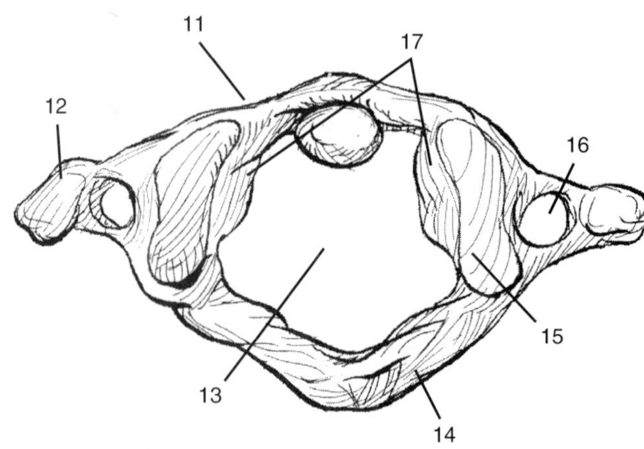

FIGURE 7.2 Diagram of first cervical vertebra, superior view.

For questions 18–29, identify the anatomy of the second cervical vertebra in Figure 7.3.

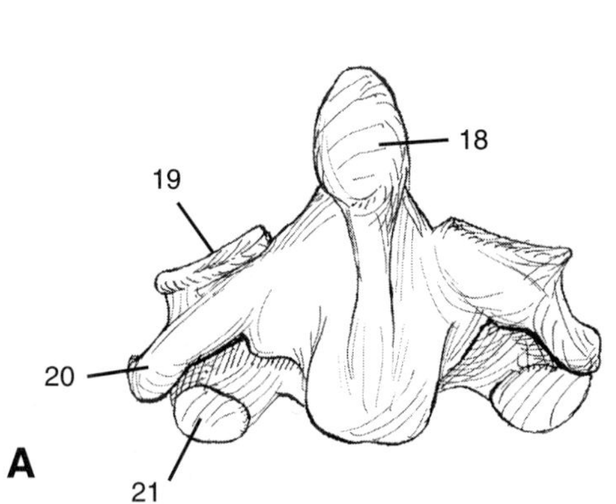

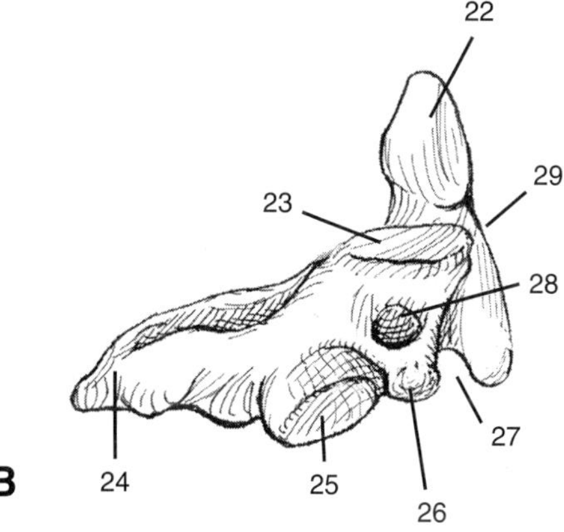

FIGURE 7.3 Diagram of second cervical vertebra, (A) anterior and (B) lateral views.

18. ______________________

19. ______________________

20. ______________________

21. ______________________

22. ______________________

23. ______________________

24. ______________________

25. ______________________

26. ______________________

27. ______________________

28. ______________________

29. ______________________

30. The ____________ foramen is found only in cervical vertebrae.

31. The vertebral foramen provides protection for the

______________________________________.

32. Large, bulky structures on C1 that contain the articular facets are called the

______________________________________.

33. The second cervical vertebra is also called the

______________________________________.

34. The first zygapophyseal joint is called the

______________________________________.

35. The pedicles and laminae unite to form the vertebral or neural arch.

a. true

b. false

36. The facet on the superior articular process faces anteriorly.

a. true

b. false

37. Which structure passes through the transverse foramen?

a. vertebral artery

b. spinal nerve

c. spinal cord

d. cauda equina

38. Which vertebrae is called the atlas?

a. C1

b. C2

c. C5

d. C7

39. The first cervical vertebra is atypical because it does not possess a:

a. body

b. posterior arch

c. facet

d. anterior arch

40. The atlanto-occipital joint allows for _____ of the head.

1. flexion

2. rotation

3. lateral tilt

a. 1 and 2

b. 1 and 3

c. 2 and 3

d. 1, 2, and 3

41. The second cervical vertebra has a large tooth-like process projecting from it, which fits into the arch of C1. This process is called the:

a. lateral mass

b. tubercle

c. dens

d. condyle

42. The vertebral prominence of C7 derives its name from its:

a. long transverse process

b. large body

c. atypical articular process

d. large spinous process

43. The thyroid cartilage is found at the level of:

a. C1

b. C3

c. C5

d. C7

Radiographic Procedures, Analysis, and Critical Thinking

For questions 44–49, identify the radiographic anatomy of the AP cervical spine in Figure 7.4A.

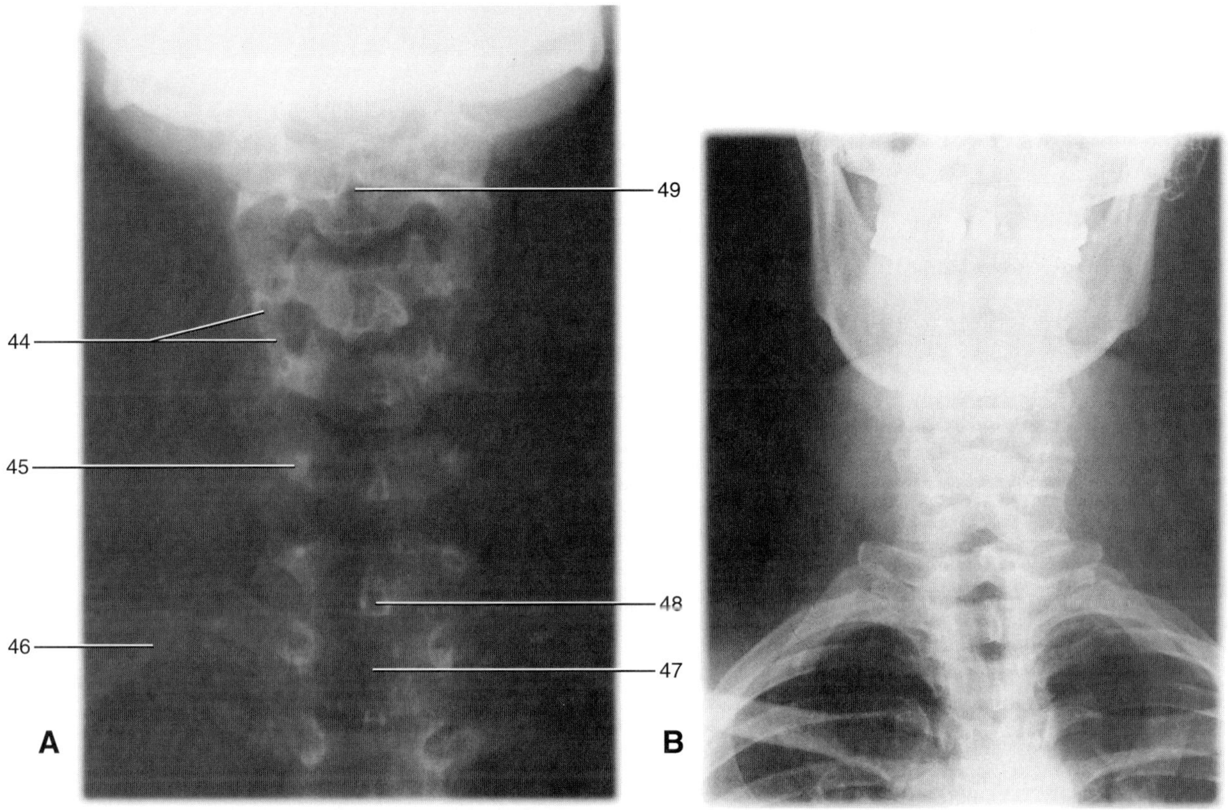

FIGURE 7.4 Radiograph of cervical spine, AP projection, (A) correct positioning and (B) incorrect positioning.

44. ______________________ **47.** ______________________

45. ______________________ **48.** ______________________

46. ______________________ **49.** ______________________

50. Compare the positioning quality of the correctly positioned radiograph in Figure 7.4A with that in Figure 7.4B. Describe the positioning error, explain what caused it, and give the step(s) necessary to correct the problem.

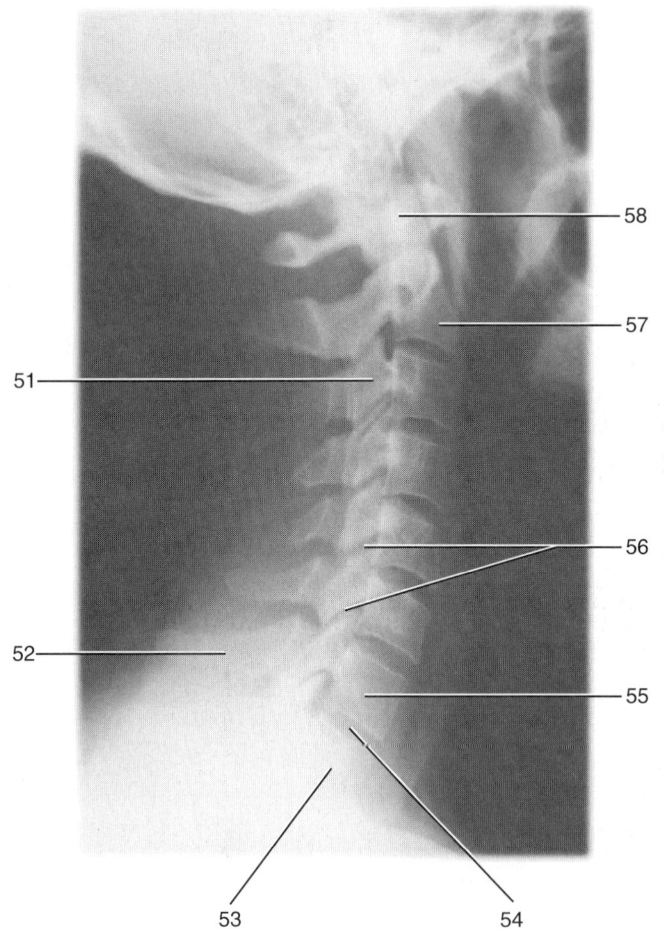

FIGURE 7.5 Radiograph of cervical spine, lateral projection.

For questions 51–58, identify the radiographic anatomy of the lateral cervical spine in Figure 7.5.

51. ____________________

52. ____________________

53. ____________________

54. ____________________

55. ____________________

56. ____________________

57. ____________________

58. ____________________

For questions 59–66, identify the radiographic anatomy of the oblique cervical spine in Figure 7.6.

59. ______________________________

60. ______________________________

61. ______________________________

62. ______________________________

63. ______________________________

64. ______________________________

65. ______________________________

66. ______________________________

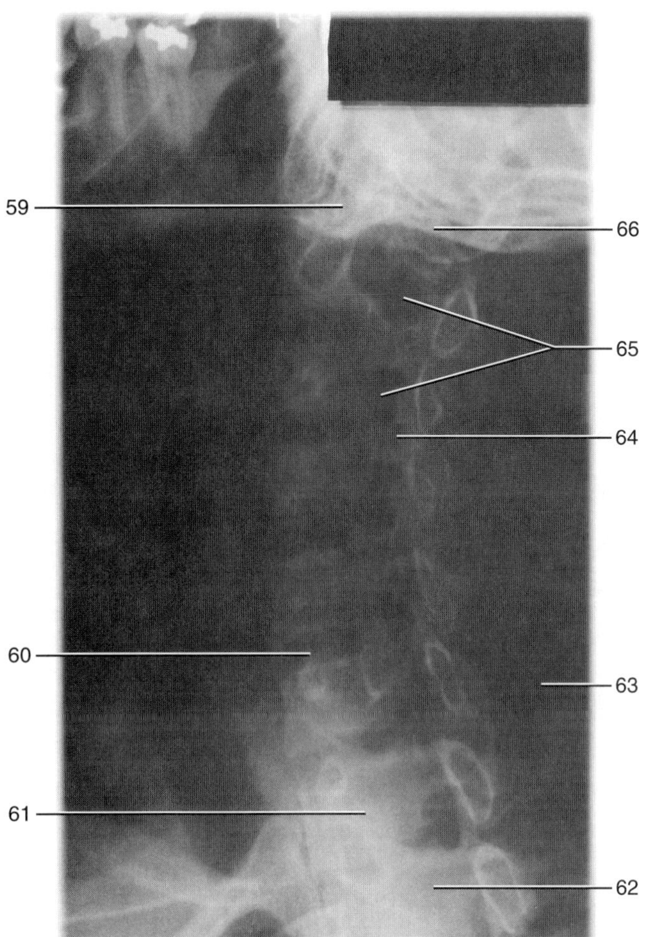

FIGURE 7.6 Radiograph of cervical spine, oblique projections

67. Can you determine the position of the patient by looking at the radiographic anatomy and the film markers on Figure 7.6? Why or why not?

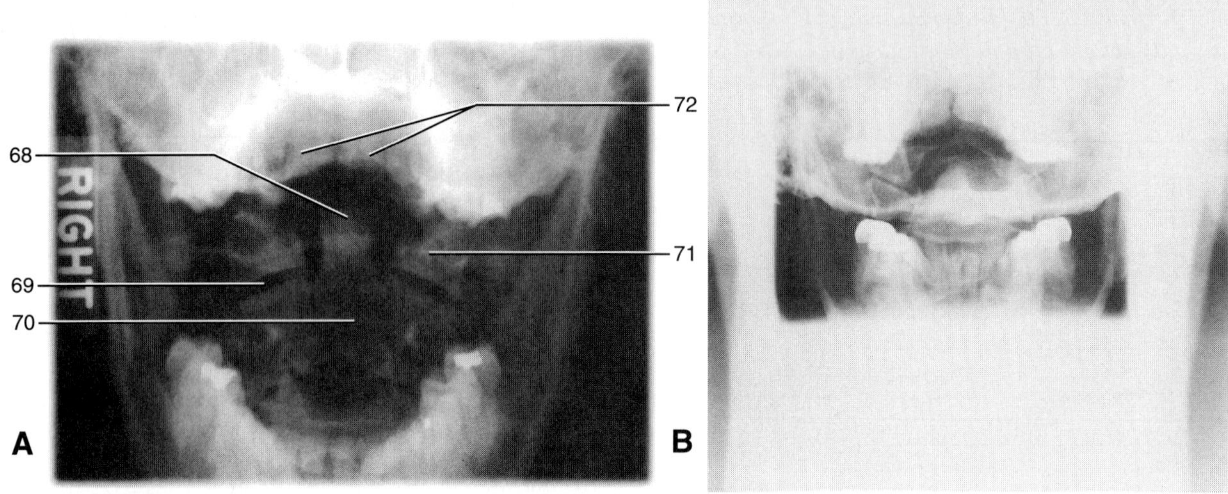

FIGURE 7.7 Radiograph of cervical spine, AP odontoid projection, (A) correct positioning and (B) incorrect positioning.

For questions 68–72, identify the radiographic anatomy of the AP open mouth projection in Figure 7.7A.

68. ______________________

69. ______________________

70. ______________________

71. ______________________

72. ______________________

73. Compare the positioning quality of the correctly positioned radiograph in Figure 7.7A with that in Figure 7.7B. Describe the positioning error, explain what caused it, and give the step(s) necessary to correct the problem.

74. For the AP open mouth projection, the __________ and the __________ should be placed in a line perpendicular to the table.

75. The __________ position best demonstrates the left intervertebral foramina of the C-spine.

76. For a lateral projection of the cervical spine, the top of the film should be placed approximately __________ inches above the EAM.

77. The advantage of the AP Otonello "wagging jaw" method over the conventional AP cervical spine is

____.

78. For the AP odontoid process using either the Fuchs or Judd method, the dens should be located __________ on the radiograph.

79. Special AP projections of the vertebral arch require that the tube be angled 25° cephalad.

a. true

b. false

80. The lateral projection of the cervical spine should be taken on deep inspiration.

a. true

b. false

81. Hyperflexion films are taken by tucking the patient's chin as close to the chest as possible.

a. true

b. false

82. For the AP odontoid process using the Fuchs method, a line from the upper incisors to the mastoid tip should be perpendicular to the table.

a. true

b. false

83. On a correctly positioned AP projection of the cervical spine, which vertebrae should be demonstrated?

a. C1–C7

b. C1–T1

c. C2–T1

d. C3–T2

84. What is the tube angle and direction for an AP projection of the cervical spine?

a. 5-10°, cephalic

b. 5-10°, caudal

c. 15–20°, caudal

d. 15–20°, cephalic

85. When performing the AP open mouth projection, if the inferior margins of the upper teeth and the mastoid tips are exactly superimposed:

a. the patient is properly positioned

b. the proper landmarks have not been used

c. the position must be corrected by dropping the chin

d. the central ray should be angled 10°

86. Which of the following should be demonstrated on an open mouth odontoid radiograph?

1. dens

2. lateral masses

3. C2

a. 1 and 2

b. 1 and 3

c. 2 and 3

d. 1, 2, and 3

87. The recommended kVp range for AP and oblique cervical spine projections is:

a. 65–70

b. 75–80

c. 85–90

d. 95–100

88. The LAO position of the cervical spine will visualize essentially the same structures as the:

a. LPO

b. RPO

c. RAO

d. lateral

89. In which projection of the cervical spine are the intervertebral foramina closest to the film (the down side) best demonstrated?

a. AP oblique

b. PA oblique

c. AP

d. lateral

90. What is the optimal tube angle and direction for AP oblique projections of the cervical spine?

a. 15–20°, caudal

b. 15–20°, cephalic

c. 25–30°, caudal

d. 25–30°, cephalic

91. Which projection best demonstrates the cervical intervertebral foramina?

a. oblique

b. lateral

c. AP

d. AP open mouth

92. The chin should be slightly extended on a lateral cervical spine to ensure that the:

a. mandible is free of superimposition on the vertebral bodies

b. occipital bone is free of superimposition on the vertebral bodies

c. head is in a true lateral position

d. midsagittal plane is parallel to the film

93. Which of the following are well visualized on a lateral radiograph of the cervical spine?

1. intervertebral foramina

2. zygapophyseal joints

3. spinous processes

a. 1 and 2

b. 1 and 3

c. 2 and 3

d. 1, 2, and 3

94. The spinous processes of the cervical vertebrae are best demonstrated by which projection?

a. AP

b. PA oblique

c. lateral

d. AP open mouth

95. Hyperflexion and hyperextension views of the cervical spine are taken to demonstrate:

a. small fractures

b. range of motion

c. dislocations

d. early arthritis

96. Some projections of the cervical spine are performed at 40 inch SID, whereas others are performed at 72 inch SID. Explain why the two different SID, are used.

Do You Remember?

97. For the AP axial projection of the sacroiliac joints, the central ray is angled 15–20° cephalic.

 a. true

 b. false

98. The longest portion of the sternum is called the:

 a. xiphoid

 b. manubrium

 c. body

 d. costochondral process

99. If a patient has sustained an injury to the right anterior ribs, which oblique position would best demonstrate the area of injury?

 a. RPO

 b. LPO

 c. RAO

 d. LAO

For questions 100–104, match the process to the bone on which it is located.

	Process	Bone
100. _____	tuberosity	a. radius
101. _____	semilunar notch	b. scapula
102. _____	tubercle	c. humerus
103. _____	acromial extremity	d. clavicle
104. _____	glenoid cavity	e. ulna

105. Which organ occupies most of the right hypochondrium?

 a. liver

 b. gallbladder

 c. stomach

 d. large intestine

106. The _____ is located at the junction of the manubrium and the body of the sternum.

 a. xiphoid process

 b. manubrial notch

 c. sternal angle

 d. sternoclavicular joint

STUDY TIP: TIME MANAGEMENT

Instructor Bob: Joe, I notice you have been doing better in my class. Have you done anything differently over the past few weeks?

Joe: You bet! When I first started the radiography program I thought that I could continue doing all the things I did before I was accepted *and* just add the new schoolwork. I never expected the program to be so labor intensive.

Instructor Bob: Didn't we tell you about that during your interview?

Joe: Of course, but I thought it applied to everyone else but me.

Instructor Bob: So you cut out all your social life?

Joe: No way! You know me better than that. What I did was manage my time more efficiently. By plotting out the hours in a day, using an inexpensive daily calendar, I found quite a bit of wasted time that I could use for study. Oh, sure I had to cut *some* social time out but ....

Instructor Bob: Let me guess, you scheduled free time in your daily plan.

Joe: How did you know? At first I was unrealistic and scheduled the whole day for classes and study but I found I was too exhausted to follow the schedule. It just didn't work.

Instructor Bob: Well, schedule in some extra time for the skull lab—I think you'll need it!

- Analyze your use of time to see where studying can best fit.
- Set a schedule, first for the entire semester, then for each day.
- Plan time for leisure, family, and social activities as well as school-related functions.
- Make daily and weekly "to do" lists. Prioritize them and check off tasks as you complete them.

> Everyone has more things to do than there is time available to do them. Time management is an essential skill for all students to learn early in the educational process.

CHAPTER **8**

Thoracic Spine

LEARNING OBJECTIVES

At the completion of this chapter, the student should be able to:

1. List and describe the bony anatomy of the thoracic spine.
2. Given drawings and radiographs, locate anatomic structures and landmarks.
3. Explain the rationale for each projection.
4. Explain the patient preparation required for each examination.
5. Describe the positioning used to visualize anatomic structures in the thoracic spine.
6. List or identify the central ray location and the extent of the field necessary for each projection.
7. Explain the protective measures that should be taken for each examination.
8. Recommend the technical factors for producing an acceptable radiograph for each projection.
9. State the patient instructions for each projection.
10. Given radiographs, evaluate positioning and technical factors.
11. Describe modifications of procedures for atypical or impaired patients to better demonstrate the anatomic area of interest.

Routine and Alternative Positions/Projections

Part	Routine	Alternative
Thoracic spine	AP	
	Lateral	Swimmer's lateral
		Oblique

QUESTIONS

Anatomy and Physiology

For questions 1–14, identify the anatomy of the thoracic vertebra in Figure 8.1.

1. ____________________

2. ____________________

3. ____________________

4. ____________________

5. ____________________

6. ____________________

7. ____________________

8. ____________________

9. ____________________

10. ____________________

11. ____________________

12. ____________________

13. ____________________

14. ____________________

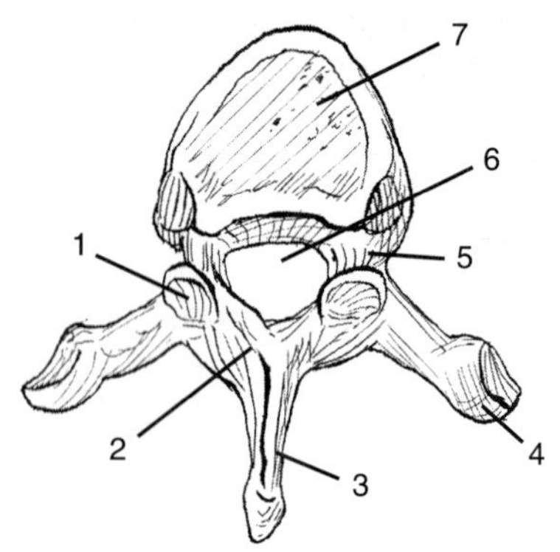

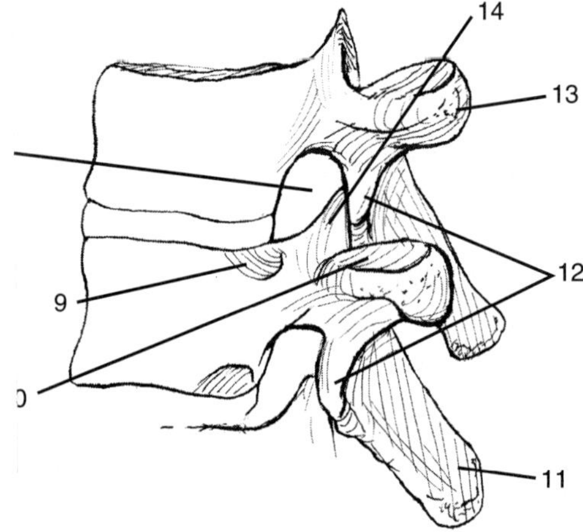

FIGURE 8.1 Diagram of typical thoracic vertebra, (A) superior and (B) lateral views.

15. The __________ lies about 2 inches below the jugular notch at the level of T4–T5.

16. The thoracic spine consists of __________ vertebrae.

17. The two types of rib articulations are called __________ and __________ joints.

18. The thoracic zygapophyseal joints form a __________ degree angle to the midsagittal plane.

19. The manubrial or jugular notch lies at the level of the __________ thoracic vertebrae.

20. The thoracic spine has a posterior convex curvature.

a. true

b. false

21. The xiphoid tip lies at the level of:

a. T6

b. T10

c. T12

d. L1

22. Compared to lumbar vertebrae, the spinous processes of thoracic vertebrae:

a. are more often bifid

b. arise anteriorly from the neural arch

c. are more blunt and point more superiorly

d. are longer and point more sharply downward

23. An abnormal posterior curvature of the spine (humpback deformity) is called:

a. lordosis

b. kyphosis

c. spondylolisthesis

d. scoliosis

24. What anatomic structure lies directly on top of the body of a thoracic vertebra?

a. pedicle

b. lamina

c. intervertebral disk

d. intervertebral foramen

25. An intervertebral foramen is formed by the _____ of one vertebra and the _____ of the vertebra below:

a. inferior vertebral notch, superior vertebral notch

b. superior vertebral notch, inferior vertebral notch

c. inferior articular process, superior articular process

d. superior articular process, inferior articular process

26. Most ribs articulate posteriorly with a thoracic vertebra at the:

1. vertebral body

2. inferior articular process

3. transverse process

a. 1 and 2

b. 1 and 3

c. 2 and 3

d. 1, 2, and 3

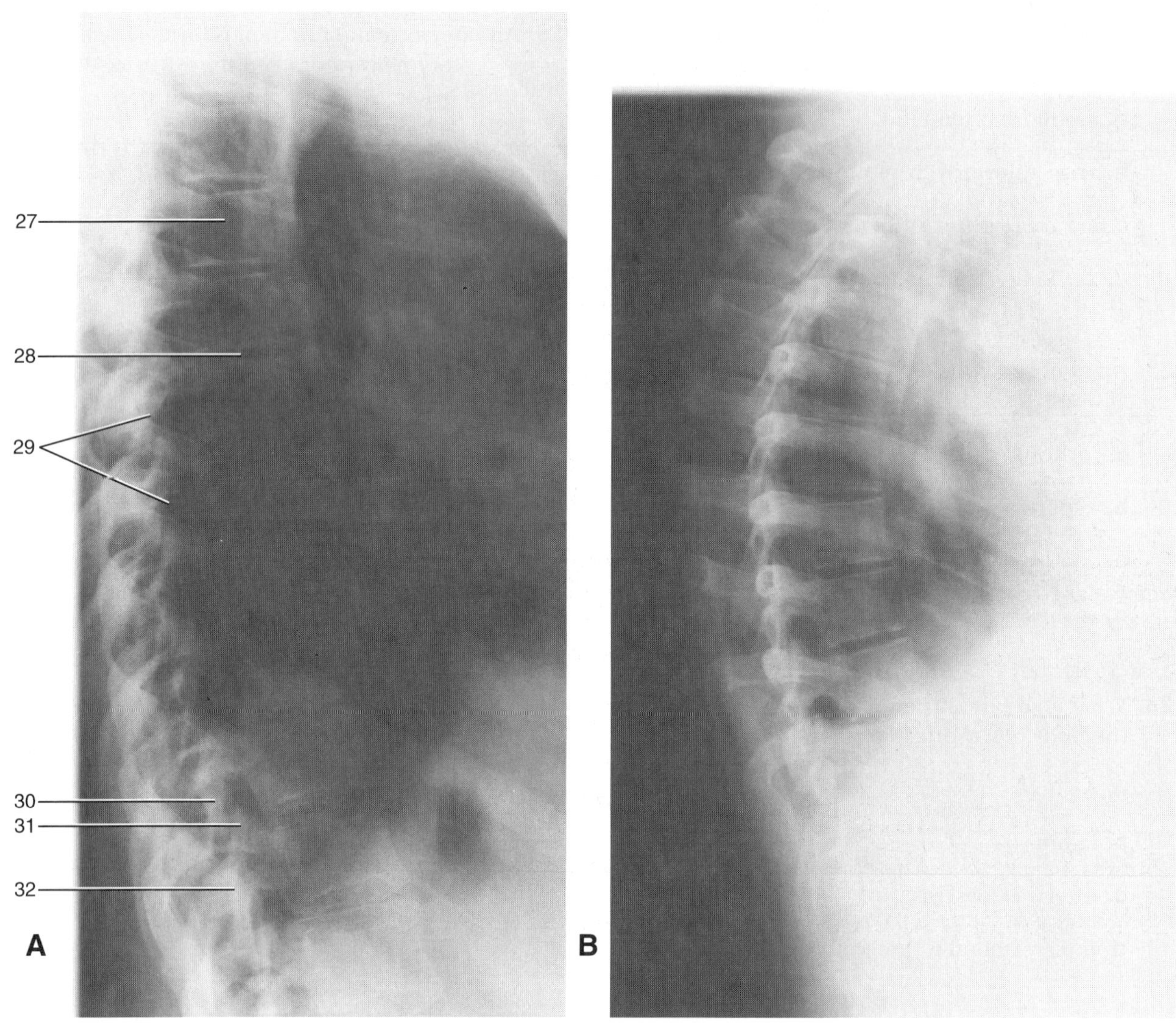

FIGURE 8.2 Radiograph of thoracic spine, lateral projection, (A) correct positioning and (B) incorrect positioning.

Radiographic Procedures, Analysis, and Critical Thinking

For questions 27–32, identify the radiographic anatomy of the lateral thoracic spine in Figure 8.2A.

27. ______________________ **30.** ______________________

28. ______________________ **31.** ______________________

29. ______________________ **32.** ______________________

33. Compare the positioning quality of the correctly positioned radiograph in Figure 8.2A with that in Figure 8.2B. Describe the positioning error, explain what caused it, and give the step(s) necessary to correct the problem.

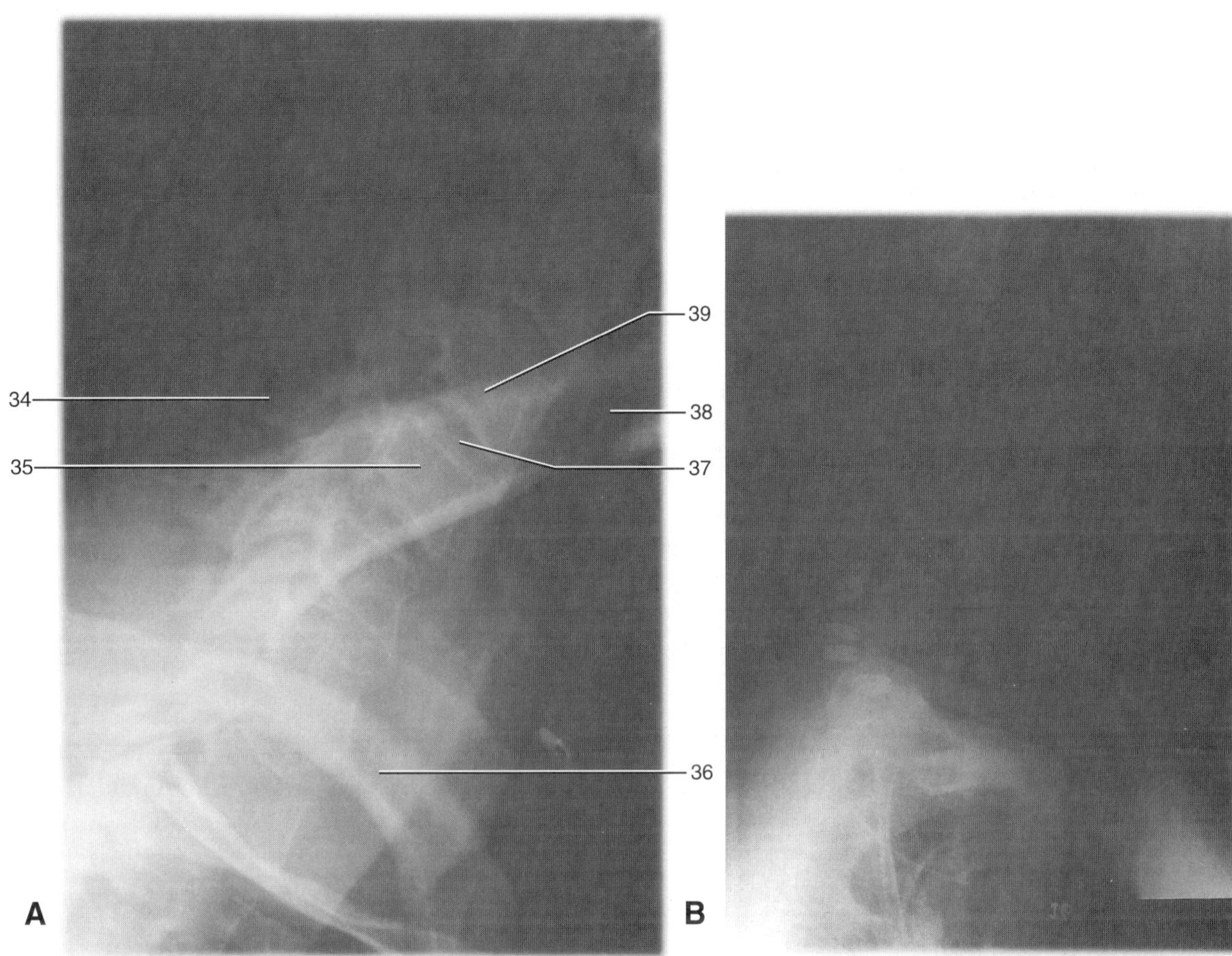

FIGURE 8.3 Radiograph of thoracic spine, Swimmers lateral projection, (A) correct positioning and (B) incorrect positioning.

For questions 34–39, identify the radiographic anatomy of the swimmer's lateral thoracic spine in Figure 8.3A.

34. ______________________

35. ______________________

36. ______________________

37. ______________________

38. ______________________

39. ______________________

40. Compare the positioning quality of the correctly positioned radiograph in Figure 8.3A with that in Figure 8.3B. Describe the positioning error, explain what caused it, and give the step(s) necessary to correct the problem.

41. The normal film size for an AP projection of the thoracic spine is __________ inches.

42. The normal kVp range for AP and lateral thoracic spine projections is __________.

43. On a lateral thoracic spine projection, the top of the cassette should be placed __________ the shoulder.

44. For oblique thoracic spine projections, patients are obliqued __________ degrees.

45. It is customary to allow the patient to breathe during exposures of the AP and lateral thoracic spine.

a. true

b. false

46. For AP thoracic spine projections, the thickest end of the wedge filter should be placed toward T1.

a. true

b. false

47. When centering for a lateral thoracic spine, the patient should be placed with the midaxillary line centered to the table.

a. true

b. false

48. The spinous processes of the thoracic spine are clearly visualized on the lateral projection.

a. true

b. false

49. Grids are not normally used for AP and lateral thoracic spine projections.

a. true

b. false

50. Because of superimposition from shoulder structures, the upper six to seven thoracic vertebrae are not normally visualized on the lateral projection.

a. true

b. false

For questions 51–54, identify the radiographic anatomy of the AP thoracic spine in Figure 8.4.

51. Pedicle

a. 1

b. 2

c. 3

d. 5

52. Transverse process

a. 3

b. 5

c. 6

d. 7

53. Spinous process

a. 1

b. 4

c. 5

d. 8

54. Costovertebral joint

a. 3

b. 4

c. 7

d. 8

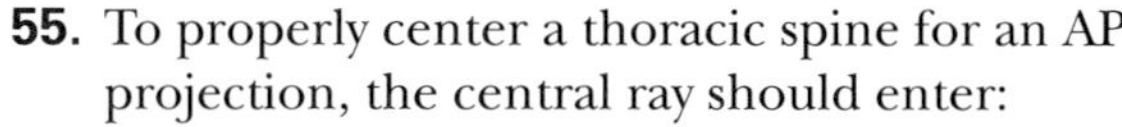

55. To properly center a thoracic spine for an AP projection, the central ray should enter:

a. 2 inches superior to the sternal angle

b. 3–4 inches below the jugular or manubrial notch

c. at the top of the iliac crest

d. 2 inches superior to the jugular or manubrial notch

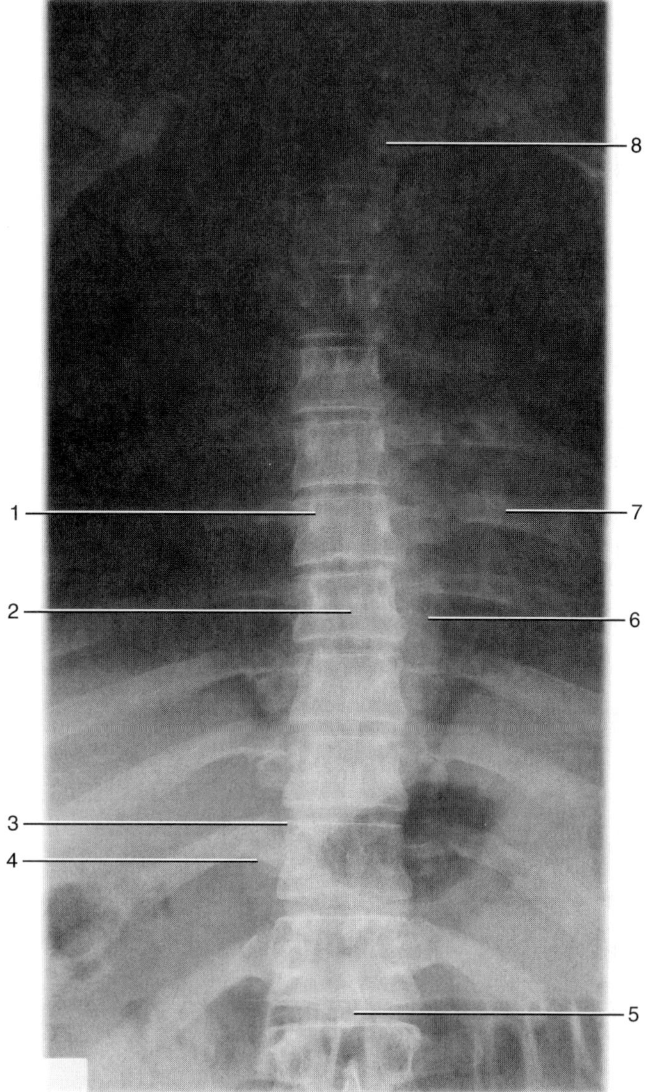

FIGURE 8.4 Radiograph of thoracic spine, AP projection.

56. The upper edge of the film for an AP projection of the thoracic spine should be

a. 1 inch below the upper border of the shoulders

b. at the level of the seventh thoracic vertebrae

c. 3 to 4 inches inferior to the manubrial notch

d. 1–2 inches above the upper border of the shoulders

57. A wedge filter is sometimes used during an AP thoracic spine examination to:

a. reduce motion

b. increase penetration

c. produce a more homogenous density throughout the T-spine

d. reduce the amount of MAS needed

58. Which structure is *not* clearly demonstrated on an AP projection of the thoracic spine?

a. disk space

b. body

c. intervertebral foramen

d. transverse process

59. When performing an AP projection of the thoracic spine, the radiographer should:

a. place the anode at the T1 end

b. place the anode at the T12 end

c. use a short SID

d. use high kVp

60. Which zygapophyseal joints are demonstrated on a PA oblique (RAO) of the thoracic spine?

a. right

b. left

c. both right and left

d. the joints furthest from the film

61. Oblique thoracic spine projections must demonstrate:

a. T1–T12

b. T1–T10

c. T7–T12

d. T4–T12

62. The patient is placed prone and the right side is rotated 70° away from the table. The patient position is best described as:

a. RPO

b. LPO

c. RAO

d. LAO

63. For a lateral thoracic spine, the arms are drawn forward at right angles to the patient to:

a. maximize patient comfort

b. place the spine parallel to the table

c. prevent the scapulae from superimposing on the vertebrae

d. place the midsagittal plane perpendicular to the film

64. What is the purpose of using a breathing technique for a lateral thoracic spine?

a. to demonstrate all 12 vertebrae

b. to better demonstrate the transverse processes

c. the motion removes lung superimposition

d. to more clearly open the intervertebral foramina

65. Which types of patients benefit most by placing a radiolucent sponge under the thoracolumbar area for lateral thoracic spine projections?

a. thin males

b. obese males

c. obese females

d. thin females

66. For a lateral thoracic spine projection a _____ can be used to blur out the images of the ribs and pulmonary structures overlying the vertebral bodies.

a. breathing technique

b. low kVp technique

c. high kVp technique

d. magnification technique

67. A radiographer examines a lateral thoracic spine radiograph and notices that T1–T4 are not visualized. What action should be taken?

a. Repeat the film centering 2–4 inches higher.

b. Repeat the film, moving the patient's arms more forward.

c. Repeat the film placing a radiolucent sponge under the thoracolumbar area.

d. Turn the film in for reading because it was accurately positioned.

68. Which vertebrae should be clearly demonstrated on a swimmer's lateral radiograph?

a. C4–T1

b. C7–T4

c. T1–T3

d. T1–T7

69. Where is the central ray placed for a swimmer's lateral?

a. C4

b. C6

c. T1

d. T3

70. For a swimmer's lateral the patient's arms are placed such that:

a. both arms are raised high above the head

b. both shoulders are depressed as much as possible

c. the arm nearest the table is raised above the head while the shoulder furthest from the table is depressed

d. the shoulder closest the table is depressed while the arm furthest from the table is raised above the head

71. When taking a swimmer's lateral you notice that the patient did not stop breathing during the exposure. What action should be taken?

a. Immediately repeat the film because the motion will degrade image quality.

b. Wait to see the film, although it is very likely it will need to be repeated.

c. Turn the film in for reading; although breathing will degrade image quality it will probably not be enough to require a repeat.

d. Turn the film in for reading; breathing may enhance image quality by obscuring overlying lung detail.

72. To better demonstrate the vertebral bodies, the central ray for a swimmer's lateral is sometimes angled:

a. 5–10° caudal

b. 5–10° cephalic

c. 15–25° caudal

d. 15–25° cephalic

73. A patient with severe kyphosis arrives for a T-spine examination. Describe how you would modify the examination for this patient's pathology.

74. Although all vertebra share certain anatomic structures, they also have unique features. Compare the structural differences between a typical cervical vertebra and a typical thoracic vertebra.

75. Some department routines require that the collimator be left open to a 14 x 17 inch square for the AP thoracic spine, whereas other departments require the radiographer to narrowly collimate to the spine. Describe the advantages and disadvantages of each.

76. A wedge filter is used for an AP thoracic spine projection but is placed in the reverse direction, with the thick end toward the bottom of the spine. Describe the appearance of the spine created by this error.

77. It is necessary to take a swimmer's lateral on a patient who has a severe spiral fracture of the right humerus. Describe the modifications in positioning, if any, that would be necessary for this patient.

78. A radiographer notices that the upper two vertebrae are clipped off the radiograph of an AP thoracic spine. Explain the positioning error that occurred and what you would do to correct it.

Do You Remember?

79. The dens and lateral masses are located on the second cervical vertebra.

    a. true

    b. false

80. PA oblique projections of the ribs require that the spine be rotated away from the side of injury.

    a. true

    b. false

81. The bony thorax is composed of the:

    1. sternum
    2. thoracic spine
    3. ribs

    a. 1 and 2

    b. 1 and 3

    c. 2 and 3

    d. 1, 2, and 3

82. The intervertebral foramina of the _____ spine are best demonstrated in the lateral projection.

    a. cervical

    b. thoracic

    c. both a and b

    d. neither a nor b

83. Which of the following would likely require the highest kVp?

    a. lateral thoracic spine

    b. lateral cervical spine

    c. swimmer's lateral thoracic spine

    d. All of the above have the same kVp range.

84. What is the largest foramen in the body?

    a. vertebral

    b. transverse

    c. obturator

    d. greater pelvic

85. Oblique PA projections of the cervical spine require a tube angle of:

    a. 15° cephalic

    b. 30° cephalic

    c. 15° caudal

    d. 30° caudal

86. The 12th pair of ribs is called _____ ribs.

    a. floating

    b. true

    c. false

    d. abdominal

87. Which bone possesses a tuberosity and a condyle?

a. femur

b. humerus

c. radius

d. ulna

88. The knee joint is located _____ to the patellar apex.

a. 1–2 cm proximal

b. 1–2 cm distal

c. 0.5 cm proximal

d. 0.5 cm distal

STUDY TIP: SUCCESSFUL TEST-TAKING—STUDYING FOR THE TEST

Kathy: I'm really depressed. I spent hours and hours studying for this test and still failed it. Instructor Bob just didn't ask anything that I studied.

Julio: Before the test, you even borrowed my notes and you seemed to know everything. What happened?

Kathy: I guess I didn't study the right material.

Juilo: You know, good notes and lots of study time are important but it's just as important to anticipate what the teacher is going to ask. When I study, I pretend I'm the teacher and make up questions to quiz myself. Let's go for a burger and I'll explain how I do it.

- If something is mentioned in the lecture and is also present in your textbook, it is probably important to know. For example, if new terms appear in bold type in the text and the teacher has written them on the board, they are probably essential to know.
- The more time the instructor spends on a topic, the more important it usually is to know.
- Lecture notes should be reviewed within 24 hours after the class and compared to the text. If there are any discrepancies, they should be brought to the attention of the teacher immediately.
- Form a study group where each person writes 10–20 possible test questions on index cards. Share the questions and answers among members of the study group.

Successful test-taking is a learned skill and sometimes the same study strategies that are successful for one test or one teacher do not apply for other tests or teachers. The essence of successful studying and, thus, test-taking is identifying what is most important and anticipating possible questions.

CHAPTER 9

Lumbar Spine, Sacrum, and Coccyx

LEARNING OBJECTIVES

At the completion of this chapter, the student should be able to:

1. List and describe the anatomy of the lumbar spine, sacrum, and coccyx.
2. Given drawings and radiographs, locate anatomic structures and landmarks.
3. Explain the rationale for each projection.
4. Explain the patient preparation required for each examination.
5. Describe the positioning used to visualize anatomic structures in the lumbar spine, sacrum, and coccyx.
6. List or identify the central ray location and the extent of the field necessary for each projection.
7. Explain the protective measures that should be taken for each examination.
8. Recommend the technical factors for producing an acceptable radiograph for each projection.
9. State the patient instructions for each projection.
10. Given radiographs, evaluate positioning and technical factors.
11. Describe modifications of procedures for atypical or impaired patients to better demonstrate the anatomic area of interest.

Routine and Alternative Positions/Projections

Part	Routine	Alternative
Lumbar Spine	AP	Lateral L5–S1
	Oblique	AP axial L5–S1 junction
	Lateral	Hyperextension/hyperflexion
		Bending exams
		Scoliosis series
Sacrum	AP	
	Lateral	
Coccyx	AP	
	Lateral	

QUESTIONS

Anatomy and Physiology

For questions 1–16, identify the anatomy of the lumbar vertebra in Figure 9.1.

1. 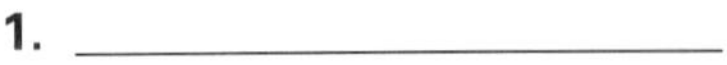

2. ______________________

3. ______________________

4. ______________________

5. ______________________

6. ______________________

7. ______________________

8. ______________________

9. ______________________

10. ______________________

11. ______________________

12. ______________________

13. ______________________

14. ______________________

15. ______________________

16. ______________________

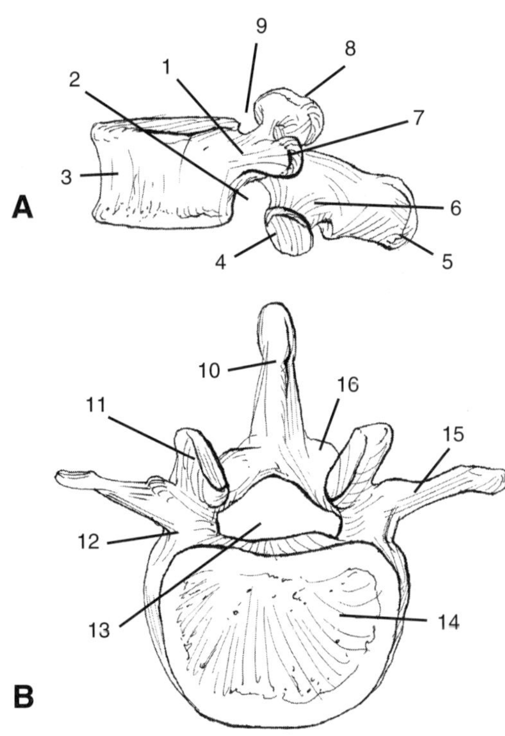

FIGURE 9.1 Diagram of lumbar vertebra, (A) lateral and (B) superior views.

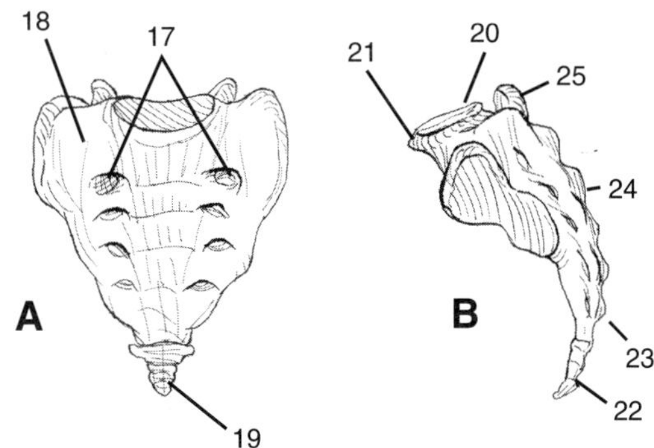

FIGURE 9.2 Diagram of sacrum and coccyx, (A) anterior and (B) lateral views.

For questions 17–25, identify the anatomy of the sacrum and coccyx in Figure 9.2.

17. ____________________

18. ____________________

19. ____________________

20. ____________________

21. ____________________

22. ____________________

23.

24. ____________________

25. ____________________

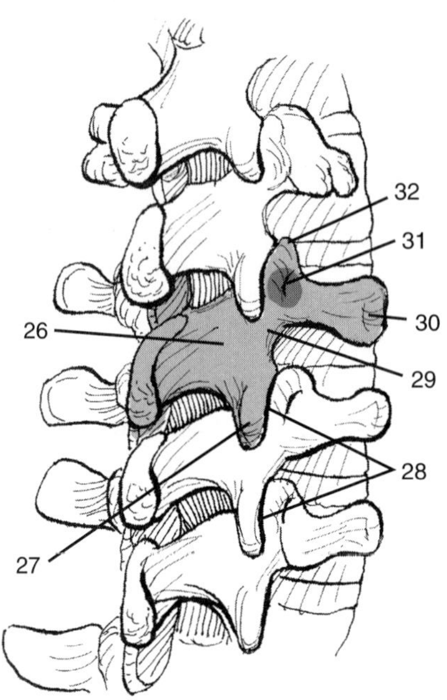

FIGURE 9.3 Diagram of oblique lumbar spine, "scotty dog."

For questions 26–32, identify the anatomy of the "Scotty dog" in Figure 9.3.

26. ____________________

27. ____________________

28. ____________________

29. ____________________

30. ____________________

31. ____________________

32. ____________________

33. The articulating surfaces of the superior and inferior articular processes are called

____.

34. The zygapophyseal joints form a __________ degree angle to the midsagittal plane.

35. The intervertebral foramen is formed by __________ and __________.

36. The posterior portion of the vertebral arch is formed by fusion of the:

a. two laminae

b. two pedicles

c. inferior articular processes

d. superior articular processes

37. The soft, semigelatinous central portion of an intervertebral disk is called the:

a. nucleus fibrosis

b. annulus pulposus

c. annulus fibrosis

d. nucleus pulposis

38. The lumbosacral junction is located at the approximate level of the:

a. iliac crest

b. symphysis pubis

c. anterior-superior iliac spine

d. pubic bone

39. An abnormal lateral curvature of the spine results in a condition called:

a. scoliosis

b. lordosis

c. subluxation

d. ankylosis

40. The iliac crest is at the approximate level of:

a. L1

b. L3

c. L4

d. sacrum

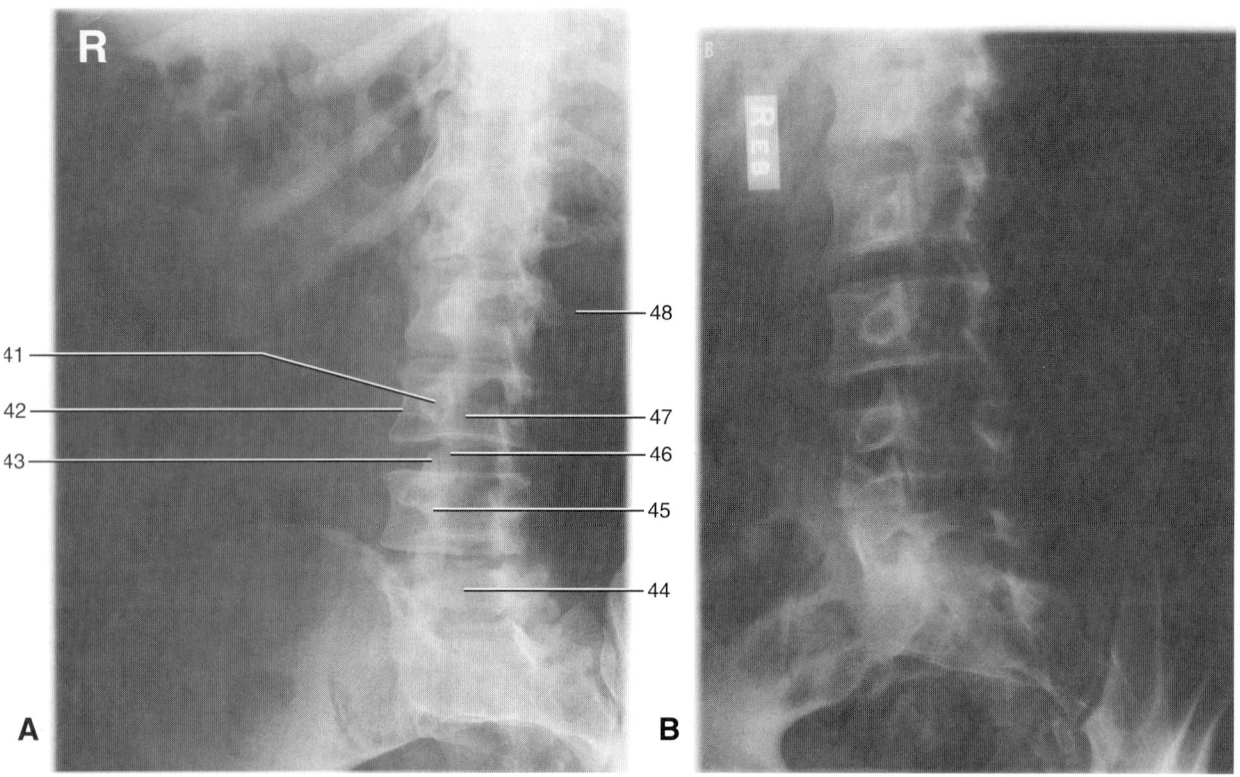

FIGURE 9.4 Radiograph of lumbar spine, oblique projection, (A) correct positioning and (B) incorrect positioning.

Radiographic Procedures, Analysis, and Critical Thinking

For questions 41–48, identify the radiographic anatomy of the oblique lumbar spine in Figure 9.4A.

41. ____________________

42. ____________________

43. ____________________

44. ____________________

45. ____________________

46. ____________________

47. ____________________

48. ____________________

49. Compare the positioning quality of the correctly positioned radiograph in Figure 9.4A with that in Figure 9.4B. Describe the positioning error, explain what caused it, and give the step(s) necessary to correct the problem.

50. Determine the position of the patient by looking at the radiographic anatomy and the film markers on Figure 9.4A. What clues led you to this answer?

For questions 51–56, identify the radiographic anatomy of the sacrum in Figure 9.5.

51. 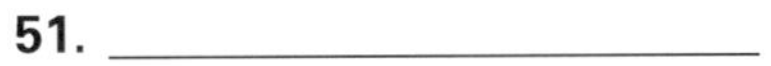

52. 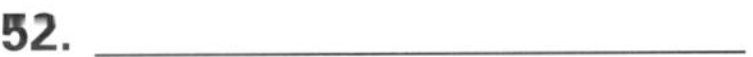

53. ____________________

54. 

55. ____________________

56. ____________________

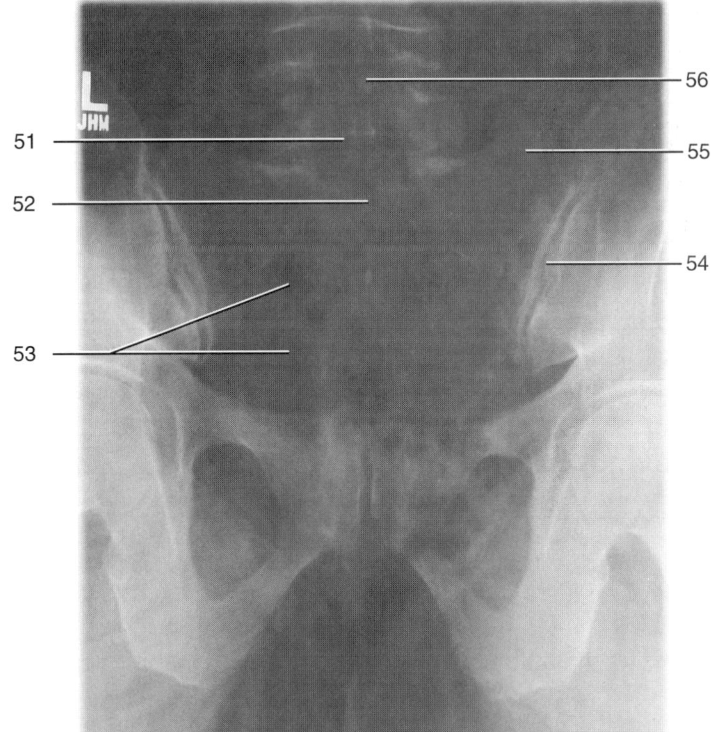

FIGURE 9.5 Radiograph of sacrum, AP projection.

57. The knees are flexed for the AP projection of the lumbar spine to

____.

58. When centering for an AP oblique projection of the lumbar spine, the sagittal plane is placed __________ inches medial to the elevated ASIS.

59. For the lateral projection of the lumbar spine, the sagittal plane is __________ and the coronal plane is __________ to the table.

60. The kVp range for a lateral projection of the L5–S1 junction is

____.

61. When centering for a lateral projection of the L5–S1 junction, the central ray should be placed __________ inches anterior to the palpated spinous processes.

62. The AP lumbar spine is the best projection for demonstrating the spinous processes.

a. true

b. false

63. If the patient cannot be placed supine, a PA projection of the lumbar spine may be substituted for the AP, provided that no acute trauma is suspected.

a. true

b. false

64. For a lateral projection of the lumbar spine, the central ray enters 1 inch anterior to the palpated spinous processes.

a. true

b. false

65. If the central ray is placed at the level of the iliac crest when using a 14 x 17 inch film for a lateral lumbar spine, L1 may not be demonstrated on the radiograph.

a. true

b. false

66. For an AP projection of the sacrum, the tube is angled 15° cephalic and enters midway between the ASIS and the iliac crest.

a. true

b. false

67. Radiographic magnification of the sacrum will be greater on a PA projection of the sacrum than on an AP sacrum.

a. true

b. false

68. The correct film size for a lateral coccyx projection is 10 x 12 inches.

a. true

b. false

For questions 69–73, identify the radiographic anatomy of the AP lumbar spine in Figure 9.6A.

69. Body of L5

a. 3

b. 5

c. 7

d. 9

70. Pedicle

a. 1

b. 6

c. 8

d. 10

71. Transverse process

a. 1

b. 2

c. 7

d. 10

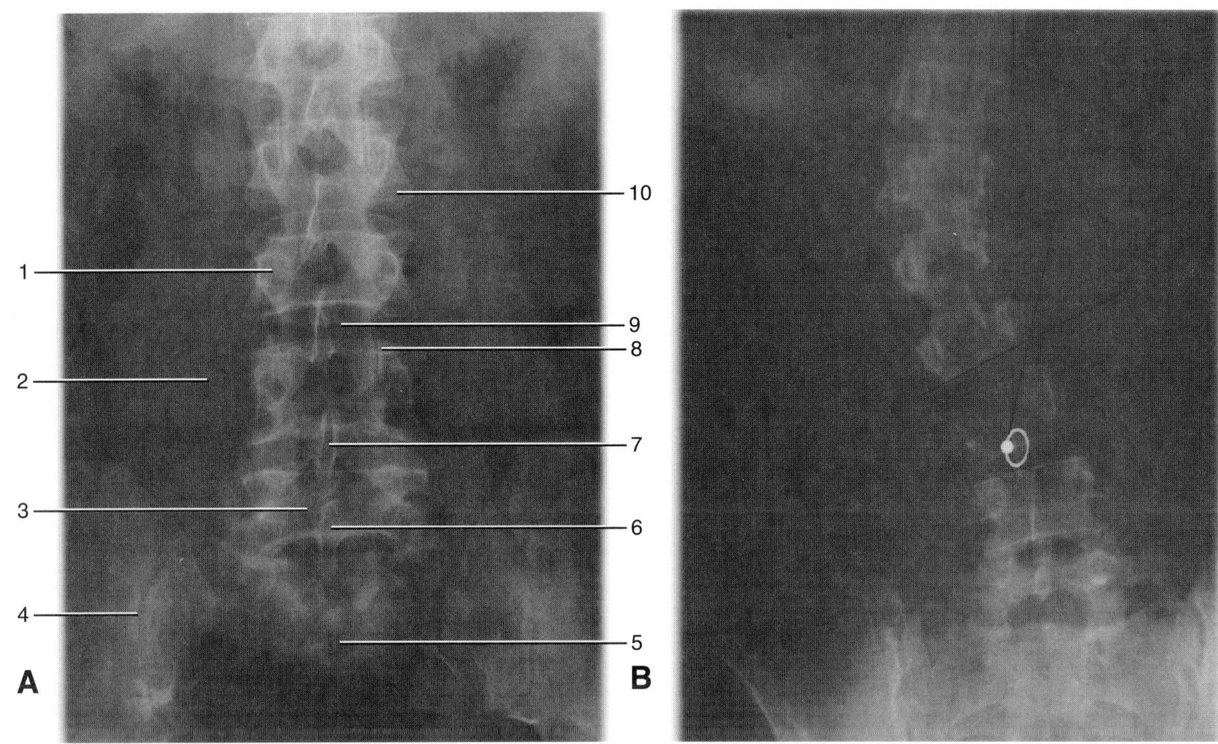

FIGURE 9.6 Radiograph of lumbar spine, AP projection, (A) correct positioning and (B) incorrect positioning.

72. Spinous process of L4

a. 3

b. 5

c. 6

d. 7

73. Intervertebral disk space

a. 4

b. 6

c. 9

d. 10

74. Compare the positioning quality of the correctly positioned radiograph in Figure 9.6A with that in Figure 9.6B. Describe the positioning error, explain what caused it, and give the step(s) necessary to correct the problem.

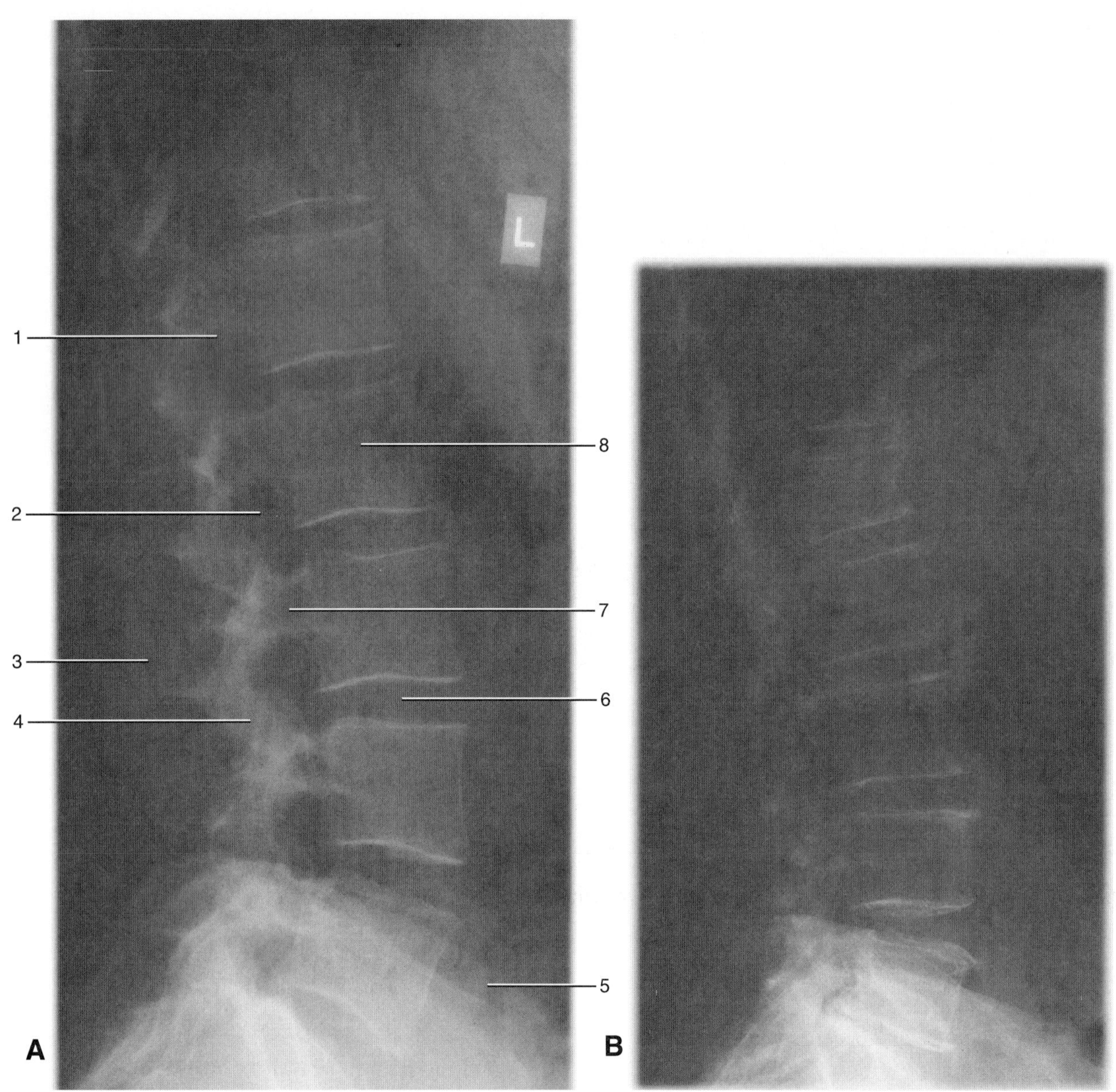

FIGURE 9.7 Radiograph of lumbar spine, lateral projection, (A) correct positioning and (B) incorrect positioning.

For questions 75–79, identify the radiographic anatomy of the lateral lumbar spine in Figure 9.7A.

75. Spinous process

a. 1

b. 3

c. 4

d. 7

76. Inferior vertebral notch

a. 1

b. 4

c. 5

d. 7

77. Pedicle

a. 3

b. 4

c. 7

d. 8

78. Iliac crest

a. 3

b. 4

c. 5

d. 6

79. Intervertebral foramen

a. 2

b. 6

c. 7

d. 8

80. Compare the positioning quality of the correctly positioned radiograph in Figure 9.7A with that in Figure 9.7B. Describe the positioning error, explain what caused it, and give the step(s) necessary to correct the problem.

81. When using a 14 x 17 inch cassette, an AP lumbar spine should be centered:

a. 1–2 inches above the iliac crest

b. at the level of the iliac crest

c. at the level of the ASIS

d. 1–2 inches below the level of the iliac crest

82. Which of the following are *not* clearly demonstrated on an AP projection of the lumbar spine?

a. spinous processes

b. transverse processes

c. pedicles

d. bodies

83. The optimal kVp range for an AP projection of the lumbar spine is:

a. 65–70

b. 68–73

c. 75–80

d. 85–90

84. For AP projections of the lumbar spine, flat contact gonad shields should not be used for _____ patients.

a. female

b. male

c. elderly

d. pediatric

85. The zygapophyseal joints *nearer* the table are clearly demonstrated when the patient is in the _____ position.

a. LAO

b. lateral

c. supine

d. RPO

86. Which of the following should be well demonstrated on an oblique lumbar spine radiograph with the patient in an RPO position?

1. right zygapophyseal joints

2. right intervertebral foramina

3. right superior and inferior articular processes

a. 1 and 2

b. 1 and 3

c. 2 and 3

d. 1, 2, and 3

87. For an oblique projection of the lumbar spine with the patient in the LAO position, the central ray is placed _____ inch(es) to the _____ of the spinous processes.

a. 2–3, right

b. 2–3, left

c. 1, right

d. 1, left

88. When examining an RPO lumbar spine radiograph, a radiographer notes that the left zygapophyseal joints are not well demonstrated and that the pedicle is quite posterior to the vertebral body. What is the most probable positioning error?

a. The patient is obliqued more than 45°.

b. The patient is obliqued less than 45°.

c. The patient was not obliqued at all.

d. There was no error—the part was properly positioned.

89. Which projection best demonstrates the intervertebral foramina of the lumbar spine?

a. AP

b. AP oblique

c. lateral

d. PA oblique

90. The optimum patient angle for an AP oblique projection of the lumbar spine is _____.

a. 15°

b. 30°

c. 45°

d. 60°

91. The proper breathing instruction for a lateral projection of the lumbar spine is:

a. suspend breathing on inspiration

b. breathe quietly during the exposure

c. take short rapid breaths during the exposure

d. suspend breathing on expiration

92. A lateral lumbar spine radiograph should clearly demonstrate the:

1. intervertebral foramina

2. spinous processes

3. disk spaces

a. 1 and 2

b. 1 and 3

c. 2 and 3

d. 1, 2, and 3

93. If the spine is not parallel to the table for a lateral lumbar spine on a female patient, the central ray should be directed:

a. perpendicular to the film

b. 5° cephalic

c. 5° caudal

d. 12° caudal

94. The routine film size for a lateral projection of the L5–S1 junction is _____ inches.

a. 14 x 17

b. 11 x 14

c. 10 x 12

d. 8 x 10

95. For a lateral projection of the L5–S1 junction, the central ray is placed:

a. 2 inches inferior to the iliac crest

b. 1/2 inch inferior to the iliac crest

c. at the level of the ASIS

d. 2 inches inferior to the ASIS

96. The tube angle for a lateral projection of the L5–S1 junction is _____, _____.

a. 10–15°, caudal

b. 10–15°, cephalic

c. 5–10°, caudal

d. 5–10°, cephalic

97. Compared to a routine lateral lumbar spine, the lateral projection of the L5–S1 junction usually requires:

a. more kVp

b. less kVp

c. less SID

d. more SID

98. To open the L5–S1 joint space in the AP axial projection, the tube should be angled _____ cephalic.

a. 5°

b. 20°

c. 35°

d. 45°

99. For scoliosis examinations of the lumbar spine, the PA projection is preferred over the AP because the PA:

a. results in less magnification

b. better demonstrates the abnormal curvature

c. opens up the joint spaces better

d. results in lower patient dose

100. Weight-bearing bending films of the lumbar spine are taken primarily to demonstrate:

a. tumors

b. degree of mobility after spinal fusion

c. trauma

d. calcium loss due to osteoporosis

101. Hyperflexion films of the lumbar spine are taken by having the patient bend ____ as much as possible.

a. forward

b. backward

c. to the right

d. to the left

102. To determine motion in the area of a spinal fusion of the lumbar spine, which of the following examinations is indicated?

a. lateral recumbent

b. lateral erect

c. AP axial L5–S1 junction

d. upright lateral flexion and extension

103. Which of the following is correct concerning the AP projection of the sacrum?

a. 10°caudal angle of central ray

b. 15° cephalic angle of central ray

c. central ray placed midway between ASIS and iliac crest

d. central ray placed at the level of the ASIS

104. For a lateral projection of the sacrum, the film is centered at the level of the:

a. greater trochanter

b. iliac crest

c. anterior-superior iliac spine

d. symphysis pubis

105. Lead blockers/shields are used to limit scatter radiation for examination of the:

1. lateral sacrum

2. lateral coccyx

3. AP sacrum

a. 1 and 2

b. 1 and 3

c. 2 and 3

d. 1, 2, and 3

106. When analyzing an AP coccyx radiograph, a radiographer observes that the coccyx is superimposed on the pubic bone. Which of the following is true?

a. The radiographer should angle the tube more caudal.

b. The radiographer should angle the tube more cephalic.

c. This superimposition is normal for this film.

d. The radiographer should use no tube angle.

107. For an AP projection of the coccyx, the central ray should enter:

a. 2 inches above the symphysis pubis

b. 2 inches below the symphysis pubis

c. 2 inches above the ASIS

d. at the iliac crest

108. For an AP projection of the coccyx, the central ray is angled _____, _____.

a. 20°, cephalad

b. 20°, caudal

c. 10°, cephalad

d. 10°, caudal

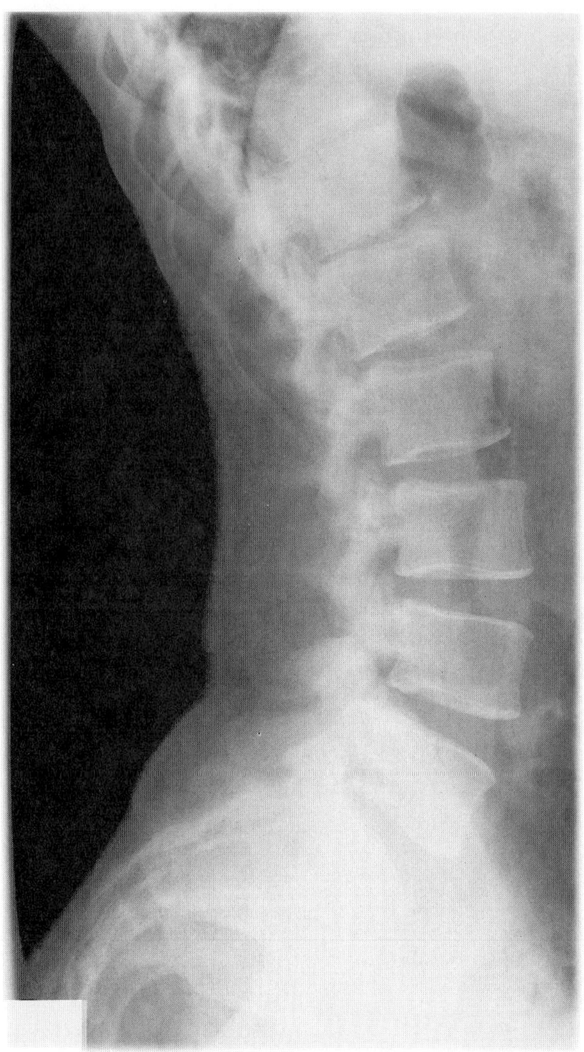

FIGURE 9.8 Radiograph of unknown lumbar spine projection.

109. Examine the radiograph in Figure 9.8. What is the name of this projection and what is the most common reason for performing the examination?

110. A radiographer notices that the upper half of L1 is clipped off the radiograph of an AP lumbar spine radiograph. Explain the positioning error that most likely occurred and what you would do to correct it.

111. It is necessary to take a lateral projection of the L5–S1 junction on a patient who has a fracture of the left hip. Describe the modifications in positioning that would be necessary for this patient.

112. Compare the appearance of the sacrum on an AP lumbar spine radiograph to that on an AP sacrum radiograph.

113. When multiple examinations are ordered for the same patient the radiographer can occasionally combine two positions on a single film. For the following, explain the advantages and disadvantages of combining two examinations.

a. lateral L5–S1 junction and lateral sacrum

b. lateral sacrum and lateral coccyx

Do You Remember?

114. Which of the following are bones that form part of the pelvic girdle?

1. ilium
2. ischium
3. sacrum

a. 1 and 2
b. 1 and 3
c. 2 and 3
d. 1, 2, and 3

115. The patella and the sacrum both have a (an):

a. cornu
b. apex
c. foramina
d. crest

116. Which of the following are diarthroidal joints?

1. zygapophyseal joint
2. metacarpophalangeal joint
3. hip joint

a. 1 and 2
b. 1 and 3
c. 2 and 3
d. 1, 2, and 3

117. The zygapophyseal joints of the ____ are best demonstrated on the oblique projection.

1. lumbar spine
2. thoracic spine
3. cervical spine

a. 1 and 2
b. 1 and 3
c. 2 and 3
d. 1, 2, and 3

118. Which of the following projections clearly demonstrate the spinous processes?

1. oblique thoracic spine
2. lateral cervical spine
3. lateral lumbar spine

a. 1 and 2
b. 1 and 3
c. 2 and 3
d. 1, 2, and 3

119. Which projections best demonstrate the intervertebral foramina?

1. oblique cervical spine
2. oblique lumbar spine
3. lateral thoracic spine

a. 1 and 2
b. 1 and 3
c. 2 and 3
d. 1, 2, and 3

120. Which of the following vertebra is characterized by a foramen in its transverse process?

a. cervical

b. thoracic

c. lumbar

d. sacral

121. In which projection is the anatomy of interest best demonstrated by instructing the patient to breathe normally during the exposure?

a. lateral thoracic spine

b. L5–S1 spot film

c. lateral cervical spine

d. AP thoracic spine

122. Which structure is present on most thoracic vertebrae but not on cervical vertebrae?

a. transverse foramen

b. vertebral notch

c. vertebral foramen

d. demifacets

123. The two AP projections of the shoulder that are usually part of a routine series are the:

a. flexion and extension

b. external and internal rotation

c. abduction and adduction

d. weight-bearing and nonweight-bearing

STUDY TIP: GENERAL TEST-TAKING STRATEGIES

Instructor Bob: Today I am going to teach the class about test-taking strategies.

Pat: Do you really think this is necessary? I mean we all needed at least a 3.0 GPA to be accepted to this class. Let's get on with trauma positioning.

Instructor Bob: I don't mean to insult anyone, but in this program we are concerned about more than GPA. Even the best students can improve their skills.

Kathy: Great, give us some tips on how to take tests. That way maybe I won't have to study so much.

Instructor Bob: Sorry. You'll still have to study.

- Always arrive on time or slightly early for a test. Arriving late always raises stress levels and decreases time allowed on the examination.
- Do not try cramming immediately before an examination. Reviewing a few difficult terms or formulae is acceptable.
- Survey the entire test before starting. Begin at the section that you feel most comfortable with, such as the multiple choice, essay, or short answer section.
- Answer the questions that you know first, skipping those for which you are unsure. Occasionally later questions will give you clues to answer those that you were unsure of.
- Plan your time wisely. Be sure you have finished about half the examination at the halfway point in time.
- Check your work carefully, rereading each question. First choices are not always correct but if you are guessing, take your initial choice.

> No test-taking strategies will substitute for adequate note-taking and studying. They can, however, raise test scores and increase performance in a course.

QUESTIONS

Anatomy and Physiology

For questions 1–4, identify the body habitus illustrated in Figure 1.1.

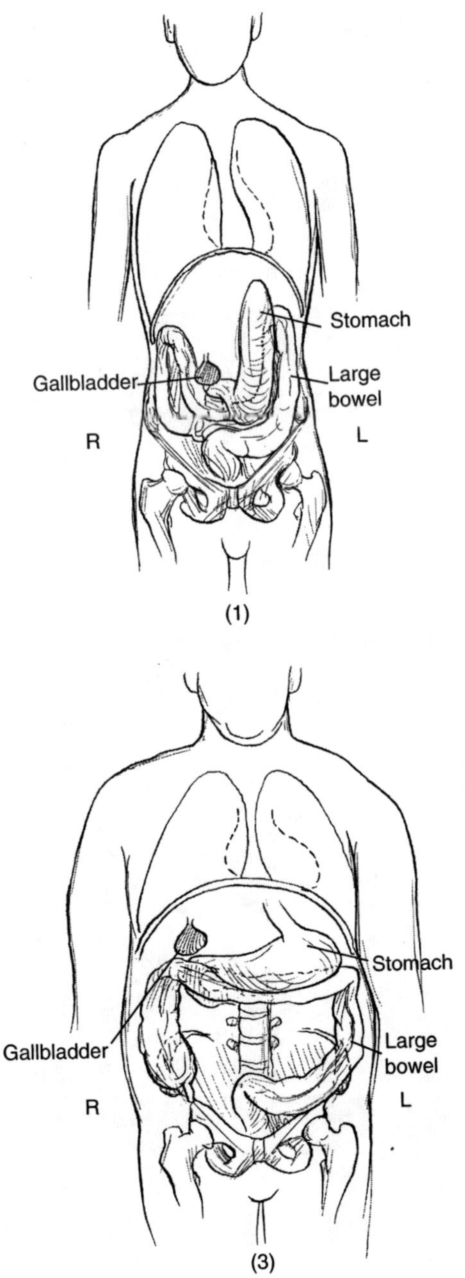

FIGURE 1.1 Body habitus.

1. ______________________________

2. ______________________________

3. ______________________________

4. ______________________________

CHAPTER 10

Trauma Spine

LEARNING OBJECTIVES

At the completion of this chapter, the student should be able to:

1. List the indications for ordering radiographs of the spine.
2. Explain the rationale for each projection used for trauma patients.
3. Describe the positioning used to visualize anatomic structures of the spine in the trauma patient.
4. Identify the location of the central ray and extent of field necessary for each projection.
5. Recommend the technical factors for producing an acceptable radiograph for each projection.
6. State the patient instructions for each projection.
7. Identify the anatomic structures that are best demonstrated on each of the trauma spine radiographs.
8. Given radiographs, evaluate positioning and technical factors.
9. Identify alternative modalities used for imaging the trauma spine.

Alternative Positions/Projections

Part	
Cervical spine (trauma)	Cross-table lateral
	AP
	AP open mouth
	Oblique
Thoracic spine (trauma)	Cross-table lateral
	Cross-table swimmer's lateral
	AP
Lumbar spine	Cross-table lateral
	AP

QUESTIONS

Radiographic Procedures, Analysis, and Critical Thinking

For questions 1–7, identify the anatomy of the trauma lateral cervical spine in Figure 10.1A.

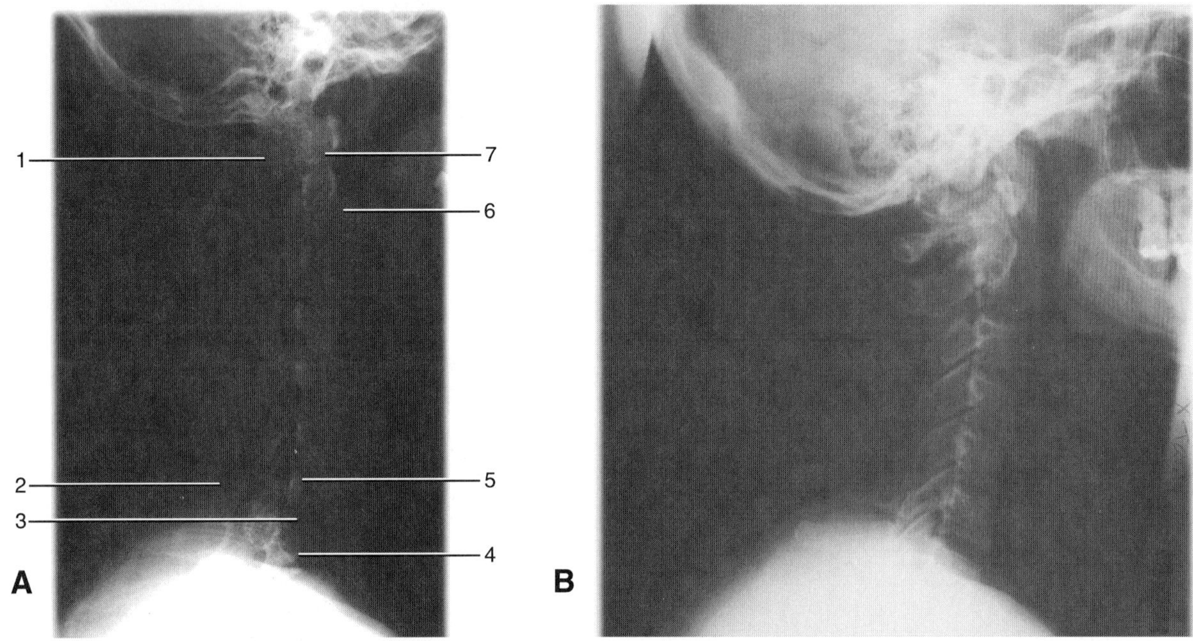

FIGURE 10.1 Radiograph of cervical spine, trauma lateral projection, (A) correct positioning and (B) incorrect positioning.

1. ____________________
2. ____________________
3. ____________________
4. ____________________
5. ____________________
6. ____________________
7. ____________________

8. Compare the positioning quality of the correctly positioned radiograph in Figure 10.1A with that in Figure 10.1B. Describe the positioning error, explain what caused it, and give the step(s) necessary to correct the problem.

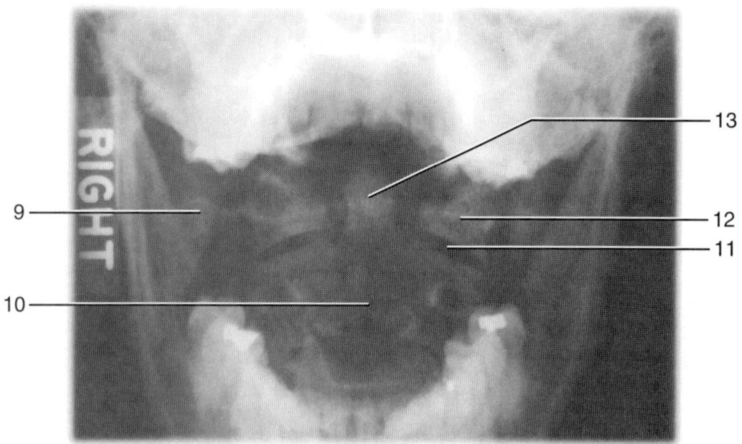

FIGURE 10.2 Radiograph of cervical spine, trauma AP open-mouth projection.

For questions 9–13, identify the anatomy of the trauma AP open-mouth cervical spine in Figure 10.2.

9. ______________________

10. ______________________

11. ______________________

12. ______________________

13. ______________________

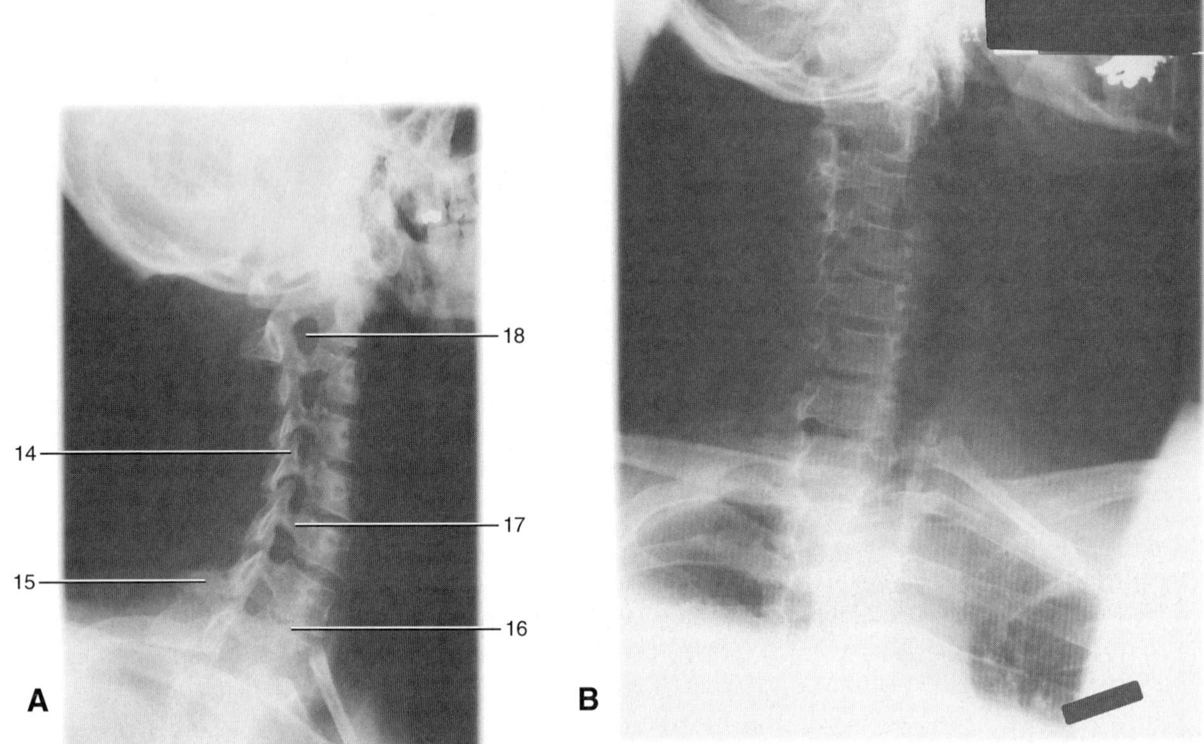

FIGURE 10.3 Radiograph of cervical spine, trauma oblique projection, (A) correct positioning and (B) incorrect positioning.

For questions 14–18, identify the anatomy of the trauma oblique cervical spine in Figure 10.3A.

14. ____________________

15. ____________________

16. ____________________

17. ____________________

18. ____________________

19. Compare the positioning quality of the correctly positioned radiograph in Figure 10.3A with that in Figure 10.3B. Describe the positioning error, explain what caused it, and give the step(s) necessary to correct the problem.

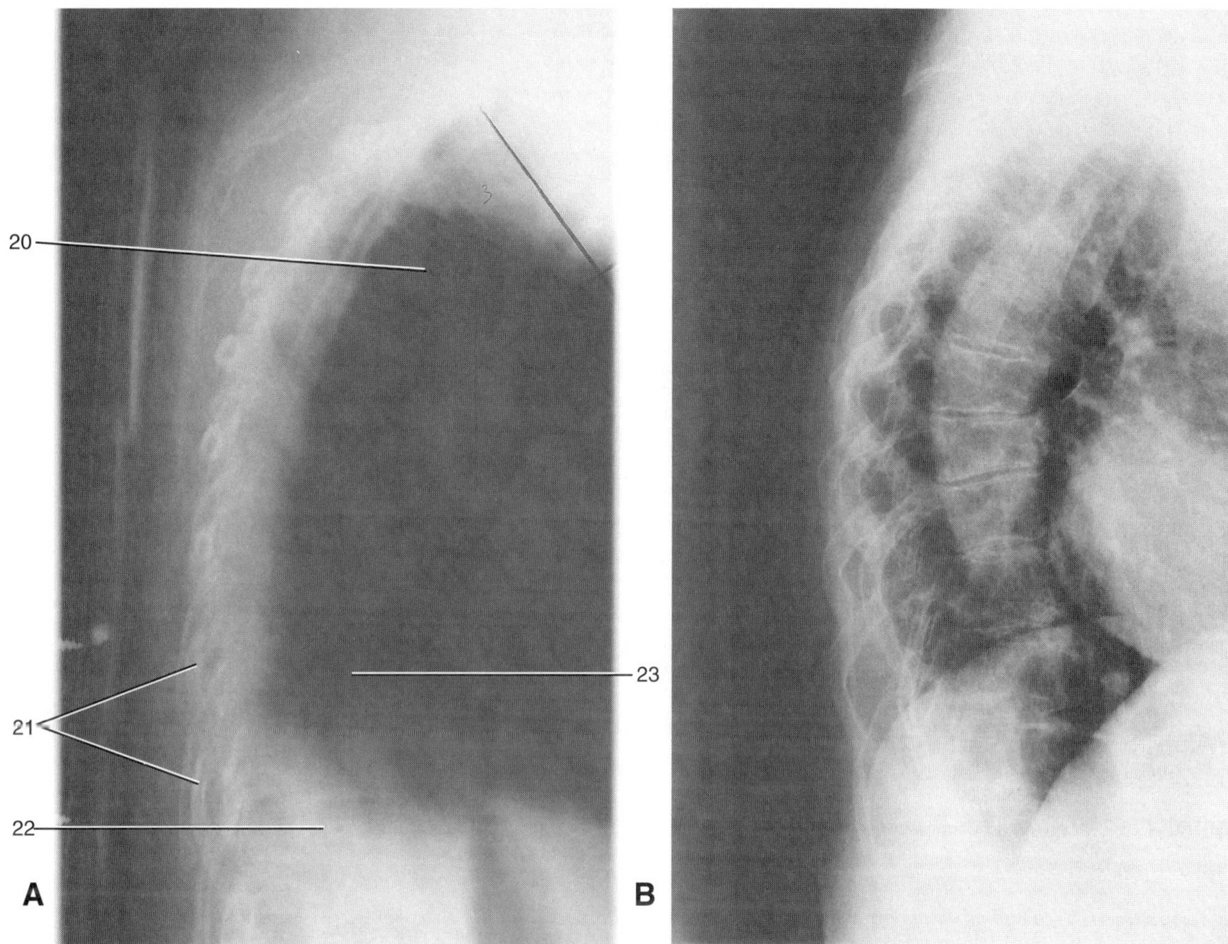

FIGURE 10.4 Radiograph of thoracic spine, trauma lateral projection, (A) correct positioning and (B) incorrect positioning.

For questions 20–23, identify the anatomy of the trauma lateral thoracic spine in Figure 10.4A.

20. ______________________

21. ______________________

22. ______________________

23. ______________________

24. Compare the positioning quality of the correctly positioned radiograph in Figure 10.4A with that in Figure 10.4B. Describe the positioning error, explain what caused it, and give the step(s) necessary to correct the problem.

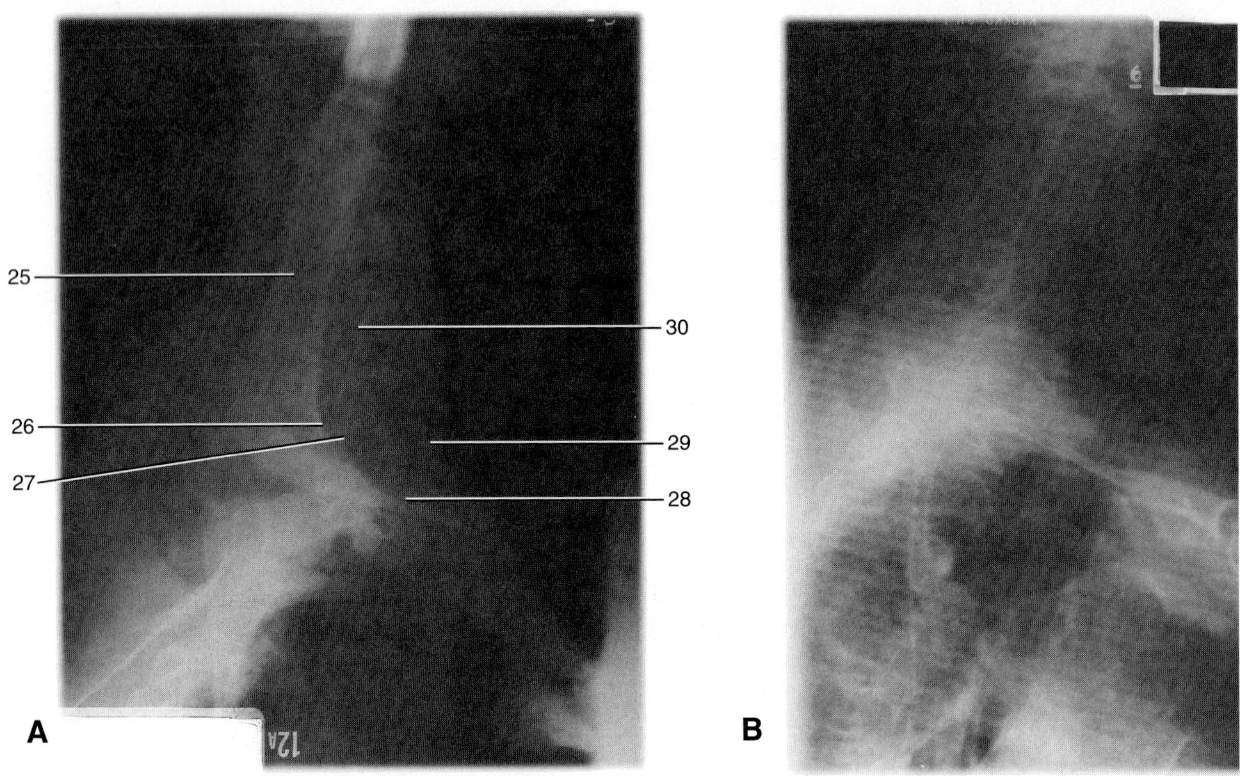

FIGURE 10.5 Radiograph of trauma swimmer's lateral thoracic spine, (A) correct positioning and (B) incorrect positioning.

For questions 25–30, identify the anatomy of the trauma swimmer's lateral thoracic spine in Figure 10.5A.

25. ______________________ **28.** ______________________

26. ______________________ **29.** ______________________

27. ______________________ **30.** ______________________

31. Compare the positioning quality of the correctly positioned radiograph in Figure 10.5A with that in Figure 10.5B. Describe the positioning error, explain what caused it, and give the step(s) necessary to correct the problem.

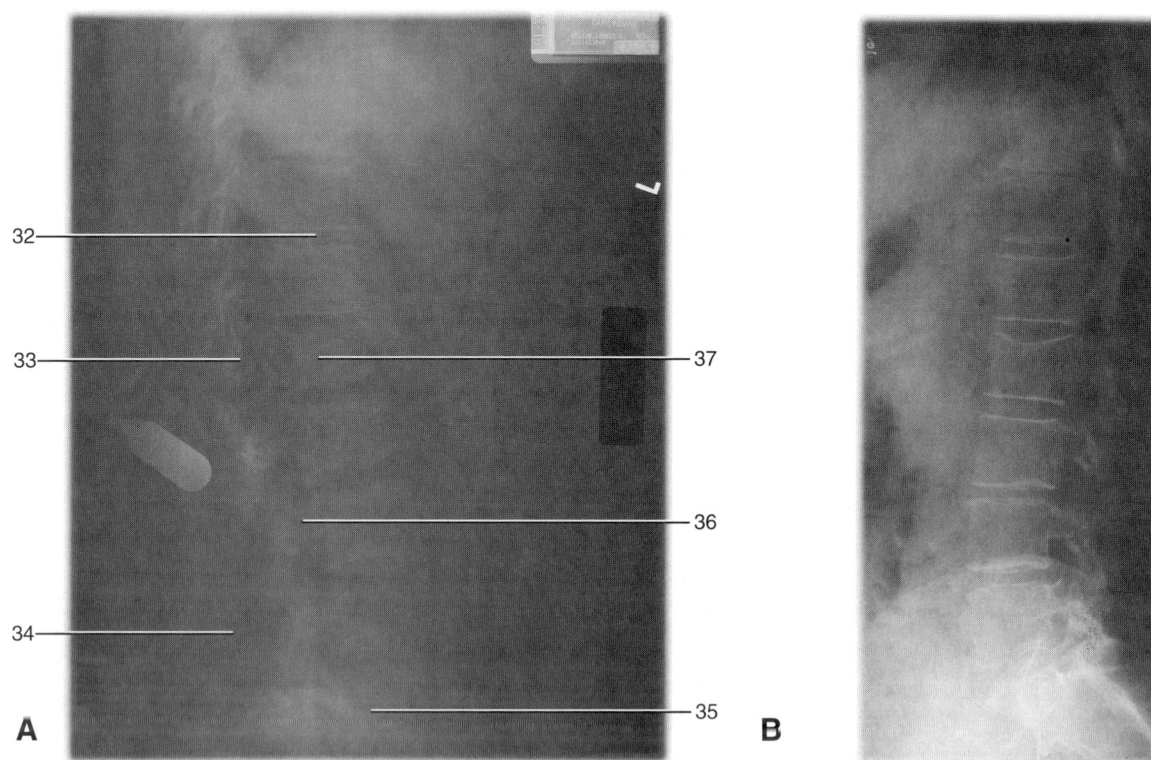

FIGURE 10.6 Radiograph of trauma lateral lumbar spine, (A) correct positioning and (B) incorrect positioning.

For questions 32–37, identify the anatomy of the trauma lateral lumbar spine in Figure 10.6A.

32. ____________________

33. ____________________

34. ____________________

35. ____________________

36. ____________________

37. ____________________

38. Compare the positioning quality of the correctly positioned radiograph in Figure 10.6A with that in Figure 10.6B. Describe the positioning error, explain what caused it, and give the step(s) necessary to correct the problem.

39. For a trauma AP open-mouth projection the __________ and the __________ should be placed in a line perpendicular to the table.

40. For a trauma lateral projection of the lumbar spine the __________ plane should be aligned to the middle of the grid cassette.

41. The kVp range for a trauma lateral projection of the lumbar spine is

__________________________________.

42. A major advantage of CT imaging of the spine is that trauma patients can be kept in cervical traction during the procedure.

a. true

b. false

43. The spinous processes of the lower thoracic spine should be visualized on a cross-table lateral of the thoracic spine.

a. true

b. false

44. The kVp for a trauma swimmer's thoracic spine is usually higher than that for a routine lateral thoracic spine.

a. true

b. false

For questions 45–49, identify the radiographic anatomy of the trauma AP lumbar spine in Figure 10.7.

45. Number 1

a. transverse process

b. pedicle

c. intervertebral disk space

d. superior articular process

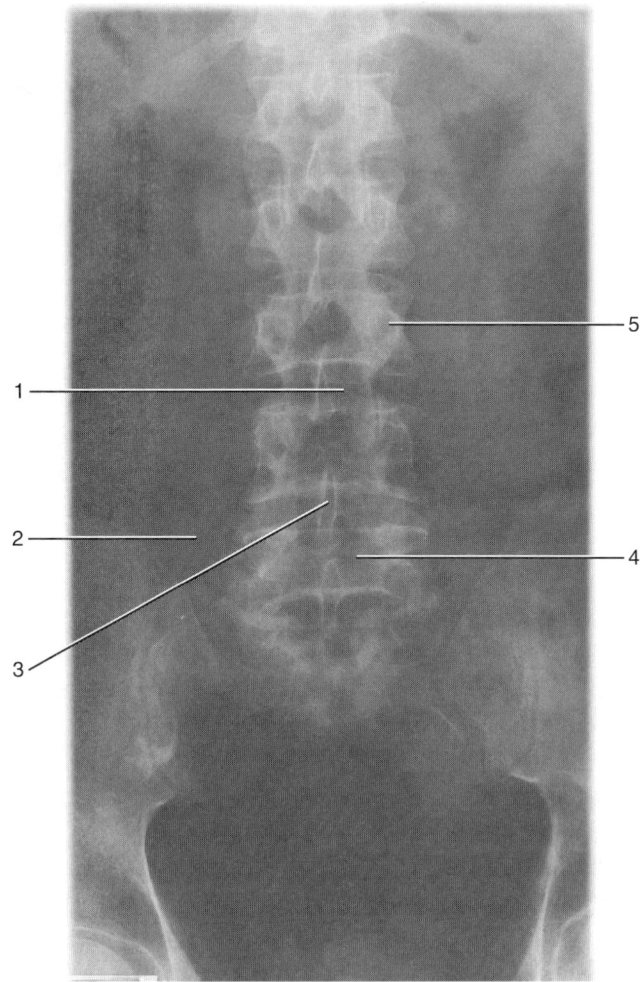

FIGURE 10.7 Radiograph of lumbar spine, trauma AP projection.

46. Number 2

a. transverse process

b. pedicle

c. spinous process

d. zygapophyseal joint

47. Number 3

a. sacrum

b. body of L5

c. spinous process of L5

d. spinous process of L4

48. Number 4

a. intervertebral disk space

b. spinous process

c. vertebral foramen

d. body of L5

49. Number 5

a. pars interarticularis

b. pedicle

c. spinous process

d. transverse process

50. The basic protocol required for severely injured patients includes:

1. AP projection

2. at least one oblique projection

3. cross-table lateral

a. 1 and 2

b. 1 and 3

c. 2 and 3

d. 1, 2, and 3

51. Which of the following is true regarding the use of CT for trauma spine evaluation?

a. CT should always be done before the plain films.

b. CT should always be done immediately after the plain films.

c. CT should be done when the plain films appear normal but symptoms still indicate spinal injury.

d. CT should never be done on spinal trauma patients.

52. Which procedure is particularly useful in the detection of trauma to nonbony structures of the spine?

a. conventional radiographs

b. CT

c. MRI

d. conventional tomography

53. The central ray for a cross-table lateral cervical spine should be placed at:

a. C2

b. C6

c. upper margin of thyroid cartilage

d. the top of the shoulders

54. For a cross-table lateral cervical spine, the neck should:

a. be placed in slight flexion

b. be placed in slight extension

c. be placed parallel to the table top

d. not be adjusted or moved

55. Cervical collars on trauma patients should:

a. be carefully removed by the radiographer for all films

b. be carefully removed by the radiographer for the lateral film only

c. be carefully removed by the radiographer only for the AP and open-mouth films

d. never be removed by the radiographer without physician consent

56. The patient position for the swimmer's lateral projection on a trauma patient is:

a. upright

b. supine

c. prone

d. recumbent lateral

57. The central ray for a swimmer's lateral of the thoracic spine should be directed to:

a. C5

b. C7

c. T2

d. T4

58. To improve visualization of the C7–T1 disk space for a lateral swimmer's position, the radiographer should angle the tube:

a. 5° caudal

b. 25° caudal

c. 5° cephalic

d. 25° cephalic

59. On a trauma AP radiograph of the cervical spine, _____ should be demonstrated.

a. all cervical vertebra

b. all cervical vertebra and T1

c. C2–T1

d. C3–T1

60. The tube angle and direction for a trauma AP projection of the cervical spine is:

a. 5–10° cephalic

b. 5–10° caudal

c. 15–20° caudal

d. 15–20° cephalic

61. Because of superimposition from shoulder structures the upper _____ thoracic vertebrae are not normally visualized on a cross-table lateral of the thoracic spine.

a. 1–2

b. 3–4

c. 5–6

d. 7–8

62. For a trauma AP projection of the thoracic spine, the central ray enters 2 inches:

a. superior to the sternal angle

b. inferior to the manubrial notch

c. inferior to the sternal angle

d. superior to the manubrial notch

63. Which of the following is *not* clearly demonstrated on a trauma AP thoracic spine?

a. disk spaces

b. vertebral bodies

c. intervertebral foramina

d. transverse processes

64. Where is the central ray directed for a trauma swimmer's lateral of the thoracic spine?

a. C4

b. C6

c. T2

d. T4

65. For a cross-table lateral of the thoracic spine, the patient's arms should:

a. be down by the sides

b. not be moved

c. be placed with hands resting on abdomen

d. be raised above the head

66. The central ray for a cross-table lateral of the lumbar spine should be directed:

a. 1–2 inches above the iliac crest

b. at the level of the iliac crest

c. at the level of the ASIS

d. 1–2 inches below the level of the iliac crest

67. Which of the following is *least* well demonstrated on a trauma AP lumbar spine?

a. spinous processes

b. transverse processes

c. pedicles

d. bodies

68. A cross-table lateral lumbar spine radiograph should clearly demonstrate the:

a. spinous processes

b. transverse processes

c. pedicles

d. laminae

69. Although MRI has become useful in trauma spine imaging, it has some important limitations. Discuss several of these limitations.

70. A radiographer observes a radiograph of a swimmer's lateral and notes that one of the humeral heads is overlying C7. Discuss at least two ways that positioning could be modified to correct this problem.

71. Occasionally, the trauma lateral cervical spine must be performed at 40 inch SID due to equipment constraints, whereas the routine lateral is performed at 72 inch SID. Describe several differences that you could expect to observe regarding the appearance of the spine on the two radiographs.

72. Multiple examinations are frequently ordered for trauma patients and the radiographer must organize the examination so that patient movement is kept to a minimum. Describe the sequence of filming for a trauma patient who needs radiographs of the cervical, lumbar, and thoracic spines.

73. Explain why a double tube angle is required for many trauma obliques of the cervical spine and why a grid cannot be used.

Do You Remember?

74. For an AP projection of the pelvis, the lesser trochanters should be clearly demonstrated without superimposition.

  a. true

  b. false

75. The series of openings in the anterior portion of the sacrum are called sacral foramina.

  a. true

  b. false

76. The normal cervical spine has a _____ curvature.

a. thoracic

b. kyphotic

c. scoliotic

d. lordotic

77. The central ray is angled for oblique cervical spines to better demonstrate the:

a. transverse foramina

b. vertebral foramen

c. intervertebral foramina

d. articular pillars

78. The symphysis pubis is located at approximately the same level as the:

a. ischial tuberosity

b. tip of the coccyx

c. iliac crest

d. greater trochanter

79. Which of the following are *not* well visualized on an AP projection of the foot?

1. calcaneus
2. fifth metatarsal
3. talus

a. 1 and 2

b. 1 and 3

c. 2 and 3

d. 1, 2, and 3

80. The first carpometacarpal joint is the articulation of the first metacarpal and the:

a. lunate

b. trapezium

c. pisiform

d. triquetrum

81. Which projection best demonstrates the coracoid process?

a. AP elbow

b. lateral elbow

c. AP shoulder

d. lateral scapula

82. For an inferosuperior axial projection of the shoulder, the central ray is directed:

a. laterally through the thorax

b. 45° through the thorax

c. through the axilla

d. perpendicular through the coracoid process

83. The patient is placed with the left side dependent. The central ray is angled 5–8° caudal, entering 1 inch below the iliac crest and 2 inches anterior to the posterior surface of the body. This position describes a lateral projection of the:

a. sacrum

b. lumbar spine

c. coccyx

d. L5–S1 junction

STUDY TIP: SUCCESSFUL TEST-TAKING—MENTAL PREPARATION

Paul: The final exam is only 2 weeks away. I always do poorly on finals.

Instructor Bob: Why is that?

Paul: I don't know, but it always happens. I just suddenly forget everything and choke.

Instructor Bob: Maybe you can change that, Paul. First, you have to stop thinking so negatively. Remember, how you did on a test last year or last month really has no relation to how you will do on this final exam. Do you want to do well?

Paul: Well, yeah, all I need is a "C" anyway.

Instructor Bob: It sounds like you need some real attitude adjustment! Let's go for some coffee to talk about it.

- Your major mental goal of test preparation should be to receive a 100%, not just a "C."
- Prepare well in advance by assembling all study notes and materials. Late test preparation greatly increases your chances of "mental block" during the test.
- Study all topics appearing on the test. Skipping topics because they are difficult or because you only need a "C" can result in panic on an examination when you encounter questions that you do not know. This panic may spread to questions that you do know.

> One of the most important factors in preparing for a test is to develop a positive attitude that you can and will be successful. Successful mental preparation never happens through last minute cramming.

SECTION V

SKULL RADIOGRAPHY

CHAPTER 11

Introduction to Skull Radiography

LEARNING OBJECTIVES

At the completion of this chapter, the student should be able to:

1. Compare and contrast cranial shapes, including differences in the degree of angle between the petrous ridges and the median plane.
2. Describe the location of cranial landmarks, lines, and planes.
3. Given radiographs, diagrams, or photographs, identify cranial landmarks, lines, and planes.
4. List the advantages and disadvantages of radiographing the cranium in the erect or recumbent position.
5. State ways of providing reasonable comfort for all patient types during cranial radiography.
6. Describe the positioning errors that result in rotation and tilt.
7. Given radiographs, recognize and differentiate between the common positioning errors of rotation and tilt.
8. Identify special considerations when radiographing the pediatric skull.

QUESTIONS

Anatomy and Physiology

For questions 1–10, identify the surface landmarks in Figure 11.1.

1. ______________________

2. ______________________

3. ______________________

4. ______________________

5. ______________________

6. ______________________

7. ______________________

8. ______________________

9. ______________________

10. ______________________

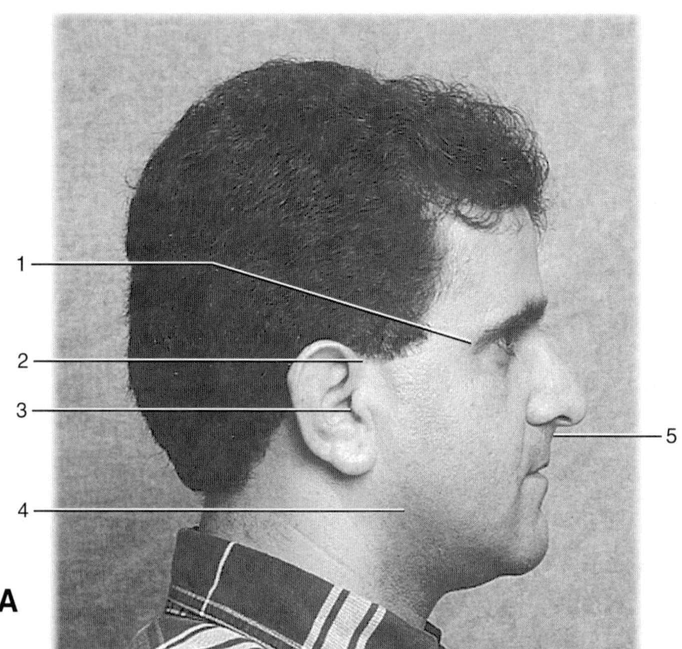

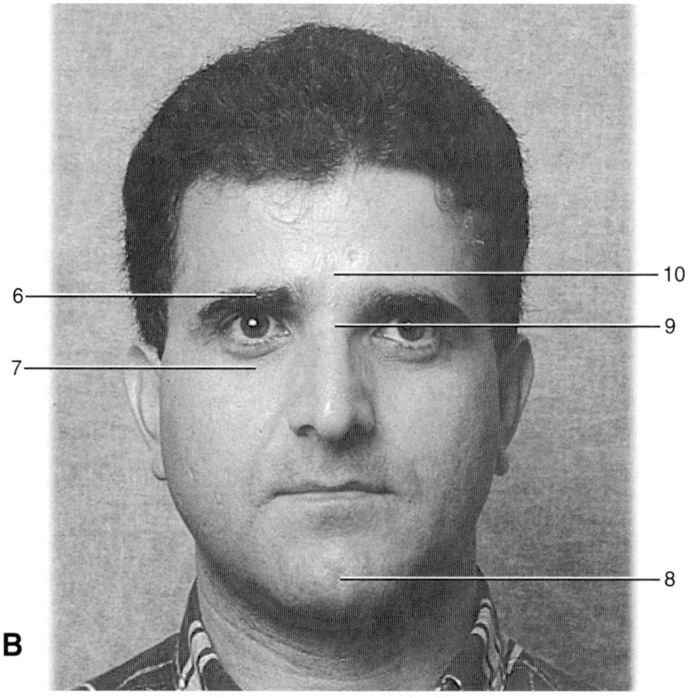

FIGURE 11.1 Surface landmarks, (A) lateral and (B) anterior.

For questions 11–15, identify the positioning lines in Figure 11.2.

11. ______________________

12. ______________________

13. ______________________

14. ______________________

15. ______________________

16. The ridge of bone just inferior to the orbit is called the

______________________________________.

17. The abbreviation TEA means _____________ ______________________________.

18. The _____________ line connects the tip of the chin with the external auditory meatus.

19. The average skull shape is known as

______________________________________.

20. The abbreviation EAM means _____________ ______________________________.

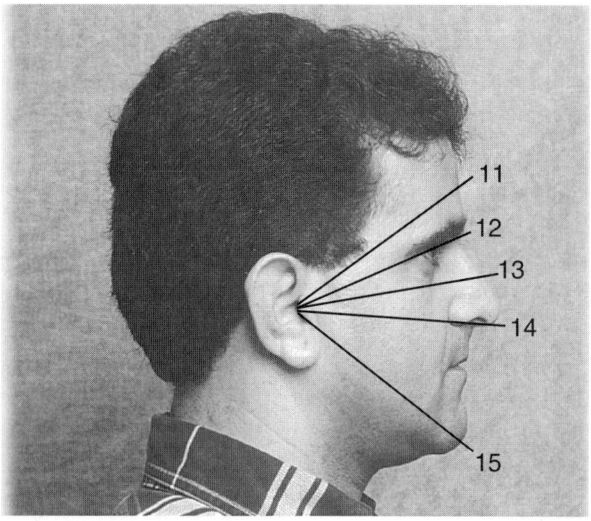

FIGURE 11.2 Positioning lines.

21. If the patient's condition allows, skull radiography should be performed upright.

a. true

b. false

22. The supraorbital line is a line drawn between both pupils.

a. true

b. false

23. In the brachycephalic skull, internal structures are generally positioned higher from the infraorbitomeatal line.

a. true

b. false

For questions 24–33, match the surface landmark with its correct description.

	Landmark	Description
24. _____	occiput	a. smooth flat surface between the eyebrows
25. _____	inion	b. most posterior surface of cranium
26. _____	vertex	c. most superior surface of cranium
27. _____	gonion	d. ridge of bone at the eyebrow
28. _____	nasion	e. depression in bone above the eyebrow
29. _____	supraorbital groove	f. point where the right and left nasal bones meet
30. _____	superciliary ridge	g. junction of the mandibular body and ramus
31. _____	mental point	h. tip of the chin
32. _____	glabella	i. external protuberance of the occipital bone
33. _____	acanthion	j. junction of upper lip and inferior nose

34. Motion of the head around the longitudinal axis is known as:

a. rotation

b. asymmetry

c. tilt

d. misalignment

35. The tragus is associated with the:

a. ear

b. eye

c. orbit

d. cranium

36. The acanthion is an anatomic reference point at the junction of the:

a. orbit and nasion

b. two parietal bones

c. upper lip and nose

d. the mandibular body and ramus

37. The positioning line connecting the external auditory meatus and the outer orbital margin is known as the:

a. acanthiomeatal line

b. orbitomeatal line

c. supraorbitomeatal line

d. infraorbitomeatal line

38. Which positioning line connects the upper lip/inferior nose to the external auditory meatus?

a. glabellomeatal

b. acanthiomeatal

c. infraorbitomeatal

d. orbitomeatal

39. The positioning error that occurs when the longitudinal axis of the head is not aligned with the longitudinal axis of the body is known as:

a. rotation

b. asymmetry

c. tilt

d. misalignment

40. A long, narrow shaped skull is known as:

a. dolichocephalic

b. mesocephalic

c. brachycephalic

d. megacephalic

41. In the average skull, the petrous ridges form a _____ angle from the midline of the body.

a. 30°

b. 40°

c. 47°

d. 54°

42. A patient arrives for a skull examination. Describe what criteria you would use to determine whether the patient should be examined recumbent or upright.

43. Why do most radiographers perform skull radiography with the patient upright rather than recumbent?

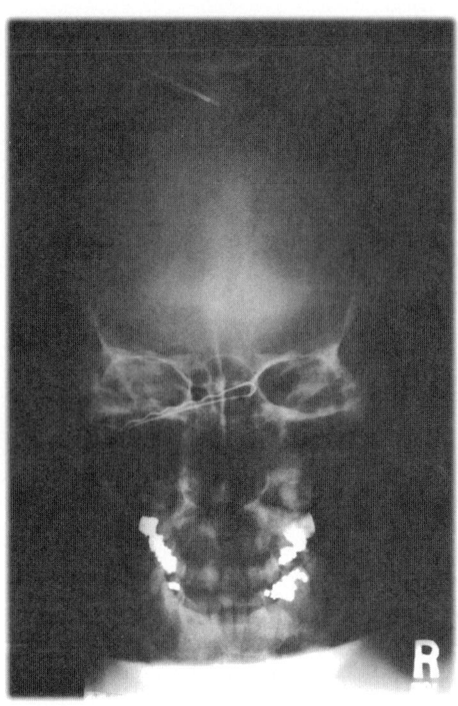

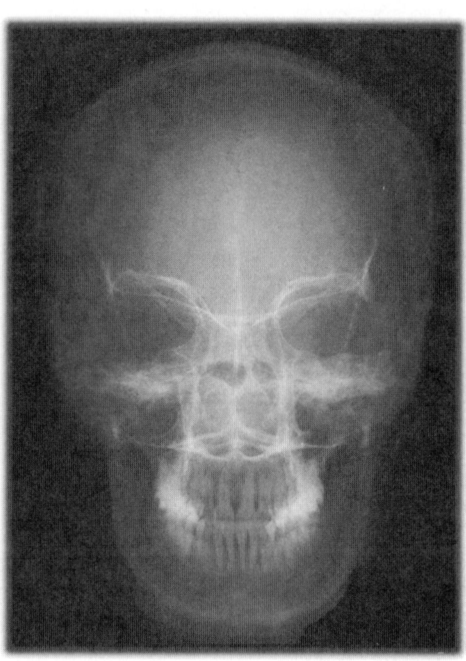

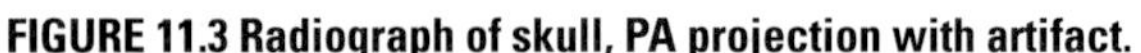
FIGURE 11.3 Radiograph of skull, PA projection with artifact.

FIGURE 11.4 Radiograph of skull, incorrect positioning.

44. Observe the skull radiograph in Figure 11.3. Explain the likely cause of this positioning error and what the radiographer could have done to prevent it.

45. Observe the radiograph of the skull in Figure 11.4. Is this an example of rotation or tilt? Give reasons for your answer.

46. Explain at least two advantages of using a collimator, cone, or diaphragm to restrict the beam to the area of interest in skull radiography.

Do You Remember?

47. Wearing gloves is the single, most important factor in the prevention of transfer of pathogens.

    a. true

    b. false

48. The RPO position of the sacroiliac joint will best demonstrate:

    a. the right joint

    b. the left joint

    c. both joints

    d. neither joint

49. Which of the following projections best demonstrates the upper portion of the talus?

    a. tangential calcaneus

    b. AP ankle

    c. plantodorsal foot

    d. oblique foot

50. The humerus and ulna articulate at the:

    a. trochlea

    b. capitellum

    c. coronoid fossa

    d. bicipital groove

51. Which projections should be taken on a patient with a suspected dislocated humerus?

    1. AP internal rotation

    2. scapular Y method

    3. transthoracic shoulder

    a. 1 and 2

    b. 1 and 3

    c. 2 and 3

    d. 1, 2, and 3

52. The atlas articulates superiorly with the:

a. axis

b. foramen magnum

c. occipital condyles

d. parietal bone

53. The patient is placed in the supine position. The central ray enters at the level of the ASIS with a 15° cephalic angle. This describes the AP projection of the:

a. coccyx

b. sacrum

c. axial L5–S1

d. lumbar spine

54. What is the tube angulation for a swimmer's lateral projection if the patient cannot separate the shoulders?

a. 5° caudal

b. 5° cephalic

c. 10° cephalic

d. 15° caudal

55. To open the joint space of the knee, the tube should be angled:

a. 5° cephalic

b. 5° caudal

c. 15° cephalic

d. 15° caudal

56. Which structures form the posterior portion of the vertebral arch?

a. one pedicle and one lamina

b. two pedicles

c. two lamina and two transverse processes

d. two laminae

STUDY TIP: ORGANIZATION

Jill and Juan have arrived at Shawn's house to study for next week's examination.

Shawn: Thanks for coming over to study because I really could use your help. I left my notes in my car, can I use yours?

Jill: Sure. Are we going to study in this room? I mean, I like your brother but it is hard to concentrate when he keeps screaming and the TV is a little loud.

Juan: I agree, can we go to the next room?

Shawn: But I always study here. Well, OK, let's go to the porch.

Jill: I hate to complain, it's very dark and cold here. Hey, Juan, did you remember to bring your book this time? I forgot mine.

Juan: Sure. Did anyone bring extra paper or pencils—mine don't have erasers on them.

Preparation for studying is essential. Although Juan, Jill, and Shawn may be able to study in this disorganized environment, a comfortable, well-lit area free from distractions will greatly improve study efficiency. Disorganization and study distractions are a common reason why students often claim to have studied for hours yet still do poorly on a test.

- If you cannot find a proper study area in your home, consider using the library or studying at a friend's house.

- Always have notes, paper, pencils, textbooks, and other class materials readily available when studying.

> Efficiency of study time is very important. By organizing the environment and your materials in advance, you can eliminate wasted time—time that should be used to accomplish the learning necessary for success in a course.

CHAPTER 12

Basic Skull Positions/Projections

LEARNING OBJECTIVES

At the completion of this chapter, the student should be able to:

1. List and describe the bony anatomy of the skull.
2. List and describe the paranasal sinuses.
3. Given drawings and radiographs, locate anatomic structures.
4. Explain the general rationale for each of the five basic projections.
5. Discuss how the five basic projections form the basis for all cranial examinations.
6. Describe the basic positioning used to visualize anatomic structures of the skull.
7. List or identify the central ray location for each projection.
8. Given radiographs, evaluate positioning.
9. Describe modifications of procedures for atypical patients to better demonstrate the anatomic area of interest.

Routine Positions/Projections

Part	Routine
Skull	Axial AP (Townes/Grashey)
	PA (and Caldwell)
	Lateral
	Submentovertical (basilar)
	Parietoacanthial (Waters)

QUESTIONS

Anatomy and Physiology

For questions 1–11, identify the anatomy of the anterior skull in Figure 12.1.

1. ______________________

2. ______________________

3. ______________________

4. ______________________

5. ______________________

6. ______________________

7. ______________________

8. ______________________

9. ______________________

10. ______________________

11. ______________________

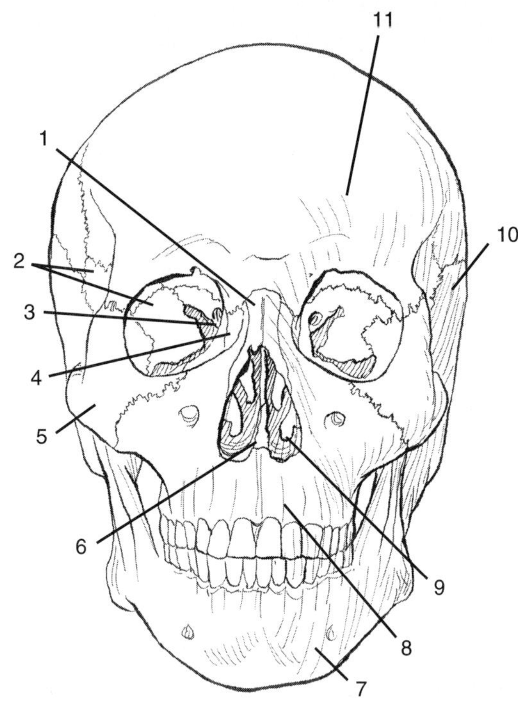

FIGURE 12.1 Diagram of skull, anterior view.

For questions 12–24, identify the anatomy of the lateral skull in Figure 12.2.

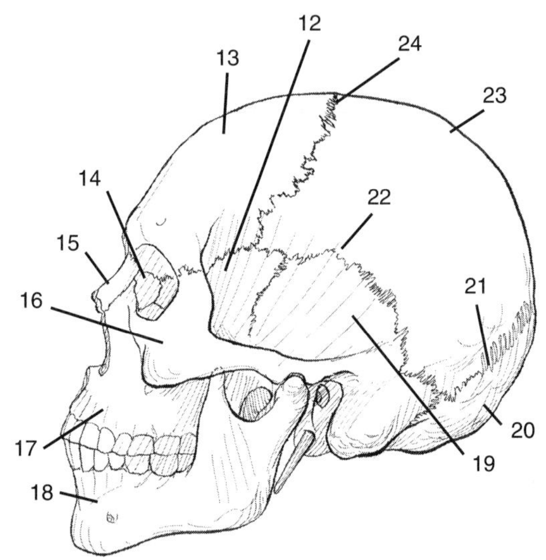

FIGURE 12.2 Diagram of skull, lateral view.

12. ______________________

13. ______________________

14. ______________________

15. ______________________

16. ______________________

17. ______________________

18. ______________________

19. ______________________

20. ______________________

21. ______________________

22. ______________________

23. ______________________

24. ______________________

For questions 25–39, identify the anatomy of the base of the skull in Figure 12.3.

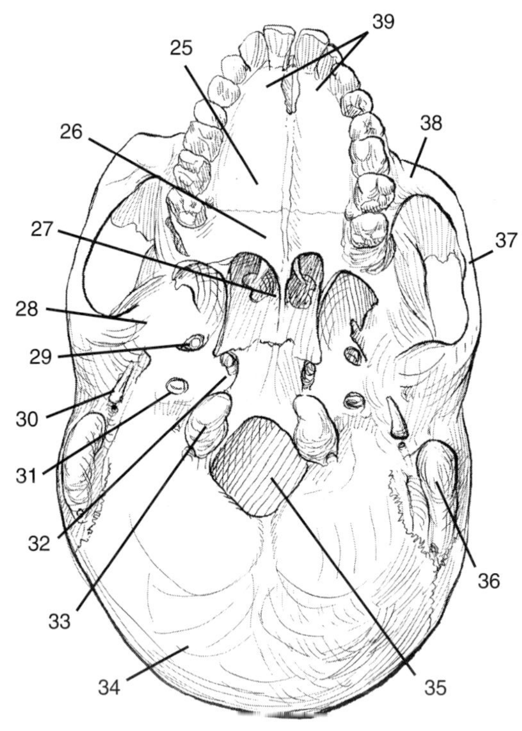

FIGURE 12.3 Diagram of skull, basal view.

25. ______________________

26. ______________________

27. ______________________

28. ______________________

29. ______________________

30. ______________________

31. ______________________

32. ______________________

33. ______________________

34. ______________________

35. ______________________

36. ______________________

37. ______________________

38. ______________________

39. ______________________

For questions 40–52, identify the anatomy of the interior aspect of the base of the skull in Figure 12.4.

40. ______________________

41. ______________________

42. ______________________

43. ______________________

44. ______________________

45. ______________________

46. ______________________

47. ______________________

48. ______________________

49. ______________________

50. ______________________

51. ______________________

52. ______________________

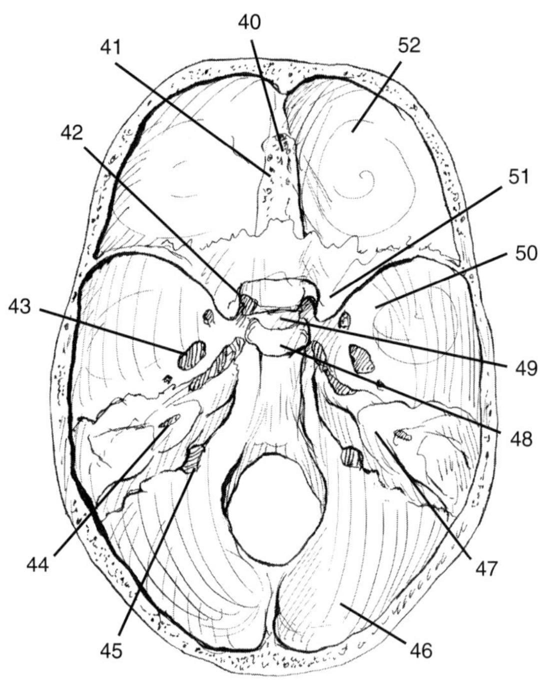

FIGURE 12.4 Diagram of skull, interior aspect of base.

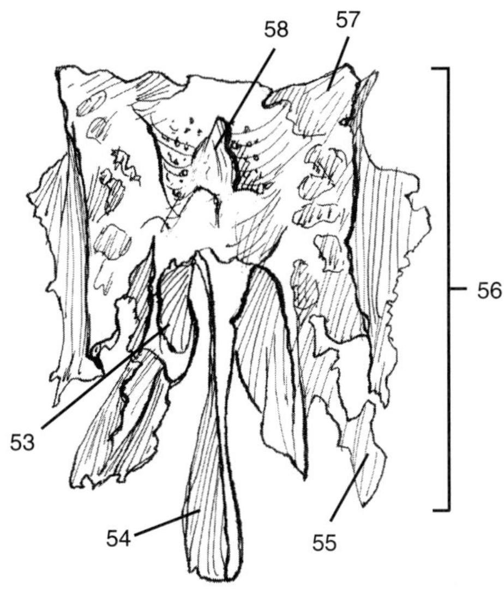

FIGURE 12.5 Diagram of ethmoid bone, anterior view.

For questions 53–58, identify the anatomy of the ethmoid bone in Figure 12.5.

53. ____________________

54. ____________________

55. ____________________

56. ____________________

57. ____________________

58. ____________________

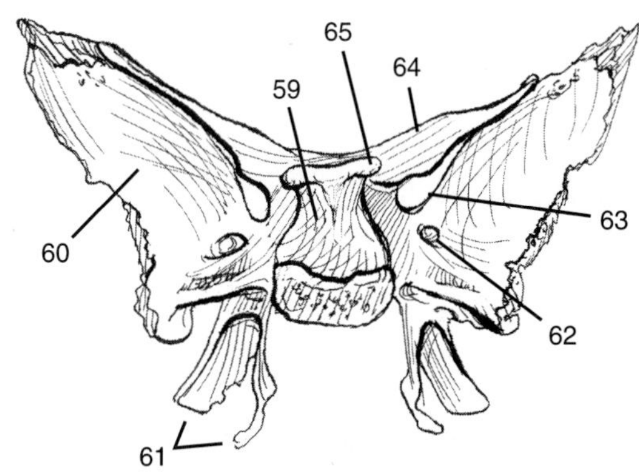

FIGURE 12.6 Diagram of sphenoid bone, posterior view.

For questions 59–65, identify the anatomy of the sphenoid bone in Figure 12.6.

59. ____________________

60. ____________________

61. ____________________

62. ____________________

63. ____________________

64. ____________________

65. ____________________

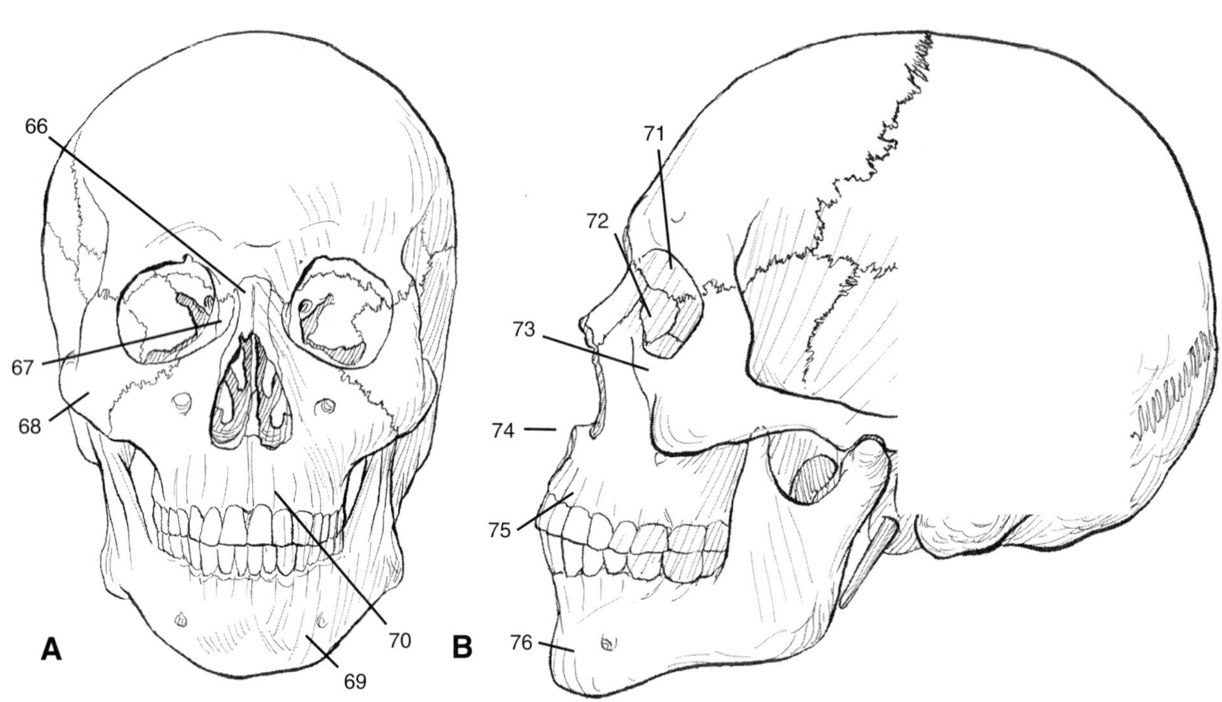

FIGURE 12.7 Diagram of facial bones, (A) anterior and (B) lateral views.

For questions 66–76, identify the anatomy of the facial bones in Figure 12.7.

66. ______________________

67. ______________________

68. ______________________

69. ______________________

70. ______________________

71. ______________________

72. ______________________

73. ______________________

74. ______________________

75. ______________________

76. ______________________

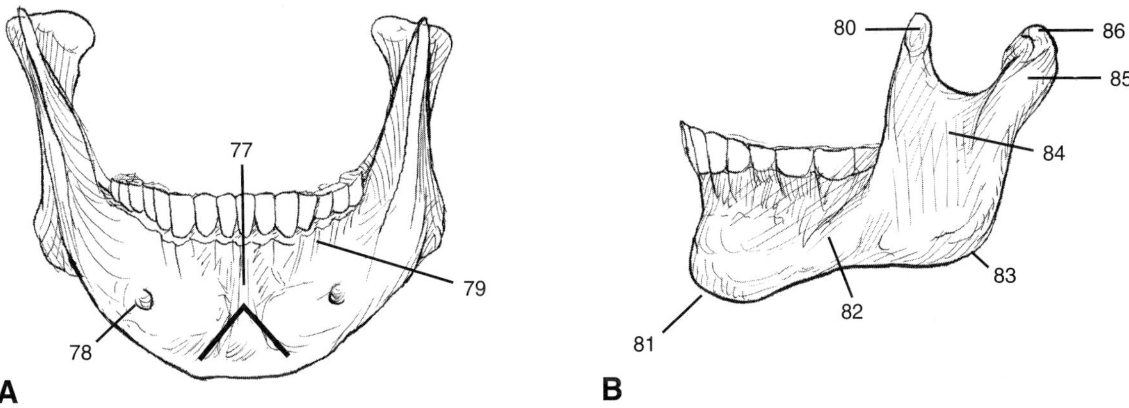

FIGURE 12.8 Diagram of mandible, (A) anterior and (B) lateral views.

For questions 77–86, identify the anatomy of the mandible in Figure 12.8.

77. ____________________

78. ____________________

79. ____________________

80. ____________________

81. ____________________

82. ____________________

83. ____________________

84. ____________________

85. ____________________

86. ____________________

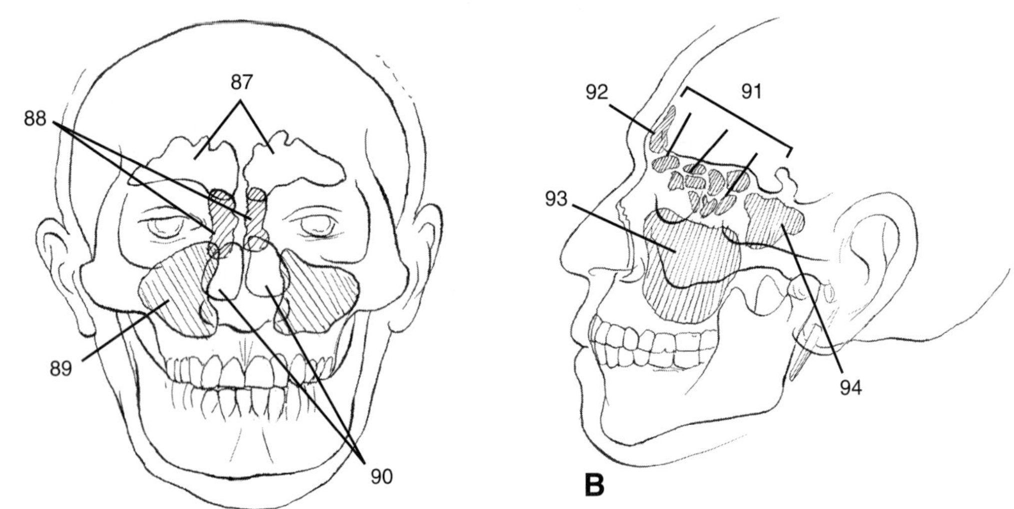

FIGURE 12.9 Diagram of paranasal sinuses, (A) anterior and (B) lateral views.

For questions 87–94, identify the anatomy of the paranasal sinuses in Figure 12.9.

87. ______________________

88. ______________________

89. ______________________

90. ______________________

91. ______________________

92. ______________________

93. ______________________

94. ______________________

95. The pituitary gland is housed in a bony structure in the sphenoid bone called the

______________________________________.

96. The ______________ articulate with the first cervical vertebra to form the occipitoatlantal joints.

97. The inion is also known as the

______________________________________.

98. The carotid artery travels through a hole in the temporal bone called the

______________________________________.

99. The bregma is the point where the ______________ and ______________ sutures meet.

100. The lateral wall of the orbit is composed of parts of the ______________ and ______________ bones.

101. The roots of the teeth can sometimes be found projecting into the ______________ sinus.

For questions 102–123, match the process to the bone on which it is found.

Process		Bone
102. _____	sella turcica	**a.** occipital
103. _____	foramen magnum	**b.** ethmoid
104. _____	external auditory meatus	**c.** temporal
105. _____	superciliary arch	**d.** sphenoid
106. _____	pars petrosa	**e.** frontal
107. _____	pterygoid process	**f.** parietal
108. _____	styloid process	**g.** maxillary
109. _____	mandibular fossa	**h.** zygomatic
110. _____	jugular foramen	**i.** lacrimal
111. _____	coronoid process	**j.** mandible
112. _____	antrum of Highmore	**k.** palatine
113. _____	foramen rotundum	
114. _____	anterior nasal spine	
115. _____	crista galli	
116. _____	mastoid process	
117. _____	temporal process	
118. _____	lesser wing	
119. _____	dorsum sellae	
120. _____	gonion	
121. _____	posterior clinoid process	
122. _____	foramen lacerum	
123. _____	superior nasal conchae	

124. The sphenoid bone articulates with all other cranial bones.

a. true

b. false

125. The majority of the nose is composed of the nasal bones.

a. true

b. false

126. The temporomandibular joint is formed by the mandibular condyle and the temporal fossa.

a. true

b. false

127. The squamous suture is the joint where the occipital and parietal bones meet.

a. true

b. false

128. Which bone forms part of the hard palate and is shaped like the letter L?

a. lacrimal

b. vomer

c. ethmoid

d. palatine

129. Which portion of the mandible contains the sockets for the teeth?

a. alveolar process

b. condyle

c. coronoid process

d. symphysis

130. Which portion of the temporal bone contains the structures of the middle and inner ear?

a. styloid

b. petrous

c. mastoid

d. squamous

131. Which term is *not* associated with the frontal bone?

a. superciliary arches

b. glabella

c. infraorbital ridge

d. sinus

132. Which bones have an alveolar process?

1. mandible

2. zygoma

3. maxillae

a. 1 and 2

b. 1 and 3

c. 2 and 3

d. 1, 2, and 3

133. Which sutures are associated with the parietal bones?

1. sagittal

2. coronal

3. squamous

a. 1 and 2

b. 1 and 3

c. 2 and 3

d. 1, 2, and 3

134. Which bone forms a portion of the floor of the orbit, the anterior portion of the hard palate and part of the floor and lateral border of the nasal cavity?

a. palatine

b. sphenoid

c. nasal

d. maxillae

135. The superior part of the mandible that articulates with the mandibular fossa of the temporal bone is the:

a. condyle

b. coronoid process

c. symphysis

d. alveolar process

136. The transverse portion of the ethmoid bone that forms the roof of the nasal cavity is the:

a. cribiform plate

b. lateral masses

c. perpendicular plate

d. crista galli

137. Which bone does *not* articulate with the right parietal bone?

a. left parietal

b. ethmoid

c. right temporal

d. sphenoid

138. Which of the following bones help form the orbit?

1. palatine

2. vomer

3. lacrimal

a. 1 and 2

b. 1 and 3

c. 2 and 3

d. 1, 2, and 3

139. Which term is *not* associated with the temporal bone?

a. mandibular fossa

b. petrous

c. pterygoid

d. mastoid

140. The zygomatic arch consists of processes from which bones?

1. zygoma

2. maxilla

3. temporal

a. 1 and 2

b. 1 and 3

c. 2 and 3

d. 1, 2, and 3

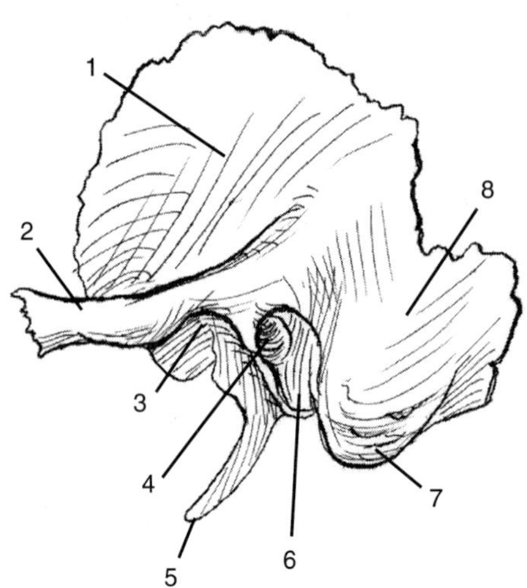

FIGURE 12.10 Diagram of temporal bone.

For questions 141–144 identify the anatomy of the temporal bone in Figure 12.10.

141. External acoustic meatus

a. 3

b. 4

c. 5

d. 7

142. Zygomatic process

a. 1

b. 2

c. 5

d. 7

143. Mastoid process

a. 5

b. 6

c. 7

d. 8

144. Mandibular fossa

a. 3

b. 4

c. 6

d. 8

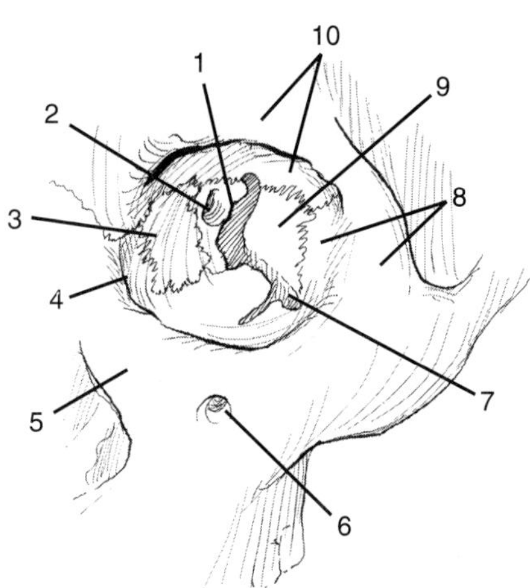

FIGURE 12.11 Diagram of orbit, anterior view.

For questions 145–151, identify the anatomy of the orbit in Figure 12.11.

145. Ethmoid bone

a. 3

b. 4

c. 9

d. 10

146. Maxilla

a. 4

b. 5

c. 8

d. 9

147. Sphenoid bone

a. 5

b. 8

c. 9

d. 10

148. Optic foramen

a. 1

b. 2

c. 6

d. 7

149. Lacrimal bone

a. 3

b. 4

c. 5

d. 9

150. Zygomatic bone

a. 5

b. 8

c. 9

d. 10

151. Inferior orbital fissure

a. 1

b. 2

c. 6

d. 7

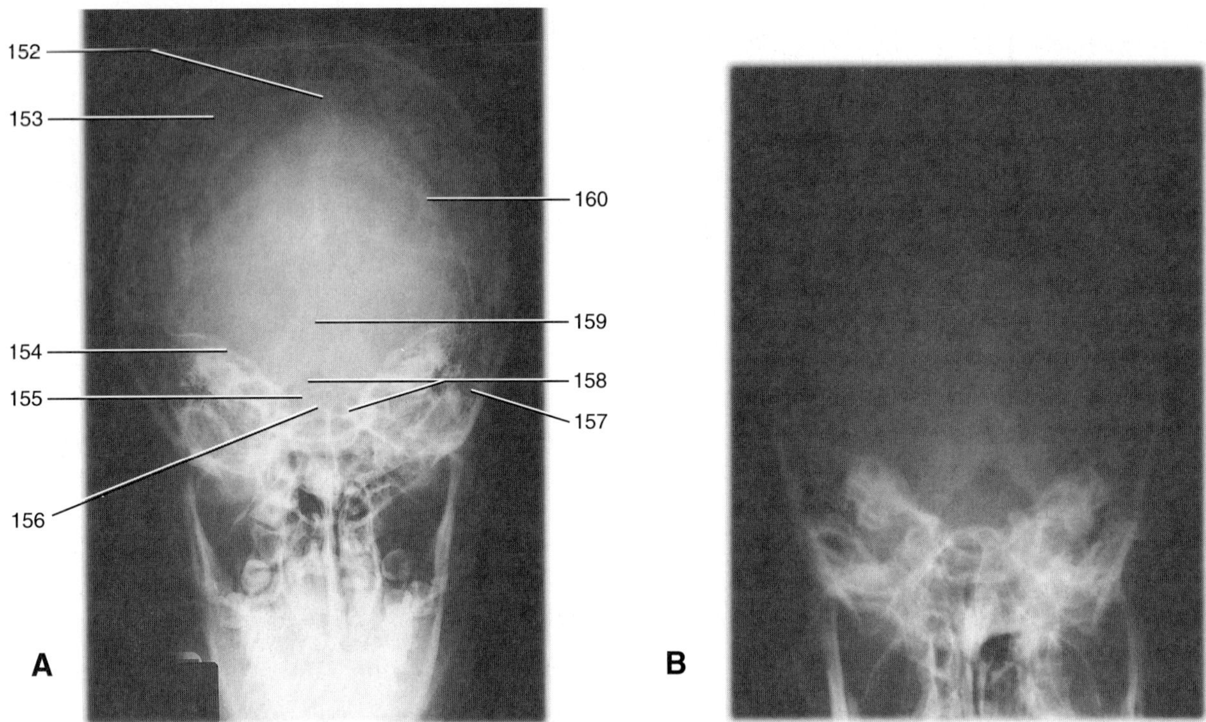

FIGURE 12.12 Radiograph of skull, AP axial (Townes) projection, (A) correct positioning and (B) incorrect positioning.

Radiographic Procedures, Analysis, and Critical Thinking

For questions 152–160, identify the radiographic anatomy on the AP axial (Townes) projection in Figure 12.12A.

152. ____________________

153. ____________________

154. ____________________

155. ____________________

156. ____________________

157. ____________________

158. ____________________

159. ____________________

160. ____________________

161. Compare the positioning quality of the correctly positioned radiograph in Figure 12.12A with that in Figure 12.12B. Describe the positioning error, explain what caused it, and give the step(s) necessary to correct the problem.

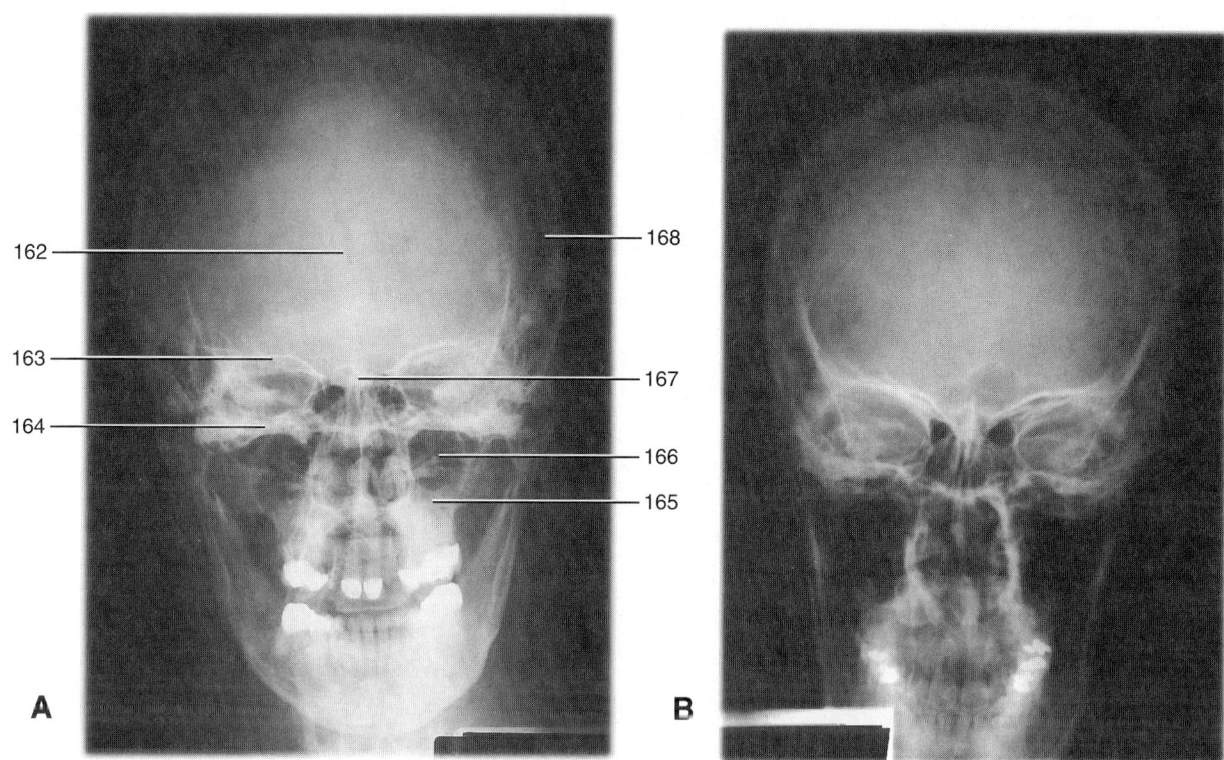

FIGURE 12.13 Radiograph of skull, PA projection, (A) correct positioning and (B) incorrect positioning.

For questions 162–168, identify the radiographic anatomy on the PA skull projection in Figure 12.13A.

162. ____________________

163. ____________________

164. ____________________

165. ____________________

166. ____________________

167. ____________________

168. ____________________

169. Compare the positioning quality of the correctly positioned radiograph in Figure 12.13A with that in Figure 12.13B. Describe the positioning error, explain what caused it, and give the step(s) necessary to correct the problem.

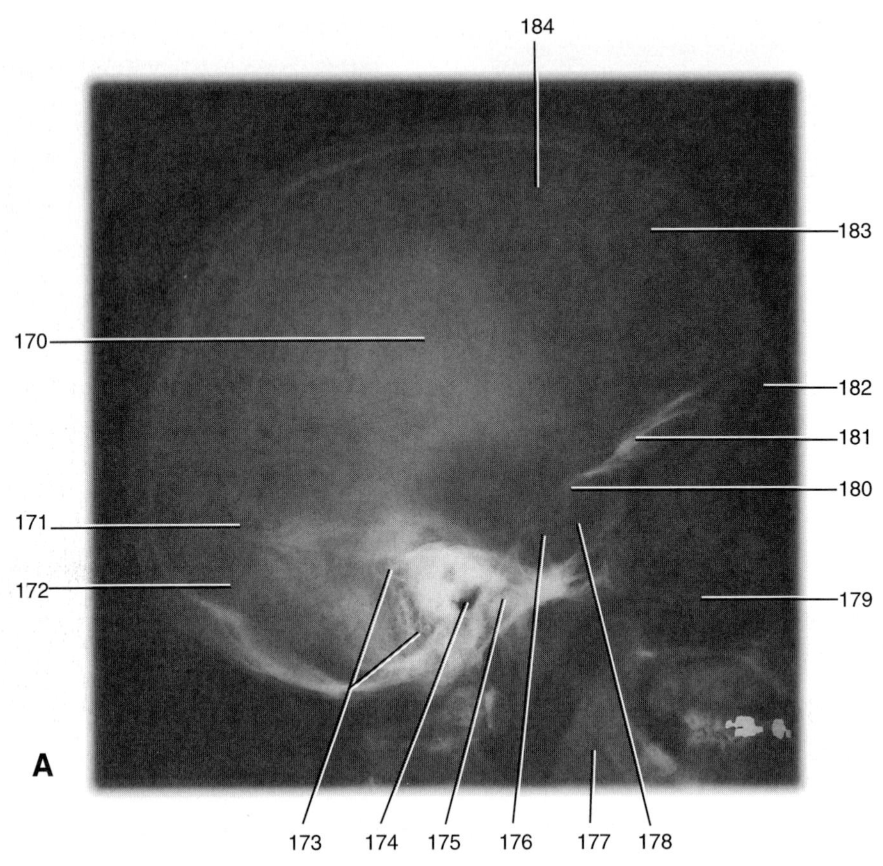

FIGURE 12.14A Radiograph of skull, lateral projection, correct positioning.

For questions 170–184, identify the radiographic anatomy on the lateral skull projection in Figure 12.14A.

170. ____________________

171. ____________________

172. ____________________

173. ____________________

174. ____________________

175. ____________________

176. ____________________

177. ____________________

178. ____________________

179. ____________________

180. ____________________

181. ____________________

182. ____________________

183. ____________________

184. ____________________

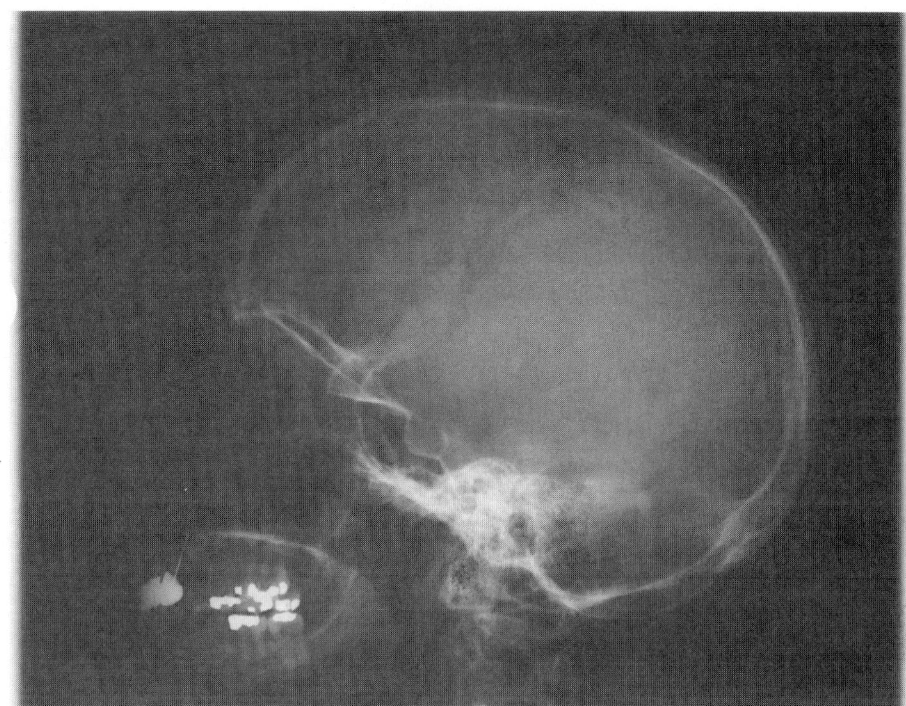

FIGURE 12.14B Radiograph of skull, lateral projection, incorrect positioning.

185. Compare the positioning quality of the correctly positioned radiograph in Figure 12.14A with that in Figure 12.14B. Describe the positioning error, explain what caused it, and give the step(s) necessary to correct the problem.

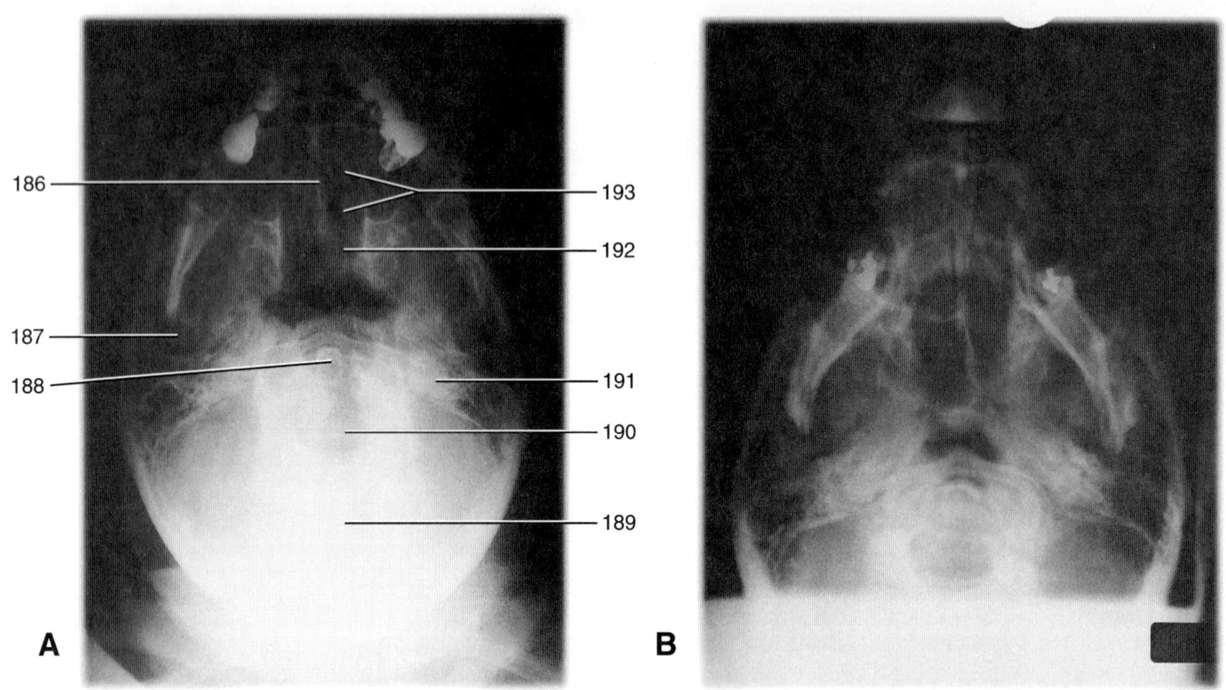

FIGURE 12.15 Radiograph of skull, submentovertical projection, (A) correct positioning and (B) incorrect positioning.

For questions 186–193, identify the radiographic anatomy on the submentovertical projection in Figure 12.15A.

186. ______________________

187. ______________________

188. ______________________

189. ______________________

190. ______________________

191. ______________________

192. ______________________

193. ______________________

194. Compare the positioning quality of the correctly positioned radiograph in Figure 12.15A with that in Figure 12.15B. Describe the positioning error, explain what caused it, and give the step(s) necessary to correct the problem.

195. Positioning accuracy of the parietoacanthial (Waters) projection is evaluated by observing

_______________________________________.

196. The central ray for a submentovertical projection of the skull is directed perpendicular to the

_______________________________________.

197. The two primary areas on the radiograph used to evaluate the positioning accuracy of a lateral skull are _______________ and _______________.

198. For a PA Caldwell projection, the central ray is angled _______________ degrees in the _______________ direction.

199. The _______________ sinuses are located between the orbit and the nasal cavity.

200. Skull radiography is the procedure of choice for demonstrating subdural hematomas.

a. true

b. false

201. The orbitomeatal line (OML) is the primary baseline used in positioning both the PA and the axial AP (Townes) projections of the skull.

a. true

b. false

202. For a PA projection of the skull with no tube angulation, the petrous ridges should completely fill the orbits.

a. true

b. false

203. The dorsum sellae should be located within the shadow of the foramen magnum on a PA Caldwell radiograph of the skull.

a. true

b. false

204. The patient is placed in the correct position for a PA projection for the skull. If the radiographer were to tuck the patient's chin further down, the petrous ridges would be projected lower in the orbits.

a. true

b. false

205. For nontrauma studies, the patient is placed into an LPO position to obtain a left lateral skull radiograph.

a. true

b. false

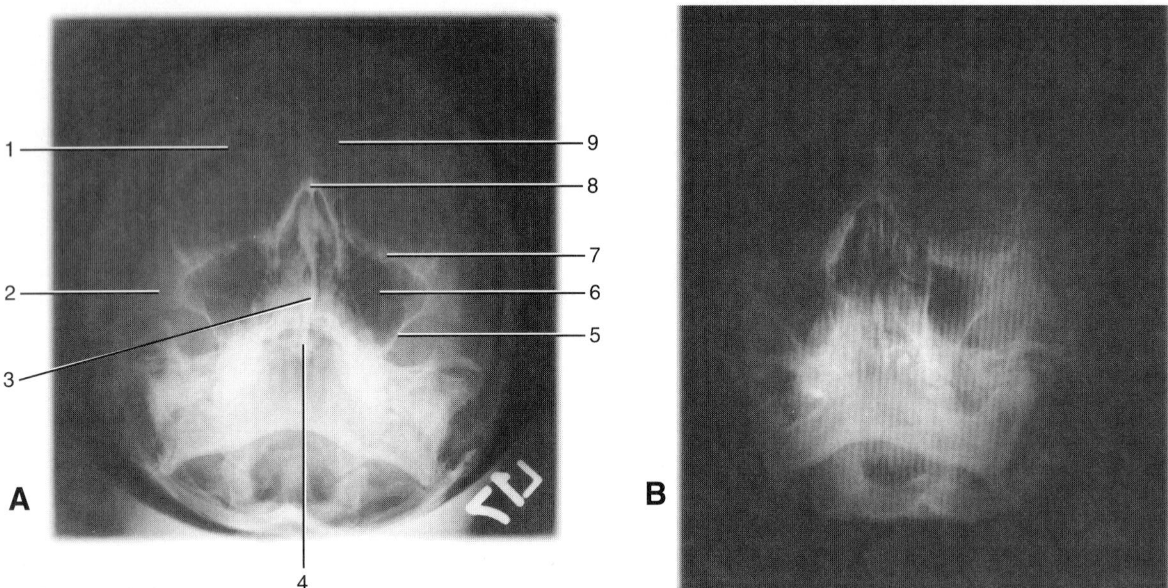

FIGURE 12.16 Radiograph of skull, parietoacanthial (Waters) projection, (A) correct positioning and (B) incorrect positioning.

For questions 206–209, identify the radiographic anatomy on the parietoacanthial (Waters) projection in Figure 12.16A.

206. Anterior nasal spine

a. 3

b. 4

c. 5

d. 8

207. Zygoma

a. 2

b. 6

c. 7

d. 8

208. Maxillary sinus

a. 5

b. 6

c. 8

d. 9

209. Inferior orbital margin

a. 1

b. 5

c. 7

d. 8

210. Compare the positioning quality of the correctly positioned radiograph in Figure 12.16A with that in Figure 12.16B. Describe the positioning error, explain what caused it, and give the step(s) necessary to correct the problem.

211. If the infraorbital line is perpendicular to the film, how many degrees should the tube be angled for an AP axial (Townes) projection?

a. 15

b. 28

c. 30

d. 37

212. The foramen magnum is demonstrated on which projection?

1. AP axial (Townes)

2. parietoacanthial (Waters)

3. PA Caldwell

a. 1 and 2

b. 1 and 3

c. 2 and 3

d. 1, 2, and 3

213. Which of the following is the best criterion to use when evaluating the positioning accuracy of an AP axial (Townes) projection?

a. Petrous ridges should be seen in profile.

b. Lamdoidal suture should be in the center.

c. Parietal bones should be symmetrical.

d. Petrous ridges should be symmetrical.

214. Medial or lateral displacement of the bony nasal septum can be demonstrated on which projections?

1. PA Caldwell

2. AP axial (Townes)

3. parietoacanthial (Waters)

a. 1 and 2

b. 1 and 3

c. 2 and 3

d. 1, 2, and 3

215. On a PA Caldwell projection of the skull, the petrous ridges:

a. completely fill the orbits

b. fill the upper third of the orbits

c. fill the lower third of the orbits

d. are free from superimposition with the orbits

216. If the midsagittal plane is parallel with the table top and the interpupillary line is perpendicular to the film, the projection is the:

a. PA

b. submentovertical

c. lateral

d. parietoacanthial (Waters)

217. Which of the following structures is *not* demonstrated on a lateral skull radiograph?

a. posterior clinoid processes

b. parietal bones

c. lambdoidal suture

d. occipital condyles

218. Of the following projections, which *best* demonstrates the occipital bone?

a. PA Caldwell

b. parietoacanthial (Waters)

c. PA

d. submentovertical

219. The orbitomeatal line (OML) is used to position all of the following projections *except* the:

a. PA Caldwell

b. submentovertical

c. AP axial (Townes)

d. AP

220. The best single radiograph for demonstrating a basal skull fracture is the:

a. submentovertex

b. AP axial (Townes) projection

c. cross-table lateral

d. Caldwell

221. For the submentovertical projection of the skull, the central ray is directed at right angles to the _____ line.

a. acanthiomeatal

b. glabellomeatal

c. infraorbitomeatal

d. orbitomeatal

222. For which projection is the patient's head extended as much as possible?

a. submentovertex

b. AP axial (Townes) projection

c. parietoacanthial

d. Caldwell

223. On a correctly positioned submentovertical projection, the mandibular symphysis is:

a. projected approximately 2 inches anterior to the frontal bone

b. projected approximately 2 inches posterior to the frontal bone

c. projected approximately 2 inches lateral to the frontal bone

d. superimposed on the frontal bone

224. If the midsagittal plane and the IOML are perpendicular to the table and a 37° caudal tube angle is used, the projection is the:

a. AP axial (Townes)

b. AP Caldwell

c. AP

d. parietoacanthial (Waters)

225. If a kyphotic patient cannot tuck the chin down far enough for an AP axial (Townes) projection, which of the following should be done?

a. Angle tube more cephalad than usual.

b. Do not angle tube at all.

c. Angle tube more caudal than usual.

d. Substitute a PA Caldwell projection.

226. If the orbitomeatal line is *slightly less* than 37° to the plane of the film when doing a parietoacanthial (Waters) projection the resultant film will show:

a. adequate demonstration of the antra

b. the petrosal shadows projected onto the lower antra

c. the petrosal shadows projected well below the antra

d. the petrosal shadows projected into the lower orbits

227. A radiographer observes the petrous ridges in the bottom third of the maxillary sinuses on a parietoacanthial (Waters) projection. What action should the radiographer take?

a. Repeat the film tucking the chin further down toward chest.

b. Repeat the film moving the chin further up, away from chest.

c. Repeat the film, aligning the IOML perpendicular to the cassette.

d. No positioning correction is necessary.

228. The radiographer often has to distinguish among types of positioning errors. Compare the radiographic appearance of a lateral skull that has (1) tilt and (2) rotation.

229. The submentovertical projection is challenging to both the patient and the radiographer. Describe some steps the radiographer can take to minimize patient stress and obtain a diagnostic film.

Do You Remember?

230. The RAO position of the cervical spine demonstrates the left apophyseal joints.

a. true

b. false

231. For the RAO sternum the patient should be rotated approximately 55°.

a. true

b. false

232. For an AP projection of the clavicle the tube is angled:

a. 25° caudal

b. 25° cephalic

c. 10° caudal

d. 10° cephalic

233. Which of the following is an example of an amphiarthrotic joint?

a. elbow

b. carpal-carpal

c. skull suture

d. pubic symphysis

234. For cross-table lateral films of the hip, which of the following are placed perpendicular to the film?

a. central ray

b. femoral neck

c. both a and b

d. neither a nor b

235. The large opening in the vertebral column that provides protection for the spinal cord is the _____ foramen.

a. vertebral

b. intervertebral

c. spinal

d. transverse

236. The articulation between a posterior rib with the body of a thoracic vertebra is a/an _____ joint.

a. costotransverse

b. zygapophyseal

c. costovertebral

d. intervertebral

237. Fibrous or immovable joints are called:

a. synarthrotic

b. amphiarthrotic

c. diarthrotic

d. osteoarthrotic

238. On a lateral projection of the wrist, which carpal bone lies closest to the film?

a. scaphoid

b. trapezium

c. pisiform

d. hamate

239. Which projection of the foot demonstrates the cuboid and metatarsal bases free from superimposition?

a. AP

b. medial oblique

c. lateral (mediolateral)

d. lateral (lateromedial)

STUDY TIP: USING CLASS TIME EFFECTIVELY

John: I can't believe you fell asleep in class again. Instructor Bob is going to lose his patience with you.

Chi: I know all this stuff anyway. Besides do you really think he noticed me? I hid behind Jill.

John: I think he noticed. He called on you twice and you never responded.

Chi: No way!

- Ask questions during class. If you do not understand the material, there is a good possibility that others in the class are also confused.
- Attend all classes. Be on time or early. Although it may not be in the syllabus, attendance always counts in the realm of subjective grading.
- Sit away from all distractions and where the action is occurring. This is usually at or near the front of the room.
- Stay awake and alert during class time, focusing on the course material.

One of best ways to prepare for a course is to use class time efficiently. Learning as much as possible during class will save considerable time in test preparation later.

CHAPTER 13

Skull and Facial Bones

LEARNING OBJECTIVES

At the completion of this chapter, the student should be able to:

1. Given radiographs, locate anatomic structures and landmarks.
2. Explain the rationale for each projection.
3. Describe the positioning used to visualize anatomic structures of the skull and facial bones.
4. List or identify the central ray location and identify the extent of the field necessary for each projection.
5. Recommend the technical factors for producing an acceptable radiograph.
6. State the patient instructions for each projection.
7. Given radiographs, evaluate positioning and technical factors.
8. Describe modifications of procedures for atypical or impaired patients to better demonstrate the anatomic area of interest.

Routine and Alternate Positions/Projections

Part	Routine	Alternative
Skull	axial AP	
	PA	
	Lateral	
	Submentovertical	
Facial bones	PA Caldwell	
	Parietoacanthial (Waters)	
	Lateral	
Nasal bones	PA Caldwell	
	Parietoacanthial (Waters)	
	Lateral	
	Superoinferior (axial)	
Orbits	PA	
	Modified parietoacanthial (modified Waters)	
	Lateral	
Optic foramen	Parieto-orbital oblique (Rhese)	Orbitoparietal oblique (reverse Rhese)
Zygomatic arches	Axial AP (Townes/Grashey)	
	Submentovertical	Oblique axial (May)
Mandible	Axial AP (Townes/Grashey)	
	PA	
	Axiolateral	
Temporomandibular joints	Axiolateral transcranial (Schuller)	
	Transcranial lateral	
	Pantomography	
Sinuses	PA Caldwell	
	Parietoacanthial (Waters)	
	Lateral	
	Submentovertical	
	Axial transoral (Pirie)	

Temporal bones	Axial AP (Townes/Grashey)	
	Axiolateral oblique (Law)	
	Posterior profile (Stenvers/Arcelin)	
	Axioposterior oblique (Mayer)	
	Submentovertical	
Sella turcica	Axial AP (Townes/Grashey)	Axial PA (Haas)
	Lateral	

QUESTIONS

Radiographic Procedures, Analysis, and Critical Thinking

For questions 1–5, identify the radiographic anatomy on the parietoacanthial (Waters) projection for nasal bones in Figure 13.1A.

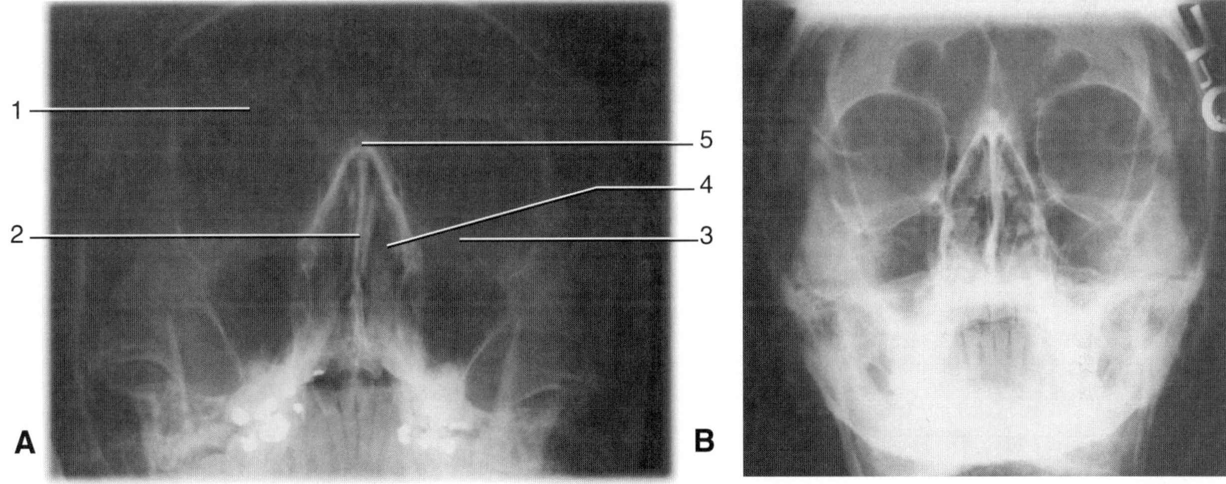

FIGURE 13.1 Radiograph of nasal bones, parietoacanthial (Waters) projection, (A) correct positioning and (B) incorrect positioning.

1. ____________________
2. ____________________
3. ____________________
4. ____________________
5. ____________________

6. Compare the positioning quality of the correctly positioned radiograph in Figure 13.1A with that in Figure 13.1B. Describe the positioning error, explain what caused it, and give the step(s) necessary to correct the problem.

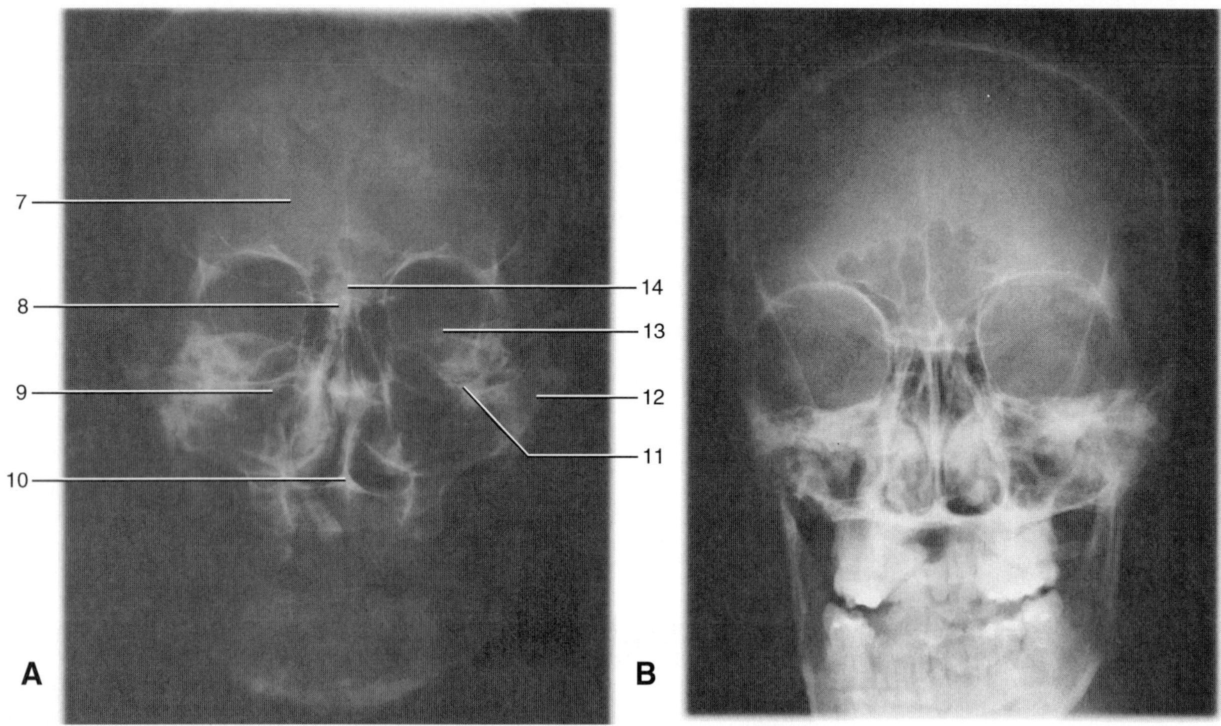

FIGURE 13.2 Radiograph of facial bones, PA Caldwell projection, (A) correct positioning and (B) incorrect positioning.

For questions 7–14, identify the radiographic anatomy on the PA Caldwell projection for facial bones in Figure 13.2A.

7. ____________________

8. ____________________

9. ____________________

10. ____________________

11. ____________________

12. ____________________

13. ____________________

14. ____________________

15. Compare the positioning quality of the correctly positioned radiograph in Figure 13.2A with that in Figure 13.2B. Describe the positioning error, explain what caused it, and give the step(s) necessary to correct the problem.

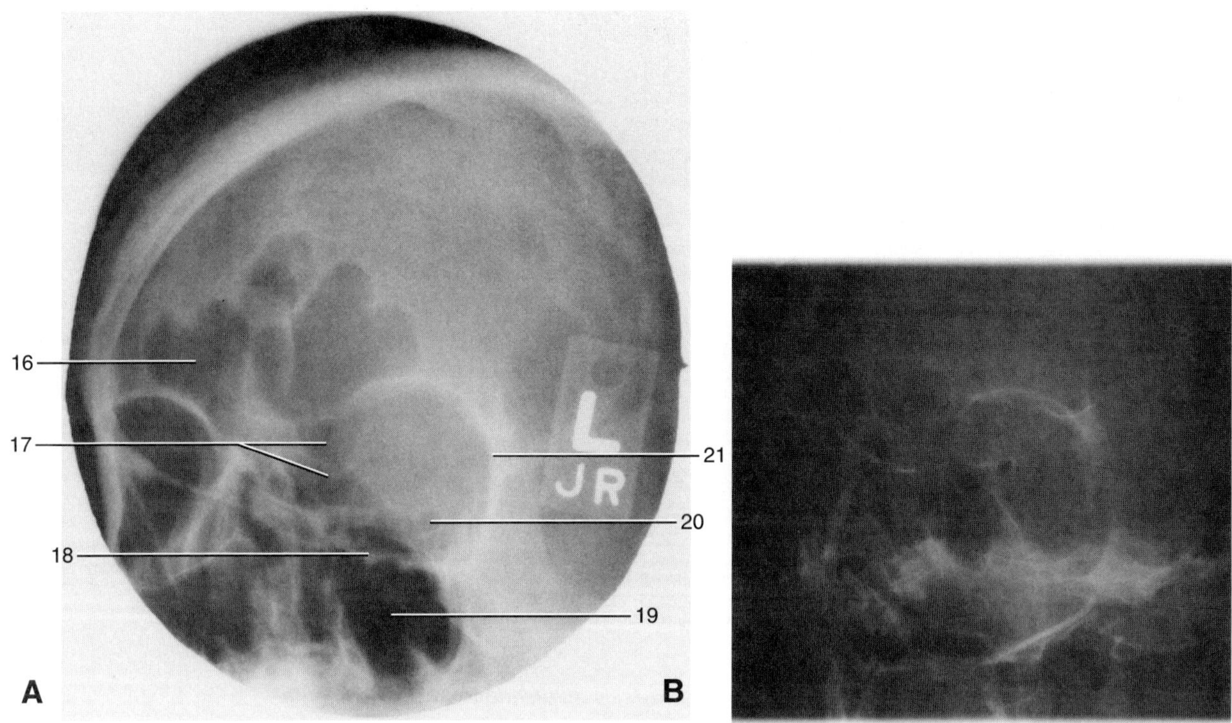

FIGURE 13.3 Radiograph of orbits, parieto-orbital oblique (Rhese) projection, (A) correct positioning and (B) incorrect positioning.

For questions 16–21, identify the radiographic anatomy on the parieto-orbital oblique (Rhese) projection in Figure 13.3A.

16. ______________________

17. ______________________

18. ______________________

19. ______________________

20. ______________________

21. ______________________

22. Compare the positioning quality of the correctly positioned radiograph in Figure 13.3A with that in Figure 13.3B. Describe the positioning error, explain what caused it, and give the step(s) necessary to correct the problem.

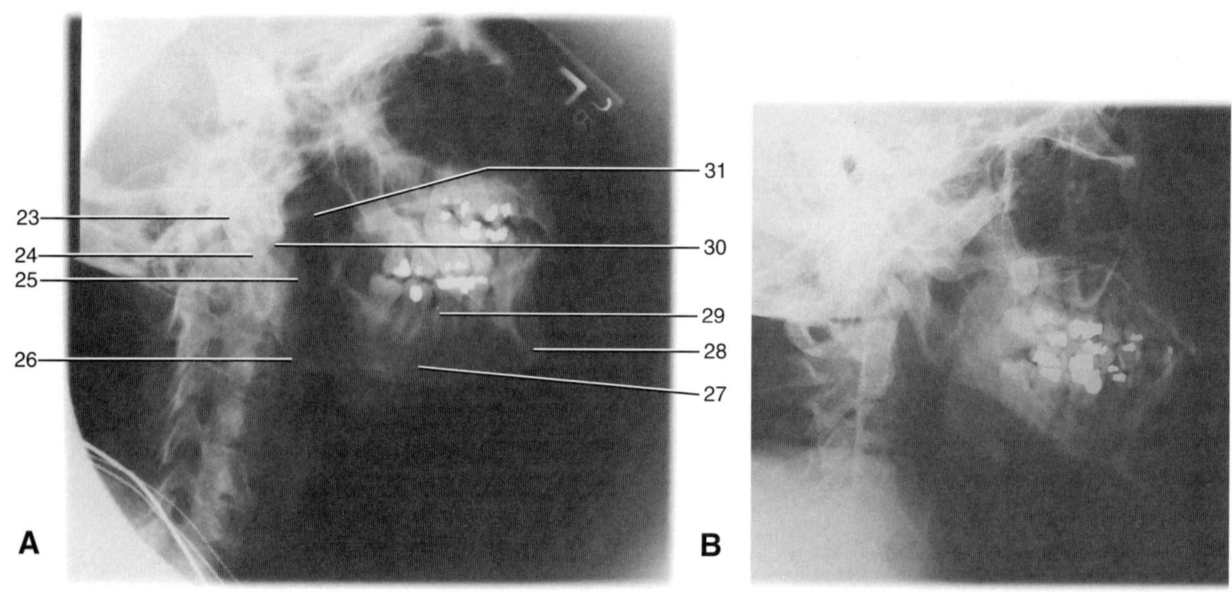

FIGURE 13.4 Radiograph of mandible, axiolateral projection, (A) correct positioning and (B) incorrect positioning.

For questions 23–31, identify the radiographic anatomy on the axiolateral mandible projection in Figure 13.4A.

23. ____________________

24. ____________________

25. ____________________

26. ____________________

27. ____________________

28. ____________________

29. ____________________

30. ____________________

31. ____________________

32. Compare the positioning quality of the correctly positioned radiograph in Figure 13.4A with that in Figure 13.4B. Describe the positioning error, explain what caused it, and give the step(s) necessary to correct the problem.

33. The central ray for a PA Caldwell projection of the nasal bones exits at the

_______________.

34. The central ray for lateral nasal bones enters

_______________.

35. The _______________ projection of the nasal bones is commonly taken without a grid.

36. When positioning superoinferior/axial nasal bones, the _______________ line is placed perpendicular to the film.

37. The parieto-orbital oblique projection is commonly called the _______________ position.

38. The kVp range for routine films of the mandible is

_______________.

39. With the mouth *open,* the mandibular condyle will be located

_______________.

40. With the mouth *closed,* the mandibular condyle will be located

_______________.

41. Pantomography is used to demonstrate anatomic structures on the

_______________.

42. For the lateral projection of the paranasal sinuses, the central ray enters

_______________.

43. The reverse submentovertical is called the _______________ projection.

44. The axiolateral oblique (Law) projection requires a tube angle of _______________ degrees in the _______________ direction.

45. The posterior profile (Stenvers) projection requires a tube angle of _______________ degrees in the _______________ direction.

46. The Haas position is called the _______________ projection.

47. On lateral nasal bones, the kVp is increased to better demonstrate soft tissue detail in the region.

a. true

b. false

48. On a modified parietoacanthial (modified Waters) projection for orbits, the petrous ridges should appear just below the maxillary antra.

a. true

b. false

49. On an AP axial (Townes) projection, the zygomatic arches should be directly superimposed on the mandibular rami.

a. true

b. false

50. The axiolateral transcranial (Schuller) projection demonstrates the temporomandibular joint closest to the table.

a. true

b. false

51. On a PA Caldwell radiograph the ethmoid sinuses should appear just superior to the nasal bones.

   a. true

   b. false

52. The central ray for the axiolateral oblique (Law) projection enters 2 inches anterior and 2 inches superior to the uppermost EAM.

   a. true

   b. false

53. The posterior profile (Stenvers) projection of the temporal bone demonstrates the petrous portion *farthest* from the film.

   a. true

   b. false

54. The axioposterior oblique (Mayer) projection of the temporal bone demonstrates the mastoid air cells *farthest* from the film.

   a. true

   b. false

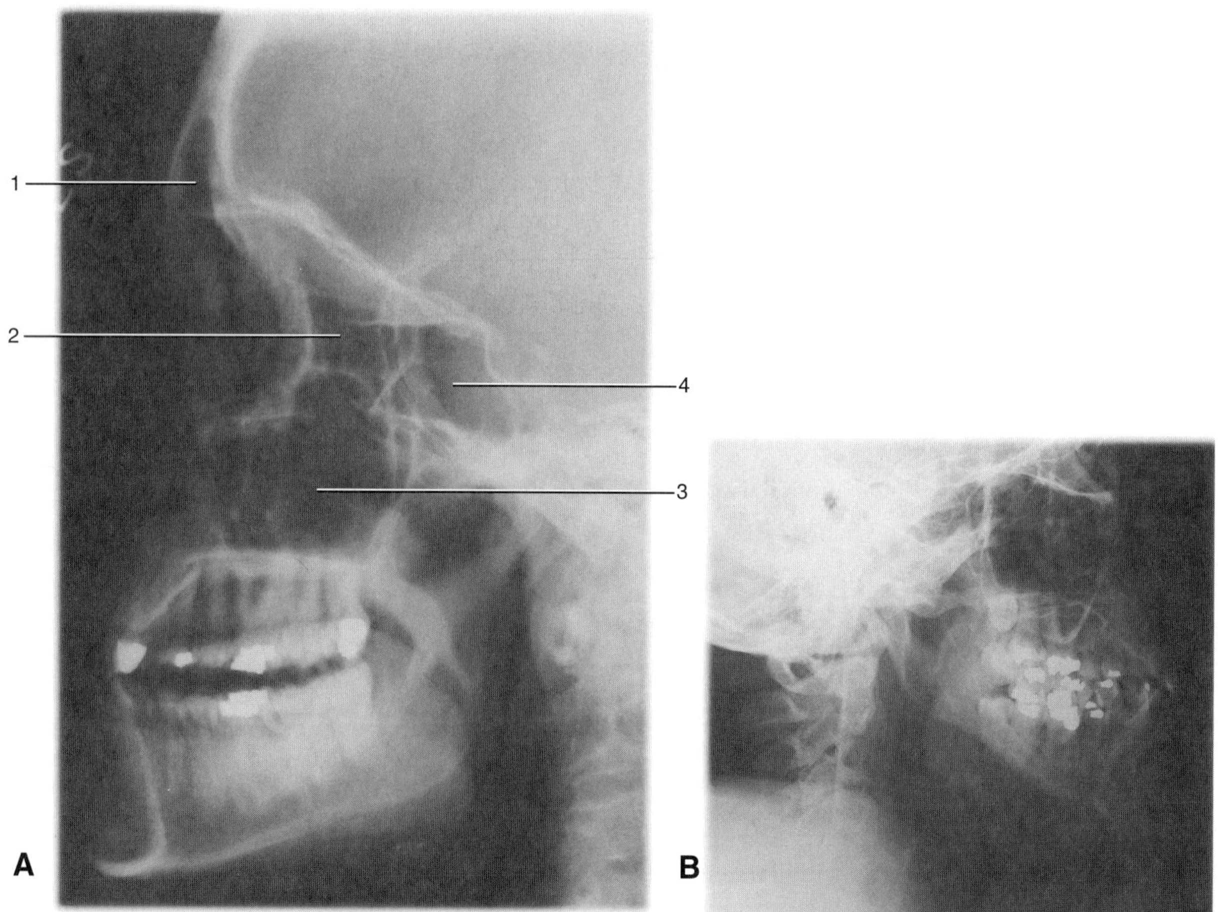

FIGURE 13.5 Radiograph of sinuses, lateral projection, (A) correct positioning and (B) incorrect positioning.

For questions 55–58, identify the radiographic anatomy on the lateral projection of the sinuses in Figure 13.5A.

55. Number 1

a. maxillary sinus

b. sphenoid sinus

c. ethmoid sinus

d. frontal sinus

56. Number 2

a. maxillary sinus

b. sphenoid sinus

c. ethmoid sinus

d. frontal sinus

57. Number 3

a. maxillary sinus

b. sphenoid sinus

c. ethmoid sinus

d. frontal sinus

58. Number 4

a. maxillary sinus

b. sphenoid sinus

c. ethmoid sinus

d. frontal sinus

59. Compare the positioning quality of the correctly positioned radiograph in Figure 13.5A with that in Figure 13.5B. Describe the positioning error, explain what caused it, and give the step(s) necessary to correct the problem.

For questions 60–63, identify the radiographic anatomy on the posterior profile (Arcelin) projection in Figure 13.6.

60. Mandibular condyle

a. 1

b. 4

c. 5

d. 6

61. Mastoid process

a. 1

b. 2

c. 3

d. 4

62. Petrous ridge

a. 2

b. 5

c. 6

d. 7

63. Internal auditory canal

a. 1

b. 5

c. 6

d. 7

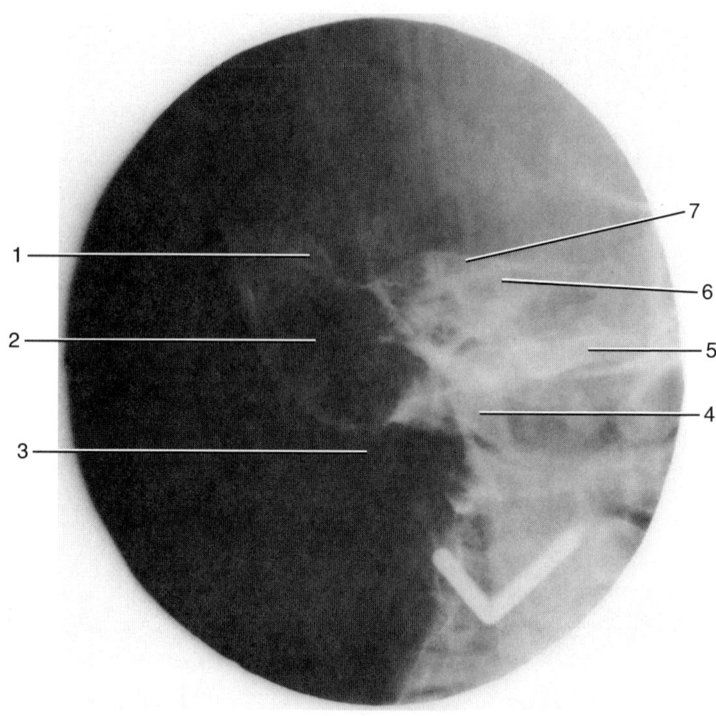

FIGURE 13.6 Radiograph of temporal bone, posterior profile (Arcelin) projection.

For questions 64–67, match each radiograph in Figure 13.7 with its name.

	Radiograph	Name
64. _____	Figure 13.7A	**a.** axioposterior (Mayer)
65. _____	Figure 13.7B	**b.** axiolateral oblique (Law)
66. _____	Figure 13.7C	**c.** orbitoparietal (Rhese)
67. _____	Figure 13-.7D	**d.** superoinferior
		e. oblique axial (May)

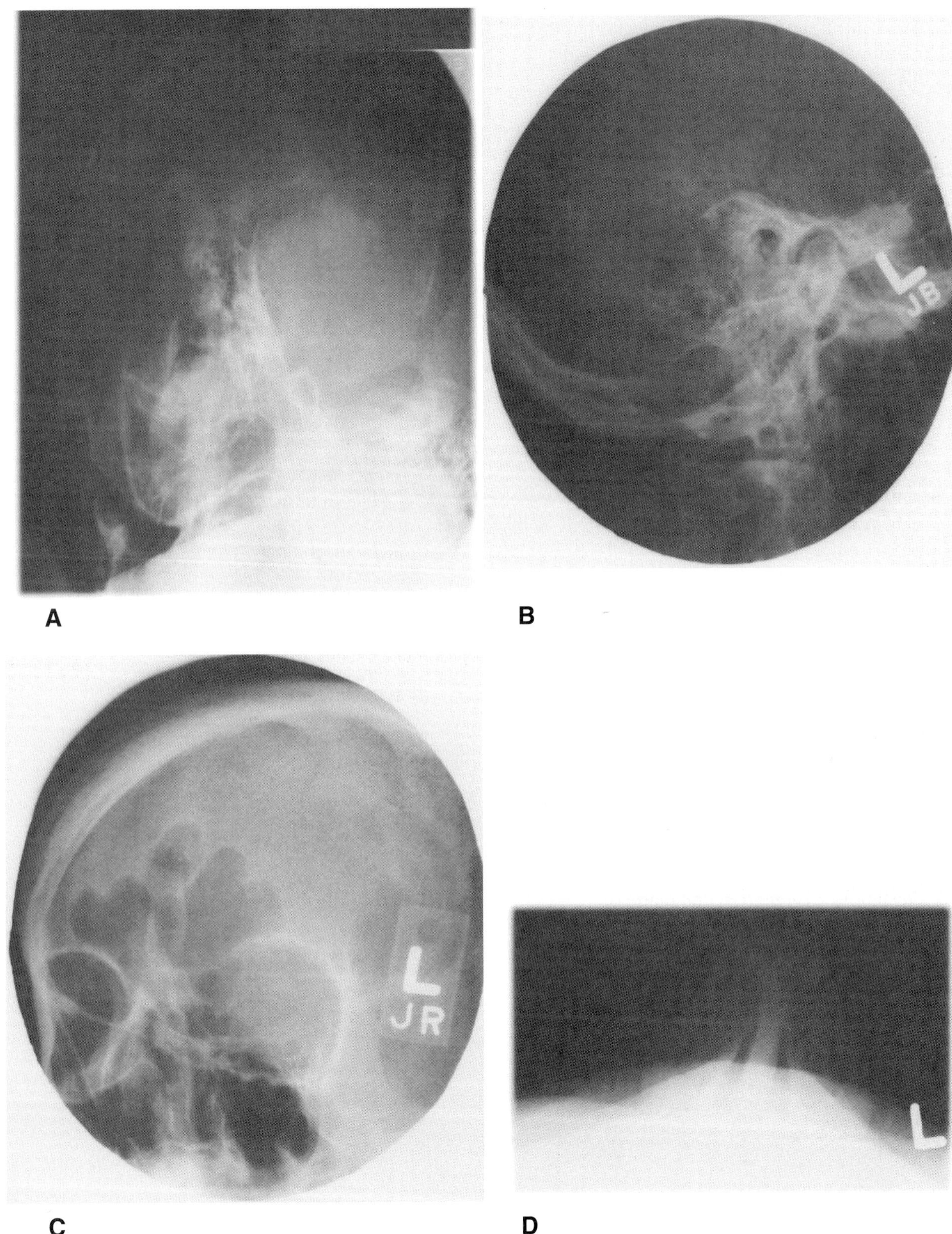

FIGURE 13.7 Multiple unknown projections (A), (B), (C), (D).

68. The central ray for a lateral projection of the cranium enters _____ the external auditory meatus.

a. 4 inches above

b. 2 inches above

c. at

d. 2 inches below

69. The central ray for a parietoacanthial (Waters) projection for facial bones exits at the:

a. mentum

b. glabella

c. nasion

d. acanthion

70. The central ray for a PA Caldwell projection for facial bones exits at the:

a. vertex

b. glabella

c. nasion

d. acanthion

71. When positioning a PA Caldwell projection for facial bones, the midsagittal plane is:

a. parallel to the cassette

b. perpendicular to the cassette

c. at a 15° angle to the cassette

d. parallel to the orbitomeatal line

72. Which projection is particularly useful for demonstrating depressed fractures of the frontal sinus?

a. PA Caldwell

b. submentovertical

c. parietoacanthial (Waters)

d. lateral

73. On a modified parietoacanthial (Waters) projection for facial bones, the petrous ridges should:

a. completely fill the orbits

b. fill the upper third of the orbits

c. fill the lower third of the orbits

d. lie below the maxillary antra

74. When positioning lateral facial bones, the midsagittal plane is placed:

a. at an angle of 15° to the film

b. at an angle of 15° to the central ray

c. perpendicular to the film

d. parallel to the film

75. The central ray for a lateral projection of the facial bones enters at the:

a. zygoma

b. glabella

c. nasion

d. acanthion

76. For the parietoacanthial projection of the nasal bones, the orbitomeatal line forms an angle of _____ with the plane of the film.

a. 15°

b. 30°

c. 37°

d. 55°

77. Which of the following are commonly included in a departmental protocol for nasal bones?

1. lateral
2. submentovertical
3. parietoacanthial (Waters)

a. 1 and 2

b. 1 and 3

c. 2 and 3

d. 1, 2, and 3

78. Lateral displacement of the bony nasal septum is demonstrated on which projections?

1. lateral
2. PA Caldwell
3. parietoacanthial (Waters)

a. 1 and 2

b. 1 and 3

c. 2 and 3

d. 1, 2, and 3

79. For which projection of the orbits is the midsagittal plane perpendicular to the midpoint of the cassette and the orbitomeatal line perpendicular to the film?

a. PA

b. modified parietoacanthial (modified Waters)

c. lateral

d. parieto-orbital oblique (Rhese)

80. Which of the following *best* demonstrates the floor of the orbits?

a. parieto-orbital oblique (Rhese)

b. PA Caldwell

c. parietoacanthial (Waters)

d. modified parietoacanthial (modified Waters)

81. Which of the following is perpendicular to the plane of the film for the parieto-orbital oblique (Rhese) projection of the orbits?

a. infraorbitomeatal line

b. orbitomeatal line

c. acanthiomeatal line

d. glabellomeatal line

82. In the parieto-orbital oblique (Rhese) projection, the head is positioned so that the _____ are in contact with the table.

a. forehead, nose, and chin

b. nose, zygoma, and chin

c. forehead, zygoma, and nose

d. forehead and lips

83. When positioning a parieto-orbital oblique (Rhese) projection, the head is adjusted so that the midsagittal plane forms an angle of _____ with the plane of the film.

a. 55°

b. 53°

c. 37°

d. 90°

84. On a properly positioned parieto-orbital oblique (Rhese) projection, the optic foramen is located in the _____ _____ quadrant of the orbital shadow.

a. upper, outer

b. lower, outer

c. upper, inner

d. lower, inner

85. For the submentovertical projection for the zygomatic arches, the central ray is directed at right angles to the _____ line.

a. infraorbitomeatal

b. orbitomeatal

c. acanthiomeatal

d. glabellomeatal

86. Which of the following are commonly performed to demonstrate the zygomatic arches?

1. modified parietoacanthial (modified Waters)

2. submentovertical

3. AP axial (Townes)

a. 1 and 2

b. 1 and 3

c. 2 and 3

d. 1, 2, and 3

87. When positioning the oblique axial (May) projection for zygomatic arches, the patient's head is turned _____ _____ the affected side.

a. 25°, away from

b. 15°, toward

c. 25°, toward

d. 15°, away from

88. The oblique axial (May) projection is a variation of which projection?

a. parieto-orbital oblique (Rhese)

b. PA Caldwell

c. parietoacanthial (Waters)

d. submentovertex

89. The central ray for a PA projection of the mandible is directed:

a. perpendicular to the film

b. 20° cephalic

c. 20° caudal

d. 35° cephalic

90. For an axiolateral projection of the mandibular body, the head is tilted _____ .

a. 0°

b. 10°

c. 30°

d. 45°

91. Which projection *best* demonstrates a fracture of the mandibular condyle?

a. AP

b. submentovertex

c. axiolateral

d. lateral

92. For an AP axial (Townes) projection of the mandible, the _____ line is perpendicular to the film.

a. infraorbitomeatal

b. orbitomeatal

c. acanthiomeatal

d. glabellomeatal

93. If the head is placed in a true lateral position, an axiolateral mandible requires a tube angle of:

a. 10–15° caudal

b. 10–15° cephalic

c. 25–35° caudal

d. 25–35° cephalic

94. For the axiolateral transcranial (Schuller) projection of the temporomandibular joints, the central ray is angled:

a. 10–15° cephalic

b. 10–15° caudal

c. 25–30° cephalic

d. 25–30° caudal

95. For the lateral transcranial projection of the temporomandibular joints, the head is rotated _____ the plane of the film.

a. 25° away from

b. 15° toward

c. 25° toward

d. 15° away from

96. Demonstration of the temporomandibular articulation is *best* performed using:

a. a long focal film distance

b. tomography

c. breathing technique

d. extremity cassettes with an extension cone

97. Which of the following are used for demonstration of the TMJs?

1. tomography
2. Schuller method
3. Mayer method

a. 1 and 2

b. 1 and 3

c. 2 and 3

d. 1, 2, and 3

98. On a PA Caldwell projection of the paranasal sinuses, the petrous ridges should:

a. completely fill the orbits

b. fill the upper third of the orbits

c. fill the lower third of the orbits

d. be free from superimposition with the orbits

99. The PA Caldwell projection primarily demonstrates which paranasal sinuses?

1. sphenoid

2. ethmoid

3. frontal

a. 1 and 2

b. 1 and 3

c. 2 and 3

d. 1, 2, and 3

100. The parietoacanthial (Waters) projection best demonstrates the _____ sinus group.

a. sphenoid

b. ethmoid

c. maxillary

d. frontal

101. The lateral projection best demonstrates the _____ sinus group.

a. sphenoid

b. ethmoid

c. maxillary

d. frontal

102. The submentovertical projection primarily demonstrates which paranasal sinuses?

1. sphenoid

2. ethmoid

3. frontal

a. 1 and 2

b. 1 and 3

c. 2 and 3

d. 1, 2, and 3

103. The submentovertical projection is used for the evaluation of the:

1. sphenoid sinus

2. mandibular condyles

3. zygomatic arches

a. 1 and 2

b. 1 and 3

c. 2 and 3

d. 1, 2, and 3

104. In the axial transoral (Pirie) projection, which sinus group is visualized through the open mouth?

a. sphenoid

b. ethmoid

c. maxillary

d. frontal

105. Which structures are demonstrated on an AP axial (Townes) projection of the temporal bones?

1. mastoid air cells
2. petrous ridges
3. internal auditory canals

a. 1 and 2
b. 1 and 3
c. 2 and 3
d. 1, 2, and 3

106. For the axiolateral oblique (Law) projection of the temporal bones, the face is rotated _____ the plane of the film

a. 25° away from
b. 15° toward
c. 25° toward
d. 15° away from

107. The axiolateral oblique (Law) projection best demonstrates the:

a. temporomandibular joint
b. petrous ridges
c. zygomatic arches
d. mastoid air cells

108. For the anterior profile (Arcelin) projection, the central ray is directed:

a. 10–12° cephalic
b. 10–12° caudal
c. perpendicular to the film
d. parallel to the film

109. In the posterior profile (Stenvers) projection, the head is rotated _____ from a PA projection.

a. 15°
b. 30°
c. 45°
d. 55°

110. In the axioposterior oblique (Mayer) projection, the head is rotated _____ from a PA projection.

a. 15°
b. 25°
c. 30°
d. 45°

111. The central ray for the axioposterior oblique (Mayer) projection requires a tube angle of _____ in the _____ direction.

a. 15°, cephalic
b. 15°, caudal
c. 45°, cephalic
d. 45°, caudal

112. For the lateral projection of the sella turcica, the central ray enters _____ to the EAM.

a. 1 inch anterior and 1 inch inferior
b. 3/4 inch anterior and 3/4 inch superior
c. 3/4 inch posterior and 3/4 inch superior
d. 1 inch posterior and 1 inch inferior

113. To demonstrate the dorsum sellae and the posterior clinoids in the AP axial (Townes) projection, the tube is angled _____ caudal.

a. 15°

c. 30°

c. 37°

d. 45°

114. To demonstrate the sella turcica in the lateral projection the central ray is directed:

a. 15° caudal

b. 25° caudal

c. 45° caudal

d. perpendicular to the film

115. If the patient cannot be placed in the prone position for a Waters position of the facial bones, a similar projection can be obtained in the supine position by positioning:

a. the orbitomeatal line perpendicular and central ray at 30° caudal angle

b. the acanthiomeatal line perpendicular and central ray at a 30° caudal angle

c. the infraorbitomeatal line perpendicular and central ray at a 30° cephalad angle

d. the infraorbitomeatal line perpendicular and central ray at a 30° caudal angle

116. One evaluation criterion for lateral orbits is that the orbits themselves are superimposed. Of what diagnostic value is this film if the structures are superimposed?

117. If the optic foramen lies in the upper quadrant of the orbital shadow for a parieto-orbital oblique (Rhese) projection, what is the likely problem?

118. Zygomatic arches are taken at a lower kVp compared to most other skull examinations. Explain why this reduced kVp is needed to properly demonstrate structures in this region.

119. Explain why three different rotations of the head are required on an axiolateral mandible to demonstrate all anatomic regions of this bone.

120. Explain why temporomandibular joint examinations include films with the mouth open and closed and why both joints are taken instead of just the affected one.

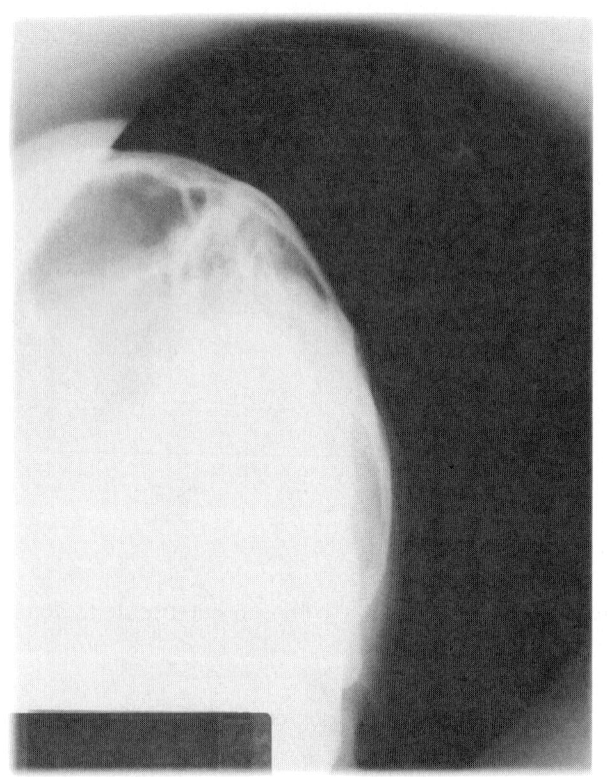

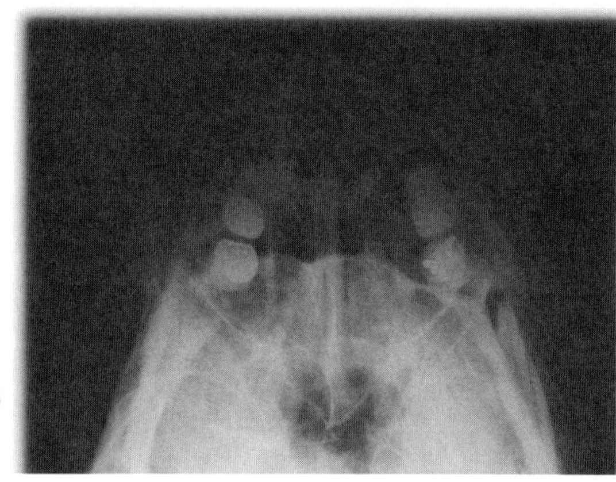

FIGURE 13.8 Zygomatic arch projections.

121. Examine the two zygomatic arch projections in Figure 13.8. Determine which of the two is the more diagnostic radiograph and defend your answer.

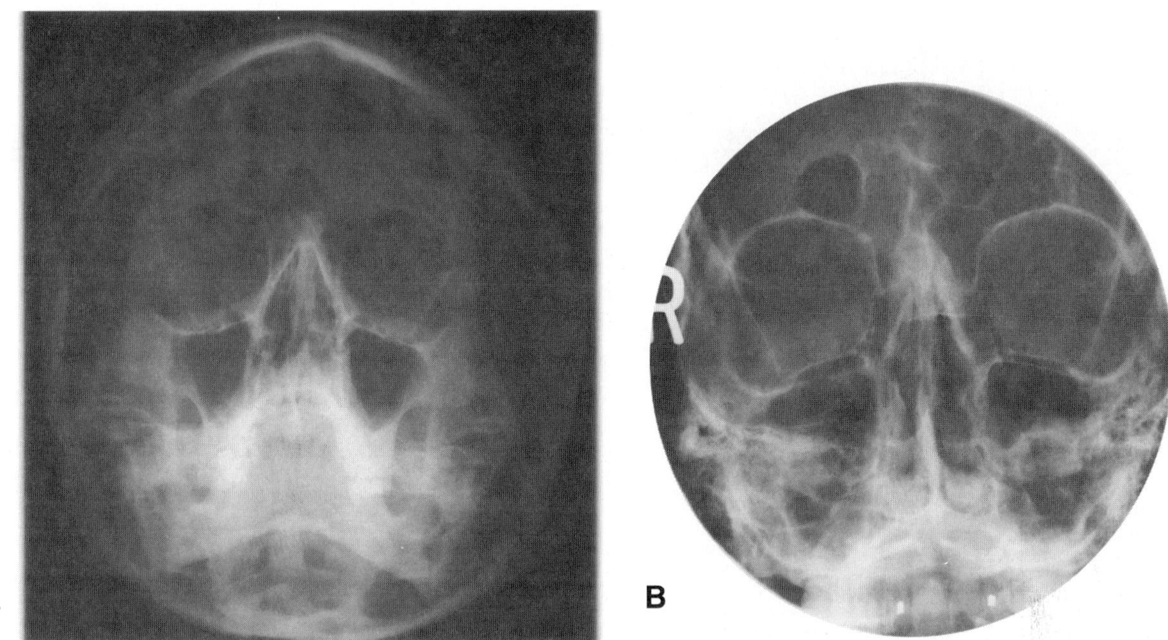

FIGURE 13.9 (A) and (B) Parietocanthial projection.

122. Examine the two parietoacanthial projections for sinuses in Figure 13.9. Determine which of the two is the more diagnostic radiograph and defend your answer.

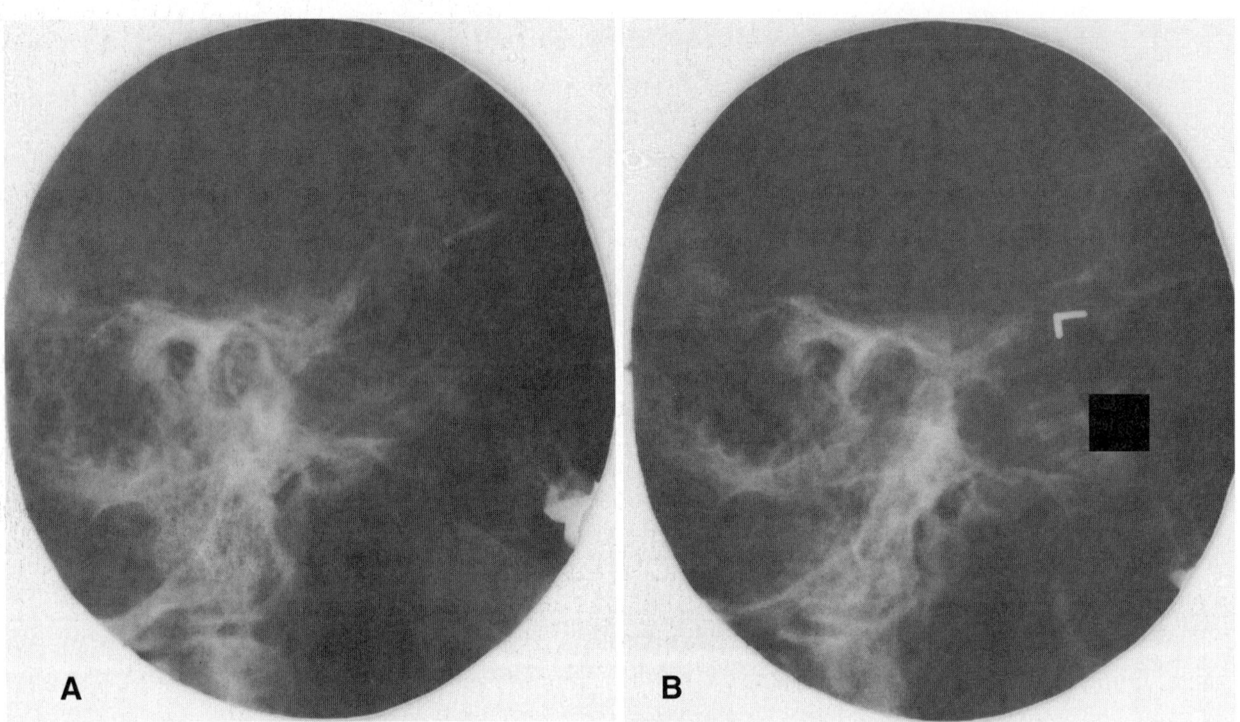

FIGURE 13.10 (A) and (B) Temporomandibular joint projection.

123. Examine the two temporomandibular joint projections in Figure 13.10. Determine which is the open-mouth view and explain the clues that led to this conclusion.

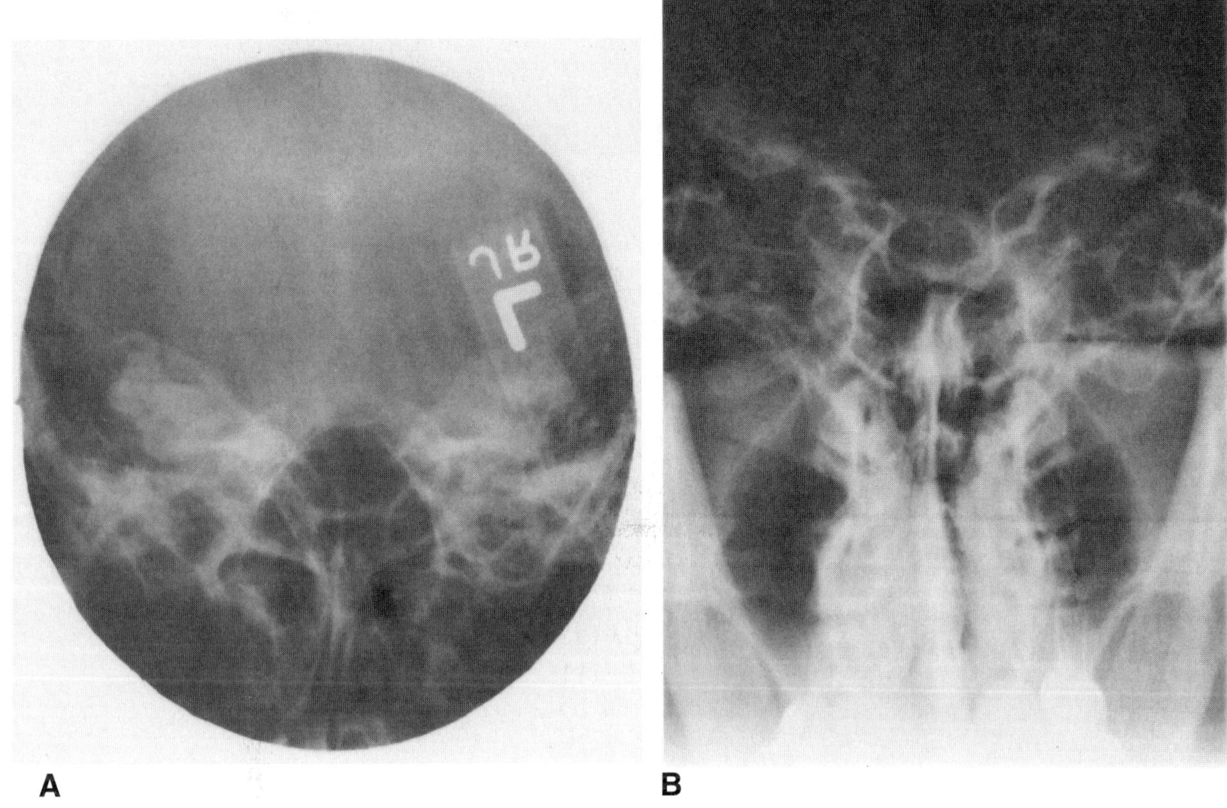

FIGURE 13.11 (A) and (B) Sella turcica projections.

124. Examine the two sella turcica projections in Figure 13.11. Determine which used a 30° tube angle and which used a 37° tube angle and explain the clues that led to this conclusion.

Do You Remember?

125. An AP ankle radiograph should demonstrate the distal fibula free of any superimposition from the distal tibia.

a. true

b. false

126. The position of the diaphragm will lower during expiration.

a. true

b. false

127. The lordotic projection of the chest primarily demonstrates the hilum portion of the lung.

a. true

b. false

128. On a lateral scapula radiograph, which structures should be exactly superimposed?

a. axillary ribs and the vertebral border

b. body of the scapula and the axillary ribs

c. coracoid and acromion processes

d. vertebral and axillary borders

129. The articulations between the superior and inferior articulating processes of the cervical vertebrae are best seen in the _____ projection.

a. lateral

b. AP

c. AP axial (Pillar)

d. AP oblique

130. Which structure makes up the nose of the "Scotty dog" on oblique lumbar spine radiographs?

a. spinous process

b. lamina

c. transverse process

d. superior articulating process

131. The xiphoid tip is at the approximate level of:

a. T8

b. T9

c. T10

d. T12

132. The semilunar notch articulates with which portion of the humerus?

a. coronoid process

b. capitellum

c. lateral condyle

d. trochlea

133. A patient arrives through the emergency room for a calcaneous examination. Her foot is slightly extended and she is unable to place the plantar surface of her foot perpendicular to the cassette. The radiographer should:

a. use a 40° tube angle

b. use less than 40° tube angle

c. use more than 40° tube angle

d. consult the emergency room physician for assistance

134. The central ray for a scaphoid view of the wrist is commonly angled _____ .

a. 5°

b. 10°

c. 15°

d. 20°

STUDY TIP: MANAGING TEST ANXIETY

Minutes before the test, students are gathering outside the classroom.

Jean: What is that tube angle for the AP axial again? And what is the best view for the cervical pedicles. Quick, before instructor Bob arrives. Darn, I should have studied this more last night.

Jill: Give it up, Jean. If you don't know it by now, you won't remember it on the test.

John: Jill is right. You are better off sitting quietly and taking some deep breaths with extended exhalations. That's what I do to help relax.

Jill: I like to think or meditate about calming places, like a waterfall or peaceful forest, before starting the test. The calming helps to clear my mind and reduce the test anxiety.

Jean: Are you guys crazy? Talking about breathing and waterfalls at a time like this. You probably don't know the tube angle anyway. Hey, Juan, what is the tube angle ....

Test anxiety is a condition that can be overcome. For many students, managing anxiety can result in greater academic success.

- Most test anxiety is caused by insufficient test preparation. Improving study habits should always be examined as a first solution to test anxiety.
- Take active steps to manage your test anxiety, whether it be through changing study habits, deep breathing, meditation, or another established method. The problem often becomes worse if ignored.

> Excessive anxiety is damaging to your health and can lead to poor performance. Because of the intensity of health education programs, identification and management of test anxiety should be an early goal of students in these programs.

CHAPTER 14

Trauma Head Positioning

LEARNING OBJECTIVES

At the completion of this chapter, the student should be able to:

1. Describe the circumstances and patient conditions that would necessitate a trauma skull series.
2. Explain the rationale for each projection used for trauma patients.
3. List or discuss the skills the radiographer should possess to perform trauma radiography.
4. Describe the positioning and cassette placement used to visualize anatomic structures in the skull of the trauma patient and describe how these differ from routine projections.
5. Identify the location of the central ray and the extent of the field necessary for producing each projection.
6. Recommend the technical factors for producing an acceptable radiograph for each projection and discuss differences from routine studies.
7. State the patient instructions for each projection.
8. Given radiographs, evaluate positioning and technical factors.

Routine Positions

Part	Routine
Skull	Trauma AP
	Trauma lateral
	Trauma AP axial (Grashey/Townes)

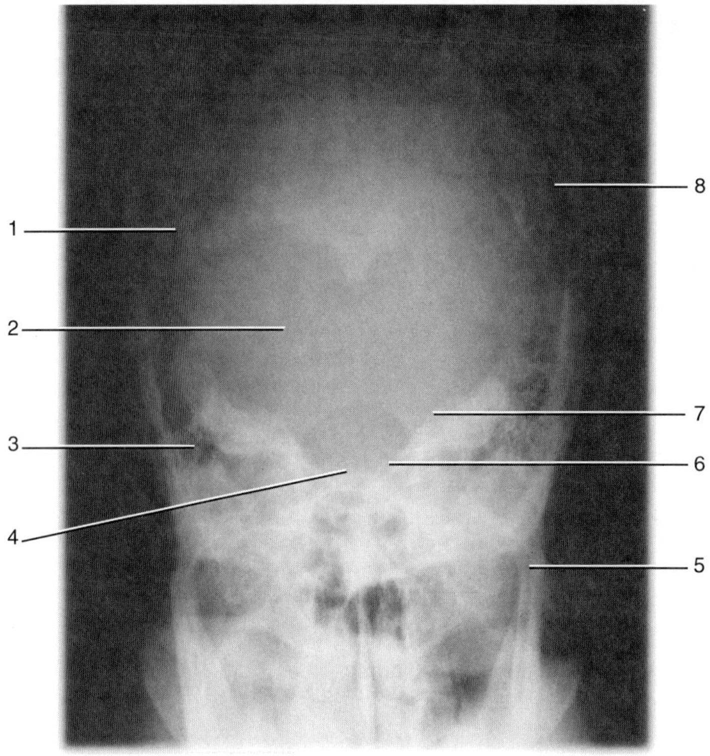

FIGURE 14.1 Radiograph of skull, trauma AP axial (Townes) projection.

QUESTIONS

Radiographic Procedures, Analysis, and Critical Thinking

For questions 1–8, identify the radiographic anatomy on the trauma AP axial (Townes) projection in Figure 14.1.

1. ______________________
2. ______________________
3. ______________________
4. ______________________
5. ______________________
6. ______________________
7. ______________________
8. ______________________

9. Analyze the positioning quality of the radiograph in Figure 14.1. Describe any positioning changes that could be done to improve the film.

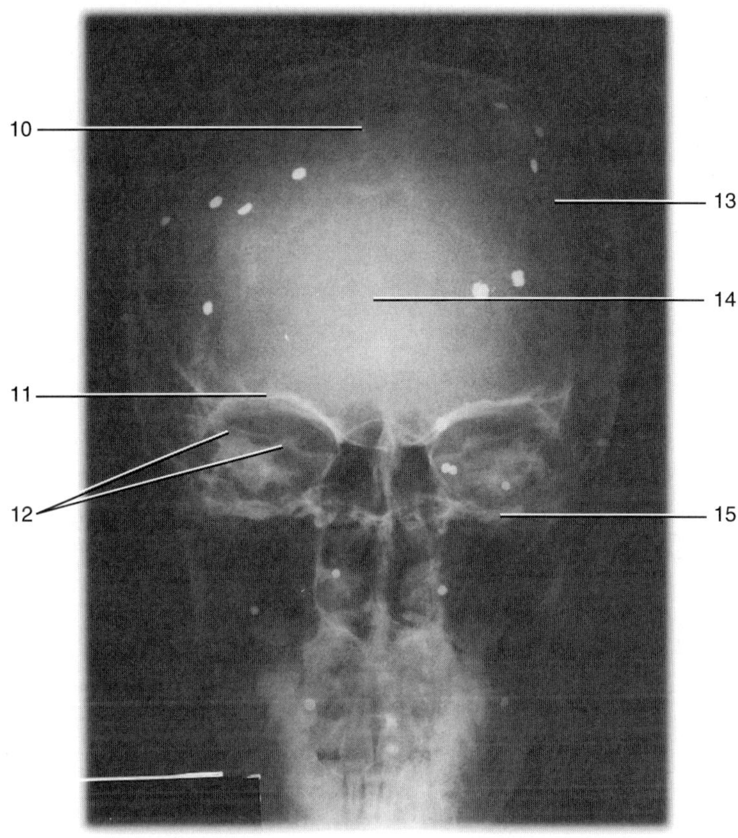

FIGURE 14.2 Radiograph of skull, trauma AP projection.

For questions 10–15, identify the radiographic anatomy on the trauma AP skull projection in Figure 14.2.

10. ____________________

11. ____________________

12. ____________________

13. ____________________

14. ____________________

15. ____________________

16. Analyze the positioning quality of the radiograph in Figure 14.2. Describe any positioning changes that could be done to improve the film.

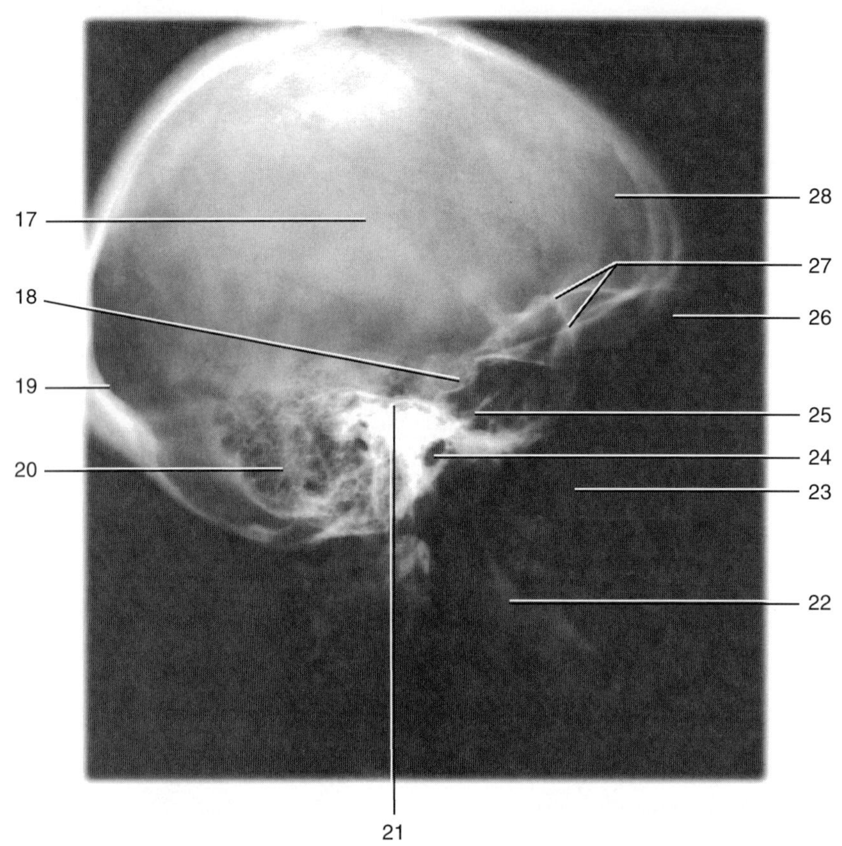

FIGURE 14.3 Radiograph of skull, trauma lateral projection.

For questions 17–28, identify the radiographic anatomy on the trauma lateral skull projection in Figure 14.3.

17. ______________________

18. ______________________

19. ______________________

20. ______________________

21. ______________________

22. ______________________

23. ______________________

24. ______________________

25. ______________________

26. ______________________

27. ______________________

28. ______________________

29. Analyze the positioning quality of the radiograph in Figure 14.3. Describe any positioning changes that could be done to improve the film.

30. High level planning and organization skills are essential skills of a trauma radiographer.

a. true

b. false

31. Which of the following is the reverse of the AP axial (Townes) projection?

a. Arcelin method

b. Grashey method

c. Haas method

d. Schuller method

32. If the infraorbitomeatal line is perpendicular to the film for an AP projection (reverse Caldwell), how many degrees cephalad should the tube be angled?

a. 7

b. 8

c. 15

d. 23

33. Describe some specific examples of nonverbal communication that would assist the radiographer in meeting the needs of a trauma patient.

34. List some organization skills that would help the radiographer to better meet the needs of a trauma patient.

35. Describe some ways that a radiographer could convey a sense of compassion to a trauma patient.

36. Explain how a radiographer assesses the level of consciousness of a trauma patient.

37. Describe how the radiographer would assess whether or not a patient's injuries warrant a trauma skull series.

38. Why is a lateral cervical spine often taken before starting a trauma skull series?

39. When performing a trauma AP axial (Townes) projection, you notice that the patient cannot tuck the chin down and that the orbitomeatal line is approximately 10° from perpendicular. What action would you take to obtain the best possible film?

40. A patient arrives in the emergency room strapped prone to a backboard. As you attempt to start the trauma skull series, you notice that the infraorbitomeatal line is perpendicular to the film. What action would you take to obtain the best possible film for each of the following projections?

a. trauma PA projection

b. trauma PA axial projection

41. When performing a trauma lateral skull on a severely injured patient, you notice that the back of the head is lying directly on the wooden backboard. What action would you take to obtain the best possible film?

Do You Remember?

42. The hilum of the chest contains the heart, trachea, and esophagus.

a. true

b. false

43. The obturator foramen is formed by which bones?

1. pubic
2. ilium
3. ischium

a. 1 and 2

b. 1 and 3

c. 2 and 3

d. 1, 2, and 3

44. For the AP projection of the forearm, the proximal radius and ulna will be partially superimposed unless the:

a. wrist is flexed

b. elbow is flexed

c. hand is pronated

d. hand is supinated

45. Which of the following are demonstrated on an AP projection of the elbow?

1. capitellum

2. medial epicondyle

3. coracoid process

a. 1 and 2

b. 1 and 3

c. 2 and 3

d. 1, 2, and 3

46. When analyzing a radiograph of an open-mouth cervical spine, a radiographer observes that two incisors are superimposed on the dens. Which of the following is true?

a. The patient should tuck her chin toward her chest.

b. The patient should close her mouth slightly.

c. The patient should raise her chin up.

d. The radiographer should apply a caudal tube angle.

47. For a lateral lumbar spine the central ray should be directed:

a. to the level of the iliac crest

b. to the level of the ASIS

c. 1–2 inches above the iliac crest

d. 1 inch below the ASIS

48. On an AP thoracic spine the heel effect may be used to advantage by placing the cathode end of the tube:

a. toward the cervical region

b. toward the lumbar region

c. directly over T6

d. angled toward the lumbar region

49. The petrous pyramid is part of the _____ bone.

a. ethmoid

b. frontal

c. temporal

d. sphenoid

50. The head of a rib articulates with the:

a. sternum

b. tubercle of an adjacent rib

c. transverse process of a vertebra

d. body of a vertebra

51. An AP projection of the femur requires the leg to be internally rotated approximately _____.

a. 5–7°

b. 10–15°

c. 20–25°

d. 45°

STUDY TIP: VISUALIZATION

Trisha: I've noticed you seem so calm about taking this class. Why aren't you panicking like the rest of us?

Pat: Because I know I am going to pass.

Trisha: How can you *know?* How can you have that much self-confidence?

Pat: For years, I have been using a technique called visualization. Each night before I fall asleep, I form a mental picture of the auditorium. I see myself walking across the front while instructor Bob waits for me. I feel him hand me my diploma and shake my hand. I see him smile and hear him congratulate me. I hear my classmates cheering as I walk to my seat. I visualize my goal.

Trisha: Wow, that sounds great. I fall asleep worrying about my next test. Do you have anything I can read about this technique?

- Try visualization for short-term as well as long-term goals.
- Be specific, graphic, and explicit in your visualizations. Use all your imaginary senses of touch, feeling, sight, and hearing.
- Be persistent. The more you visualize a goal, the more it will become part of your positive mental attitude and the greater likelihood it will improve your chances for success.

> Visualization is a powerful mental tool for developing positive attitudes. It has been proven to be successful in reducing stress and helping people focus on their immediate and long-term goals.

SECTION VI

DIGESTIVE SYSTEM and URINARY TRACT

CHAPTER 15

Upper Gastrointestinal Tract

LEARNING OBJECTIVES

At the completion of this chapter, the student should be able to:

1. List and describe the anatomy of the upper gastrointestinal (GI) tract.
2. Explain the physiology of the upper GI tract.
3. Given drawings and radiographs, locate anatomic structures and landmarks of the upper GI tract.
4. Explain the rationale for each projection.
5. Explain the patient preparation required for each examination.
6. Describe the positioning used to visualize anatomic structures of the upper GI tract.
7. List or identify the central ray location and the extent of the field necessary for each projection.
8. Explain the protective measures that should be taken for each examination.
9. Recommend the technical factors for producing an acceptable radiograph for each projection.
10. State the patient instructions for each projection.
11. Given radiographs, evaluate positioning and technical factors.
12. Describe modifications of procedures for atypical or impaired patients to better demonstrate the anatomic area of interest.

Routine and Alternative Positions/Projections

Part	Routine	Alternative
Esophagus	AP/PA	
	Lateral	
	Obliques	
		Lateral neck
Stomach	Preliminary AP	
	PA/AP	
	Oblique	
	Lateral	
Small bowel	PA/AP	
	Ileocecal valve spot filming	

QUESTIONS

Anatomy and Physiology

For questions 1–12, identify the anatomy of the upper digestive system in Figure 15.1.

1. ______________________________

2. ______________________________

3. ______________________________

4. ______________________________

5. ______________________________

6. ______________________________

7. ______________________________

8. ______________________________

9. ______________________________

10. ______________________________

11. ______________________________

12. ______________________________

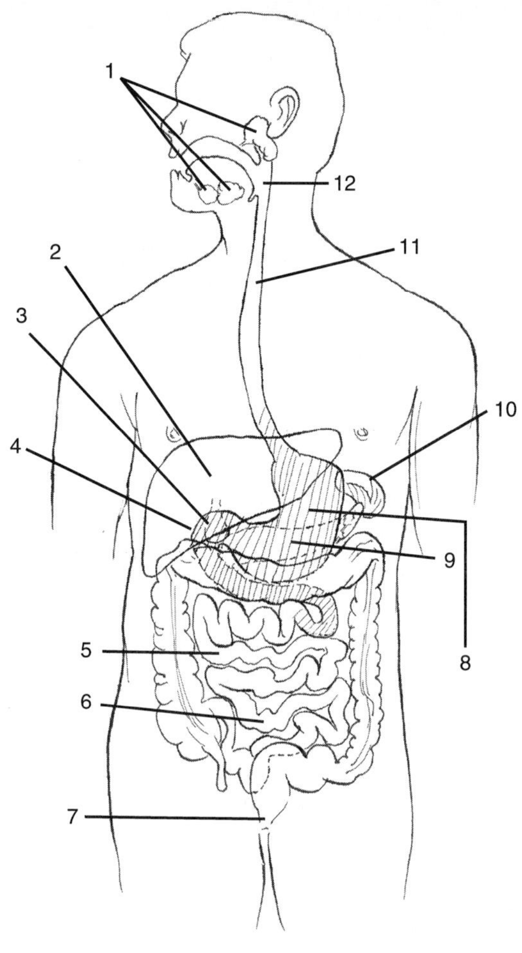

FIGURE 15.1 Diagram of the anatomy of the upper digestive system, anterior view.

For questions 13–20, identify the anatomy of the stomach in Figure 15.2.

13. ______________________________

14. ______________________________

15. ______________________________

16. ______________________________

17. ______________________________

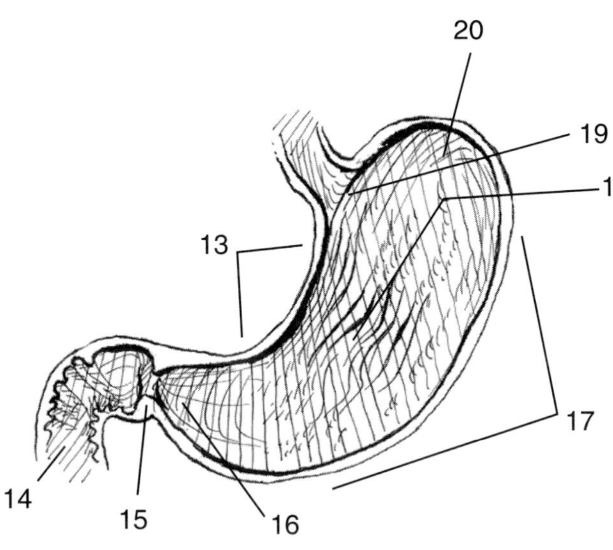

FIGURE 15.2 Diagram of stomach, anterior view.

18. ______________________

19. ______________________

20. ______________________

21. Involuntary, wave-like muscular contractions of the GI tract are called

______________________________________.

22. The final 2–5 inches of the small intestine is called the

______________________________________.

23. Dilated veins in the distal esophagus are known as

______________________________________.

24. Rugae are located in the

______________________________________.

25. The ______________ prevents food from entering the trachea.

26. The circular muscle at the end of the small bowel is called the

______________________________________.

27. Food that has undergone partial chemical and mechanical digestion is called

______________________________________.

28. The stomach normally empties in approximately ______________ hours.

29. It is recommended that patients not use tobacco before upper GI examinations because

______________________________________.

30. Crohn's disease primarily affects the duodenum.

a. true

b. false

31. Difficulty in swallowing is known as:

a. dysphonia

b. dysphagia

c. dyspepsia

d. reflux

32. Which of the following is *not* a salivary gland?

a. parotid

b. sublingual

c. subpharyngeal

d. submaxillary

33. Which of the following are considered part of the upper GI tract?

1. esophagus

2. stomach

3. ileum

a. 1 and 2

b. 1 and 3

c. 2 and 3

d. 1, 2, and 3

34. The narrow, distal portion of the stomach is the:

a. cardiac orifice

b. pylorus

c. greater curvature

d. esophageal sphincter

35. The opening at the lower end of the stomach is the:

a. cardiac orifice

b. pylorus

c. pyloric sphincter

d. esophageal sphincter

36. The stomach is primarily located in the _____ quadrant.

a. left upper

b. right upper

c. right lower

d. left lower

37. The concave right border of the stomach is called the:

a. fundus

b. lesser curvature

c. greater curvature

d. pylorus

38. After leaving the stomach, chyme enters the:

a. pylorus

b. duodenum

c. jejunum

d. ileum

39. Which organ lies within the C-loop of the duodenum?

a. spleen

b. liver

c. gallbladder

d. pancreas

40. The middle portion of the small intestine is the:

a. pylorus

b. fundus

c. jejunum

d. ileum

41. The distal portion of the small intestine that joins with the colon is the:

a. pylorus

b. ileum

c. jejunum

d. duodenum

42. The small, finger-like projections in the small intestine that vastly increase its absorptive surface area are known as:

a. plicae

b. haustra

c. rugae

d. villi

43. The process of swallowing is known as:

a. mastication

b. deglutition

c. defecation

d. salivation

44. Which structure is part of both the respiratory and digestive tracts?

a. mouth

b. larynx

c. esophagus

d. pharynx

45. Which of the following organs are located primarily in the left upper quadrant of the abdomen?

1. stomach

2. spleen

3. liver

a. 1 and 2

b. 1 and 3

c. 2 and 3

d. 1, 2, and 3

46. Compared to a sthenic patient, the *asthenic* body type will have a stomach located:

a. lower and more medial

b. lower and more lateral

c. higher and more medial

d. higher and more lateral

Radiographic Procedures, Analysis, and Critical Thinking

For questions 47–51, identify the radiographic anatomy of the esophagus and associated structures in Figure 15.3.

47. ______________________

48. ______________________

49. ______________________

50. ______________________

51. ______________________

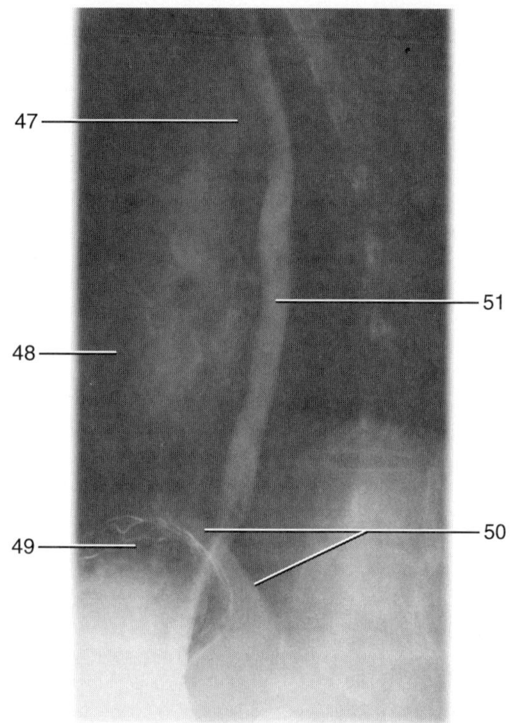

FIGURE 15.3 Radiograph of esophagus, oblique projection.

For questions 52–58, identify the radiographic anatomy of the oblique stomach in Figure 15.4A.

52. ______________________

53. ______________________

54. ______________________

55. ______________________

56. ______________________

57. ______________________

58. ______________________

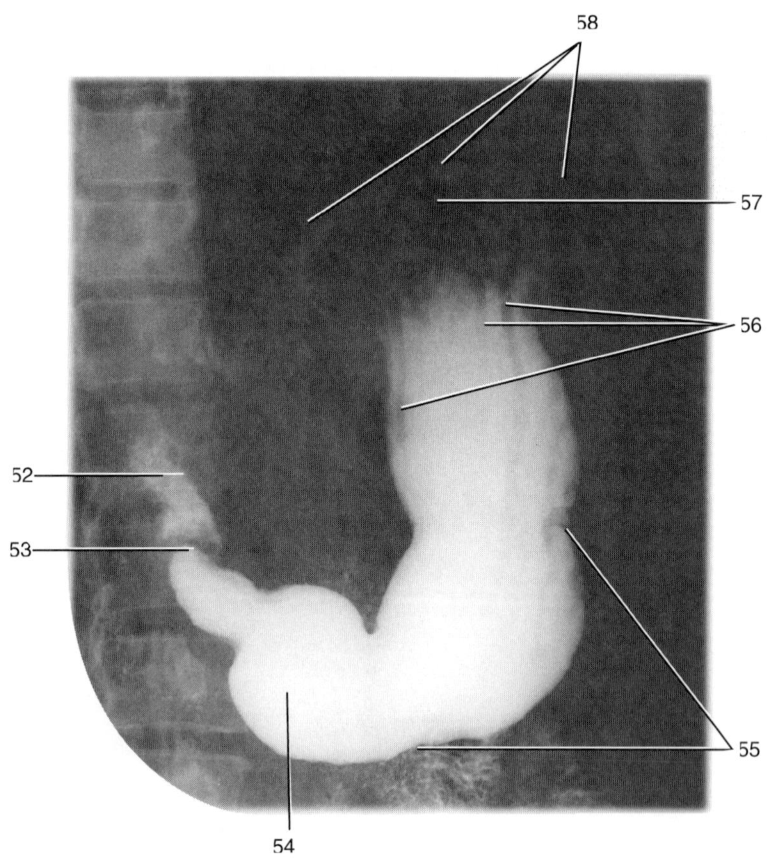

FIGURE 15.4A Radiograph of stomach, oblique projection, correct positioning.

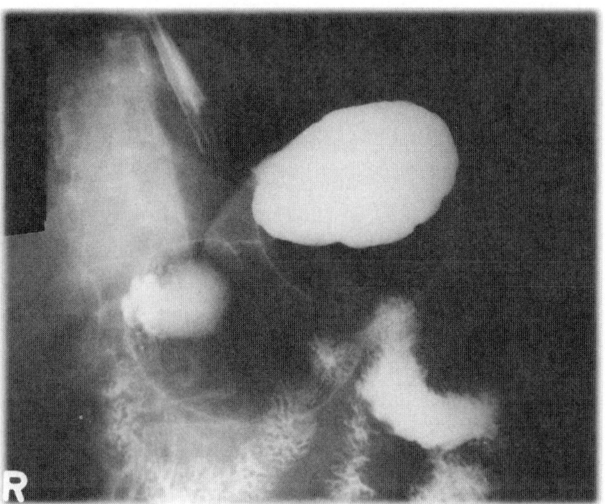

FIGURE 15.4B Radiograph of stomach, oblique projection, incorrect positioning.

59. Compare the positioning quality of the correctly positioned radiograph in Figure 15.4A with that in Figure 15.4B. Describe the positioning error, explain what caused it, and give the step(s) necessary to correct the problem.

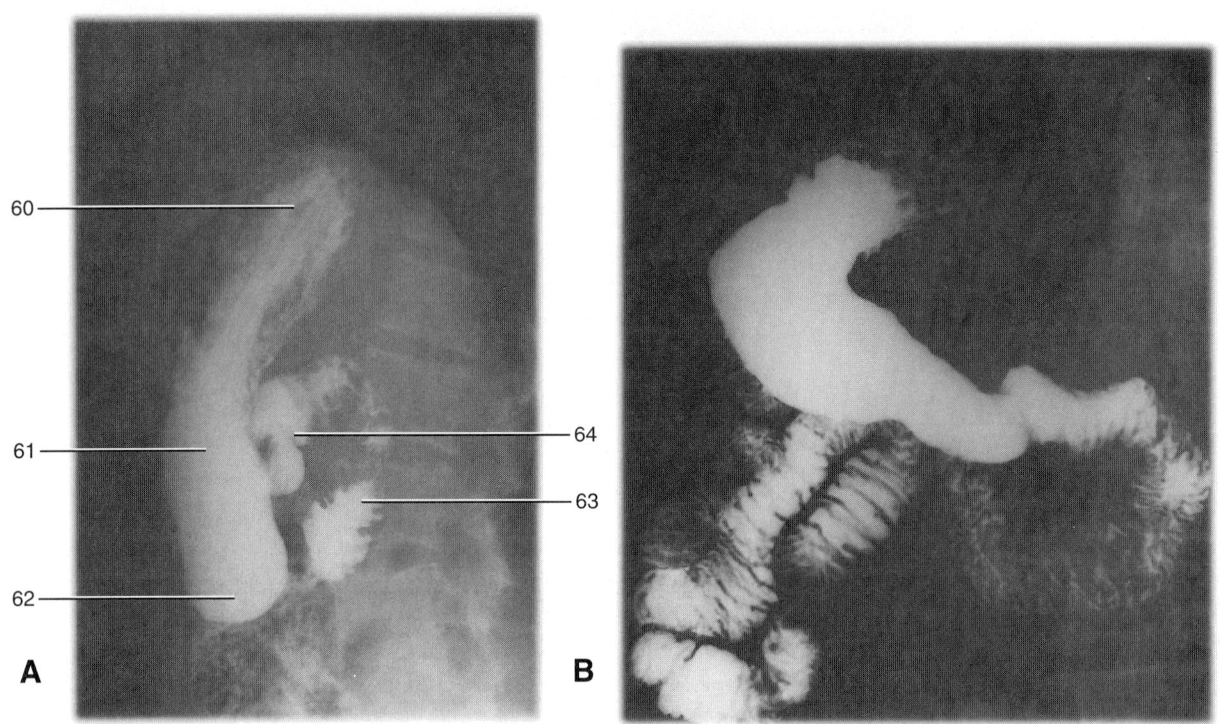

FIGURE 15.5 Radiograph of stomach, lateral projection, (A) correct positioning and (B) incorrect positioning.

For questions 60–64, identify the radiographic anatomy of the lateral stomach in Figure 15.5A.

60. ______________________

61. ______________________

62. ______________________

63. ______________________

64. ______________________

65. Compare the positioning quality of the correctly positioned radiograph in Figure 15.5A with that in Figure 15.5B. Describe the positioning error, explain what caused it, and give the step(s) necessary to correct the problem.

For questions 66–69, identify the radiographic anatomy of the small bowel in Figure 15.6.

66. ____________________

67. ____________________

68. ____________________

69. ____________________

70. Injection of barium through a catheter into the small intestine is called

____________________________.

71. The film size for esophagus examinations is ____________ inches.

72. The stomach of a hypersthenic patient is elongated, lower, and more midline in position.

a. true

b. false

73. For the RAO stomach, the central ray enters on the elevated side.

a. true

b. false

74. Esophagus films are normally taken at 70–75 kVp to produce short scale contrast.

a. true

b. false

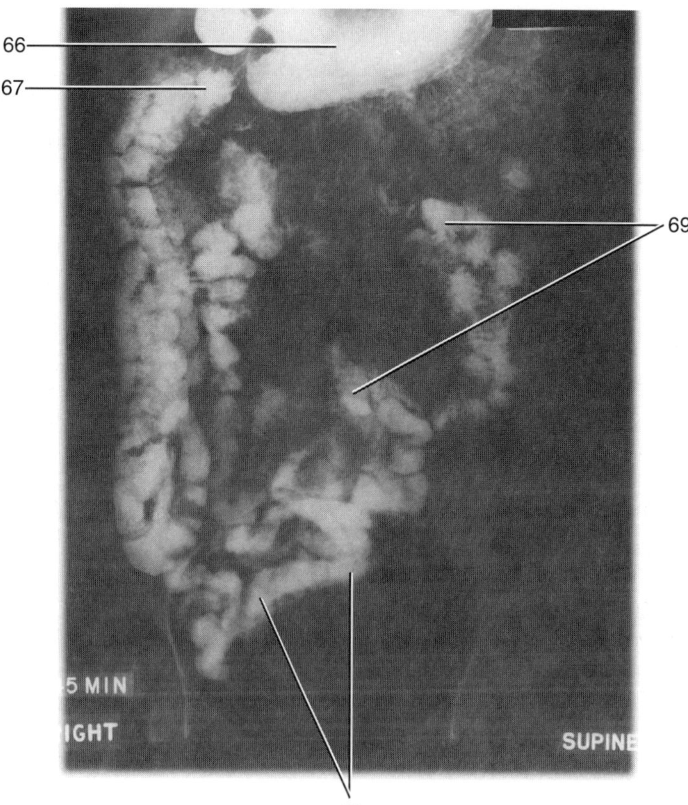

FIGURE 15.6 Radiograph of small bowel, AP projection.

75. Soft tissue films of the neck are taken at lower kVp compared to esophagus films.

a. true

b. false

76. The normal kVp range for small bowel examinations using barium is 90–100.

a. true

b. false

77. Which of the following best describes the Valsalva maneuver?

a. Hold breath on deep expiration.

b. Take a deep breath and hold it.

c. Bend over and touch one's toes while holding breath.

d. Take a deep breath and strain down.

78. Double-contrast examinations are primarily performed because they:

a. demonstrate better mucosal detail

b. are better tolerated by the patient

c. require fewer films

d. are less hazardous if perforation is present

79. The most common patient preparation for an upper GI series is:

a. only clear fluids 8 hours before the examination

b. NPO after midnight

c. enemas in the morning until clear

d. low residue diet for 2 days before the examination

80. Which of the following is true regarding barium sulfate?

a. relatively nontoxic

b. absorbed by the small intestine

c. frequently causes minor allergic reactions such as itching and hives

d. contains iodine

81. The Valsalva maneuver is performed to demonstrate small:

a. cancers

b. hiatal hernias

c. ulcers

d. diverticula

82. A patient with a suspected perforated ulcer would likely require an upper GI examination with:

a. thin barium

b. thick barium

c. iodinated water-soluble contrast

d. air contrast

83. Gonadal shielding should be used during upper GI examinations:

1. if the shield will not obscure the anatomy of interest
2. only if the radiologist requests it
3. if the patient has a reasonable likelihood of reproducing

a. 1 and 2

b. 1 and 3

c. 2 and 3

d. 1, 2, and 3

84. The kVp range for upper GI examinations using barium sulfate is:

a. 60–69

b. 70–79

c. 80–89

d. over 90

85. Obliques of the esophagus are taken with the patient rotated _____.

a. 15°

b. 30°

c. 40°

d. 60°

86. For esophagus films, the central ray is placed at the level of:

a. T2

b. T4

c. T6

d. T10

87. Which of the following is *not* normally part of the department protocol for an esophagram?

a. PA

b. LAO

c. lateral

d. LPO

88. Which of the following positioning modifications apply to filming of the stomach on a hypersthenic patient?

1. cassette placed crosswise

2. larger cassette size

3. central ray placed higher

a. 1 and 2

b. 1 and 3

c. 2 and 3

d. 1, 2, and 3

89. The central ray for a lateral stomach on an asthenic patient is placed at the level of:

a. T11

b. T12

c. L1

d. L3

90. When the patient is placed _____, the fundus of the stomach is filled with barium.

a. RAO

b. LPO

c. left lateral

d. prone

91. Which of the following are true for positioning of the lateral stomach on an average size patient?

1. Central ray enters at the mid-coronal plane.

2. Central ray enters at level of L1.

3. Patient is placed in right lateral position.

a. 1 and 2

b. 1 and 3

c. 2 and 3

d. 1, 2, and 3

92. For the LPO position of the stomach on a hypersthenic patient, the central ray enters at the level of:

a. T11–T12

b. L1

c. L3

d. L4

93. A mass lying directly behind the stomach would best be demonstrated on which projection?

a. lateral

b. AP

c. PA

d. LPO

94. Which of the following best demonstrates the duodenal bulb in hypersthenic patients?

a. AP/PA

b. RAO

c. lateral

d. LPO

95. During a double-contrast GI series, air is found in the fundus portion of the stomach when the patient is placed into which positions?

1. recumbent LPO

2. prone

3. recumbent RAO

a. 1 and 2

b. 1 and 3

c. 2 and 3

d. 1, 2, and 3

96. Which of the following best demonstrates the pylorus and duodenal bulb on a sthenic-type patient?

a. supine PA

b. erect PA

c. RAO

d. right lateral

97. Which of the following is *least* likely to be demonstrated 10 minutes after oral ingestion of barium?

a. duodenum

b. fundus

c. pylorus

d. ileum

98. A small bowel series is finished when barium reaches the:

a. ascending colon

b. cecum

c. jejunum

d. ileum

99. Timing for a small bowel series begins when:

a. the patient enters the room

b. fluoroscopy begins

c. the first radiograph is taken

d. the patient first ingests the barium

100. Film size and placement for radiographs of the small bowel are:

a. 11 x 14 inch crosswise

b. 11 x 14 inch lengthwise

c. 14 x 17 inch crosswise

d. 14 x 17 inch lengthwise

101. If radiographic studies of both the upper and lower GI tracts are ordered, which should be done first? Why should the two studies *not* be combined?

102. Describe how you would modify your positioning of a small bowel series to accommodate an obese patient.

103. A compression device and spot filming are sometimes used to examine the terminal ileum. Describe the value of using such techniques.

104. What patient symptoms would lead you to recommend to the radiologist to substitute a water-soluble contrast medium in place of barium?

Do You Remember?

105. The forehead and nose should be touching the table for a modified parietoacanthial (modified Waters) projection for the orbits.

a. true

b. false

106. Which position of the abdomen best demonstrates air/fluid levels in the intestine or free air in the abdomen?

a. supine

b. prone

c. upright

d. lateral

107. The central ray for a PA projection of the mandible exits at the:

a. lips

b. glabella

c. nasion

d. acanthion

108. Which of the following lines the wall of the abdominopelvic cavity?

a. greater omentum

b. lesser omentum

c. visceral peritoneum

d. parietal peritoneum

109. The articulations between the sacrum and the ilia open obliquely at an angle of _____.

a. 5–10°

b. 15–30°

c. 35–45°

d. 55–70°

110. On an AP axial (Townes) projection, what structure is visualized inside the foramen magnum?

a. cribiform plate

b. dorsum sellae

c. crista galli

d. sella turcica

111. The joint space of the knee is located:

a. 1 cm superior to the tibial tuberosity

b. at the midpoint of the patella

c. 1 cm inferior to the patellar apex

d. 1 cm inferior to the patellar base

112. Where should the central ray exit for a transthoracic shoulder?

a. surgical neck of the injured arm

b. midshaft of the injured arm

c. surgical neck of the unaffected arm

d. midshaft of the unaffected arm

113. The zygapophyseal articulations of the thoracic spine are best demonstrated using a patient in angle of _____.

a. 20°

b. 45°

c. 70°

d. 90°

114. For trauma cervical spine examinations, which of the following must be taken before moving the patient?

a. AP

b. both obliques

c. odontoid

d. lateral

STUDY TIP: MULTIPLE CHOICE TESTS

Maria: I think I aced that test—it was all multiple choice.

Kathy: I really bombed it even though I knew all the material. As soon as I start reading the choices, I get all confused even when I think I know the answer. Sometimes it looks like there is more than one choice and other times my answer is not there at all. The teacher makes them that way on purpose—to confuse us.

Maria: Maybe some teachers, but not instructor Bob. Maybe you need to take a different approach to the questions, like I do.

Kathy: You mean you do something besides just guess? Let's go have a bagel and give me some tips.

- Try answering each question without looking at the answers.
- The phrases "all of the above" or "none of the above" are frequently the correct response and they should be looked at very carefully.
- Statements that contain an absolute word such as always, all, every, or none are usually incorrect answers.
- If you do not know the answer but know something about the question, eliminate any that are obviously incorrect and guess at the remaining choices.
- Look for similarities in the options. Exact opposite distracters included in the same question such as up or down, right or left, and anterior and posterior often give clues that one must be the correct choice.
- If you absolutely do not have a clue guess "c". Teachers tend to choose answers in the center. Better yet, study the pattern of your instructors as the term progresses to find out what answer they most often pick. Be warned that some teachers use test banks, which tend to randomize the answers.

Multiple choice test-taking is an essential skill that should be learned early in the program.

CHAPTER 16

Lower Gastrointestinal Tract

LEARNING OBJECTIVES

At the completion of this chapter, the student should be able to:

1. List and describe the anatomy of the large intestine.
2. Explain the physiology of the lower digestive tract.
3. Given drawings and radiographs, locate anatomic structures of the lower digestive tract.
4. Explain the rationale for each projection.
5. Explain the patient preparation required for each examination.
6. Describe the positioning used to visualize anatomic structures in the large intestine.
7. List or identify the central ray location and identify the extent of the field necessary for each projection.
8. Recommend the technical factors for producing an acceptable radiograph for each projection.
9. State the patient instructions for each projection.
10. Given radiographs, evaluate positioning and technical factors.
11. Describe modifications of procedures for atypical or impaired patients to better demonstrate the anatomic area of interest.

Routine and Alternative Positions/Projections

Part	Routine	Alternative
Large intestine	PA/AP	
	Axial PA/AP	
	Obliques	
	Lateral decubitus	
	Lateral rectum	
		Oblique axial
		Axial rectosigmoid (Chassard-Lapine)
		Defecogram

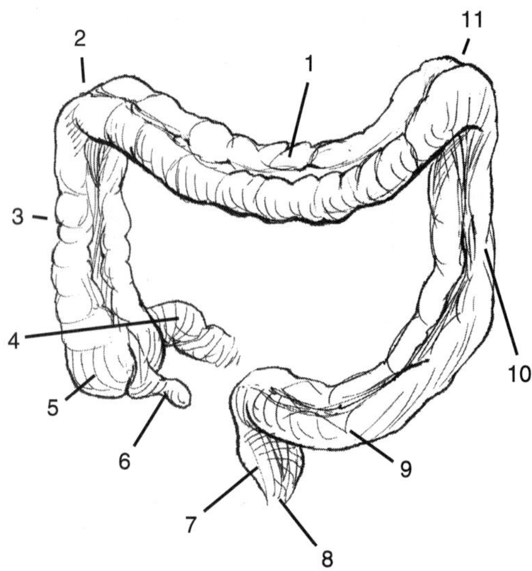

FIGURE 16.1 Diagram of large intestine, anterior view.

QUESTIONS

Anatomy and Physiology

For questions 1–11, identify the anatomy of the large intestine in Figure 16.1.

1. ______________________
2. ______________________
3. ______________________
4. ______________________
5. ______________________
6. ______________________
7. ______________________
8. ______________________
9. ______________________
10. ______________________
11. ______________________

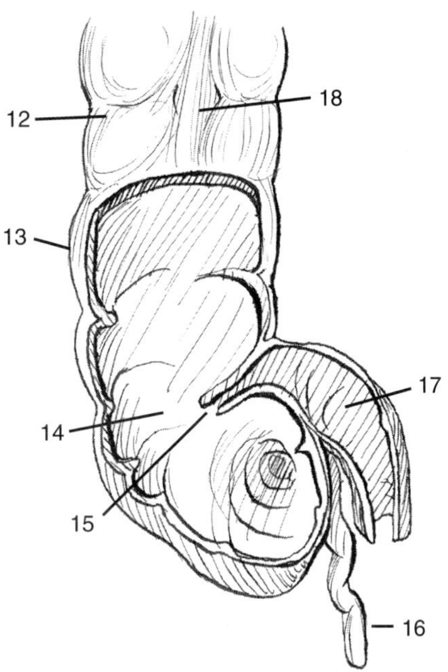

FIGURE 16.2 Diagram of ileocecal region, anterior view.

For questions 12–18, identify the anatomy of the ileocecal region in Figure 16.2.

12. ____________________

13. ____________________

14. ____________________

15. ____________________

16. ____________________

17. ____________________

18. ____________________

19. The bottom portion of the rectum curves ______________ to the anal opening.

20. The enlarged, dilated portion of the rectum is called the

____.

21. Abnormal enlargement and dilation of the veins in the rectal plexus is known as

____.

22. The vermiform process is also called the

____.

23. One important function of the large intestine is to synthesize vitamin C.

a. true

b. false

24. Pouch-like herniations of the mucosal wall of the large intestine are called diverticula.

a. true

b. false

25. Digestive matter leaving the ileum would first enter the:

a. cecum

b. rectum

c. sigmoid

d. appendix

26. Which portion of the large intestine lies between the colic flexures?

a. ascending colon

b. descending colon

c. sigmoid colon

d. transverse colon

27. The junction of the large and small intestine is called the:

a. ileocecal valve

b. ileal valve

c. sigmoid colon

d. appendix

28. The pouch-like, blind end portion of the colon is the:

a. sigmoid colon

b. rectum

c. cecum

d. appendix

29. One of the major functions of the large intestine is to:

a. secrete digestive enzymes

b. reabsorb water

c. regulate the release of bile

d. absorb vitamins and minerals

30. Folds in the mucosal wall that give the large intestine its characteristic appearance are:

a. epiploic appendages

b. taeniae coli

c. haustra

d. plicae circularis

31. An intestinal obstruction caused by the twisting of a loop of bowel is called a/an:

a. intussusception

b. volvulus

c. hiatal hernia

d. diverticulosis

32. McBurney's point is useful for locating the position of the:

a. ileocecal valve

b. proximal rectum

c. rectosigmoid junction

d. appendix

33. The junction of the transverse colon and the descending colon is the:

a. splenic flexure

b. hepatic flexure

c. sigmoid colon

d. cecum

34. Which part of the large intestine normally lies most superiorly?

a. left colic flexure

b. sigmoid colon

c. right colic flexure

d. transverse colon

35. During an enema, barium leaving the ascending colon would next enter the:

a. appendix

b. cecum

c. left colic flexure

d. right colic flexure

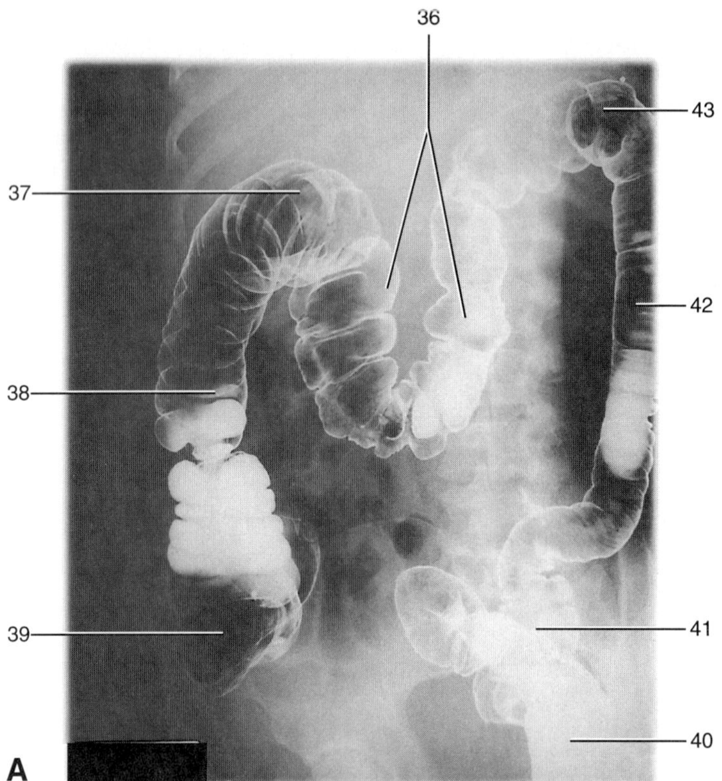

FIGURE 16.3A Radiograph of large intestine, oblique projection, correct positioning.

Radiographic Procedures, Analysis, and Critical Thinking

For questions 36–43, identify the radiographic anatomy of the oblique large intestine in Figure 16.3(A).

36. ____________________ **40.** ____________________

37. ____________________ **41.** ____________________

38. ____________________ **42.** ____________________

39. ____________________ **43.** ____________________

44. Can you determine the position of the patient by looking at the radiographic anatomy and the film markers on Figure 16.3? Why or why not?

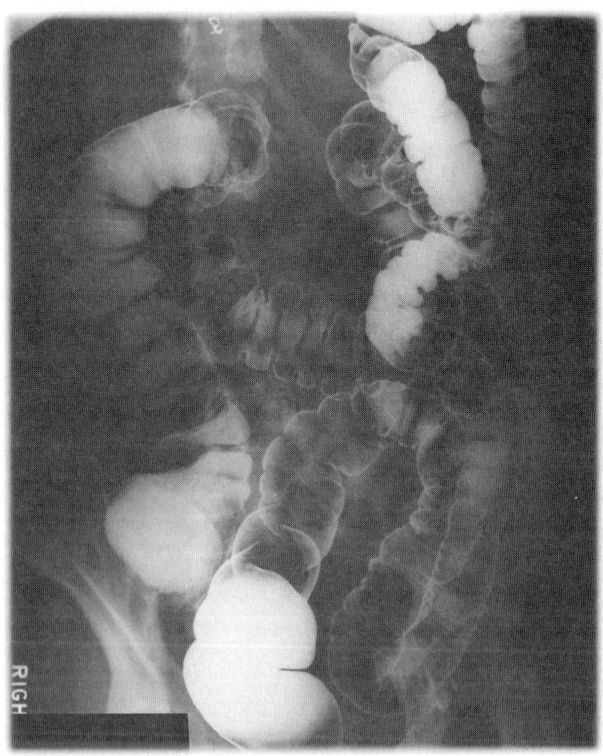

FIGURE 16.3B Radiograph of large intestine, oblique projection, incorrect positioning.

45. Compare the positioning quality of the correctly positioned radiograph in Figure 16.3A with that in Figure 16.3B. Describe the positioning error, explain what caused it, and give the step(s) necessary to correct the problem.

For questions 46–49, identify the radiographic anatomy of the lateral rectum in Figure 16.4.

46. ______________________

47. ______________________

48. ______________________

49. ______________________

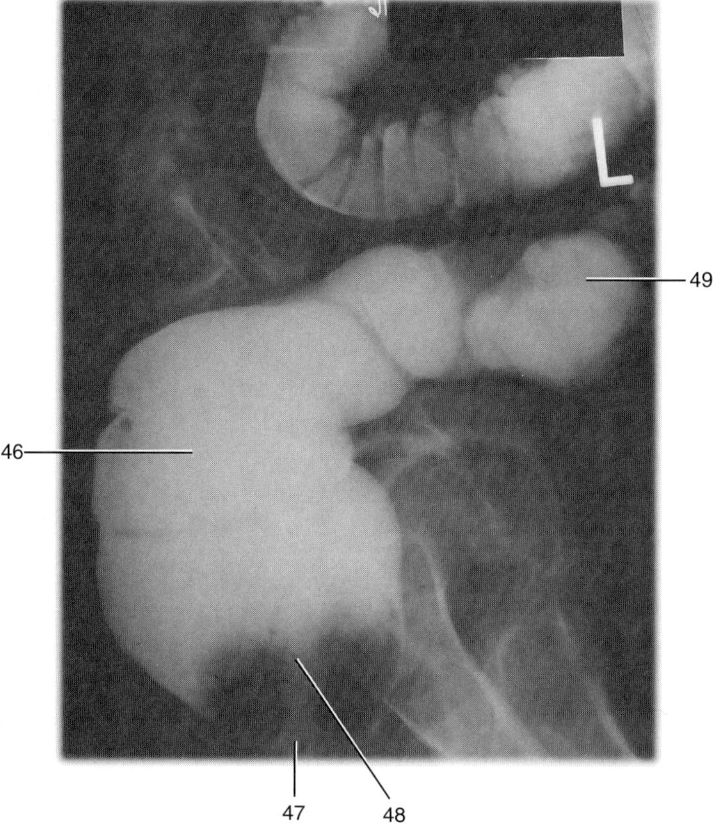

FIGURE 16.4 Radiograph of rectum, lateral projection.

For questions 50–53, identify the radiographic anatomy of the AP axial oblique large intestine in Figure 16.5.

50. ______________________

51. ______________________

52. ______________________

53. ______________________

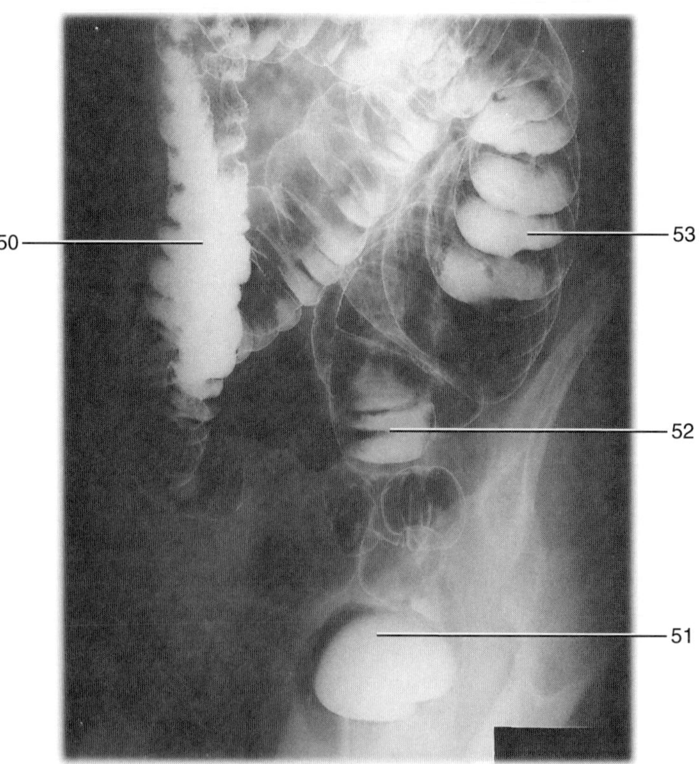

FIGURE 16.5 Radiograph of large intestine, AP axial oblique projection.

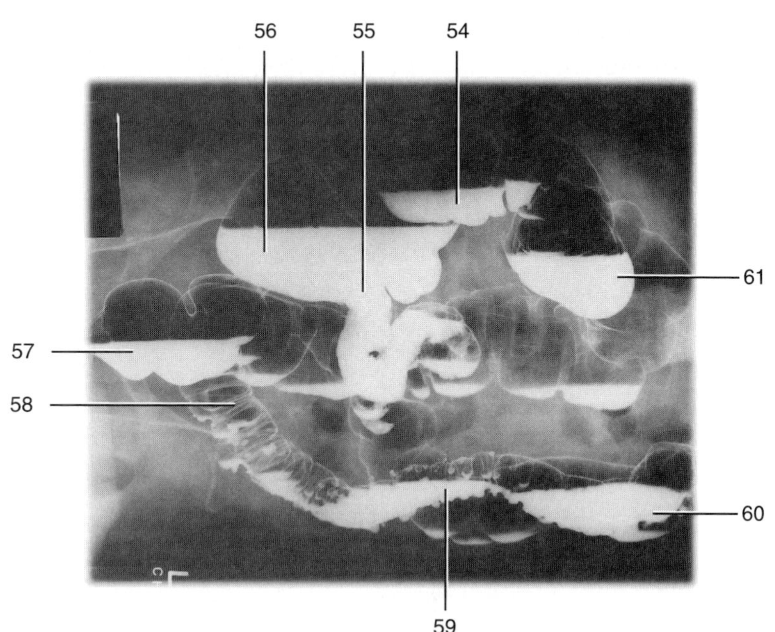

FIGURE 16.6 Radiograph of large intestine, lateral decubitus projection.

For questions 54–61, identify the radiographic anatomy of the decubitus large intestine in Figure 16.6.

54. ____________________

55. ____________________

56. ____________________

57. ____________________

58. ____________________

59. ____________________

60. ____________________

61. ____________________

62. Can you determine the position of the patient by looking at the radiographic anatomy and the film markers on Figure 16.6? Why or why not?

63. The IV pole holding the barium enema bag should be placed approximately ___________ inches above the table.

64. The enema tip should be inserted approximately ______________ inches into the rectum.

65. The inflation balloon on the retention tip should be fully inflated before the radiologist enters the room.

a. true

b. false

66. Shielding of the male gonads is not practical during barium enema fluoroscopy.

a. true

b. false

67. Barium sulfate forms a suspension in water.

a. true

b. false

68. The inflated balloon on the retention tip is normally kept in place in the patient while overhead films are taken.

a. true

b. false

69. The AP projection of the large intestine is taken on expiration.

a. true

b. false

For questions 70–74 identify the radiographic anatomy of the AP large intestine in Figure 16.7A.

70. Hepatic flexure

a. 1

b. 2

c. 4

d. 8

71. Ascending colon

a. 3

b. 4

c. 6

d. 7

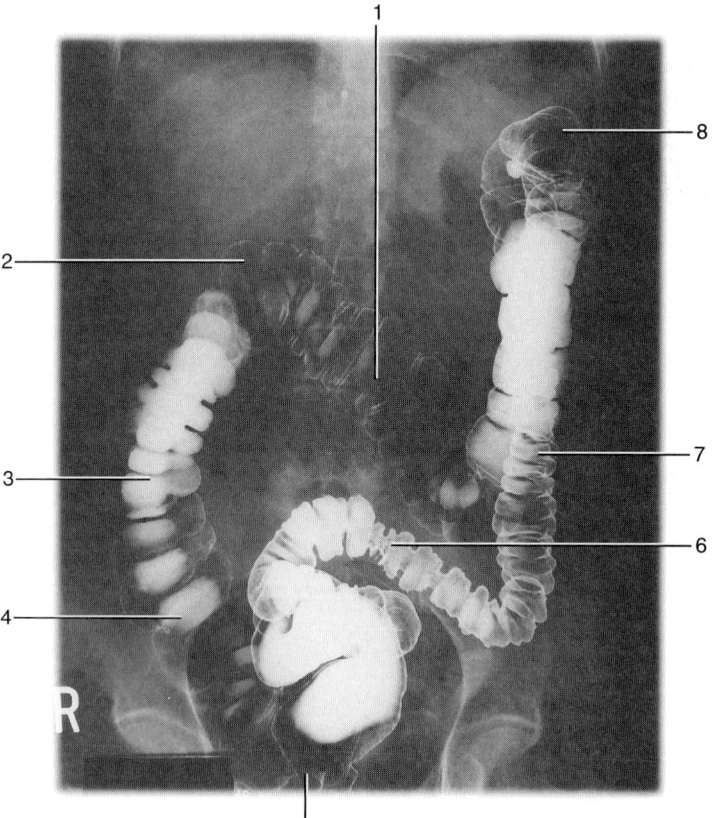

FIGURE 16.7A Radiograph of large intestine, AP projection, correct positioning.

72. Sigmoid colon

a. 4

b. 5

c. 6

d. 7

73. Transverse colon

a. 1

b. 2

c. 3

d. 8

74. Cecum

a. 3

b. 4

c. 5

d. 6

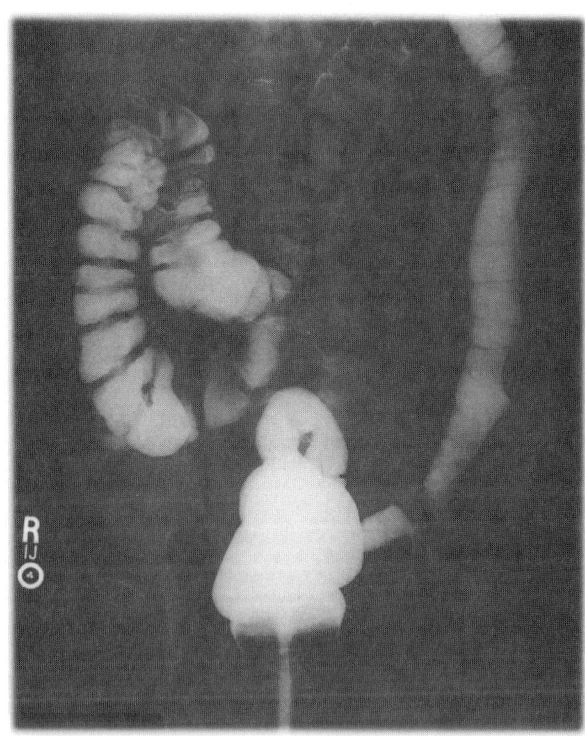

FIGURE 16.7B Radiograph of large intestine, AP projection, incorrect positioning.

75. Compare the positioning quality of the correctly positioned radiograph in Figure 16.7A with that in Figure 16.7B. Describe the positioning error, explain what caused it, and give the step(s) necessary to correct the problem.

76. Preparation for a barium enema examination would *least* likely include:

a. cleansing enemas for 2–3 days before the examination

b. laxatives 1–2 days before the examination

c. NPO after midnight

d. low residue diet for 1–2 days before the examination

77. A radiographer analyzing a barium enema radiograph notices the contrast medium has entered the terminal ileum. Which of the following is true?

a. The barium flow was stopped too soon.

b. The barium flow was left on too long.

c. The patient was unable to retain the barium.

d. Barium in the terminal ileum is a normal part of a barium enema.

78. Which of the following is a contraindication for the use of a water-soluble contrast medium for an enema?

a. the presence of a cancer

b. dehydration of the patient

c. intestinal bleeding

d. obstruction

79. A water-soluble contrast medium would likely be used for an enema in place of barium if:

a. the patient had diverticula

b. the patient had a history of allergy to barium

c. a perforation of the large intestine was suspected

d. all of the above

80. Barium is contraindicated for examinations of the large intestine when:

a. the patient has had recent colon surgery

b. cancer is suspected

c. polyps are suspected

d. colitis is suspected

81. During insertion of the enema tip, the patient is placed in the _____ position.

a. Sims'

b. Trendelenberg

c. Fowler's

d. prone

82. The double-contrast enema is particularly useful in demonstrating:

a. air/fluid levels

b. diverticuli

c. polyps

d. small cancers

83. The kVp range for single contrast barium enema films is _____ .

a. 80–90

b. 90–100

c. 100–125

d. 125–140

84. The kVp range for double-contrast enema films is _____.

a. 80–90

b. 90–100

c. 100–125

d. 125–140

85. For the AP projection of the large intestine, the central ray enters:

a. at the ASIS

b. at the iliac crest

c. at the lower margin of the ribs

d. 1–2 inches above the iliac crest

86. The RAO position of the colon best demonstrates the:

a. transverse colon

b. ileocecal valve

c. splenic flexure

d. hepatic flexure

87. The Chassard-Lapine position is taken primarily to demonstrate abnormalities of the:

a. rectum

b. rectosigmoid junction

c. right colic flexure

d. appendix

88. Which of the following positions *best* demonstrates the left colic flexure?

a. supine

b. prone

c. RPO

d. LPO

89. For obliques of the large intestine, the patient is rotated _____ .

a. 10–15°

b. 20–25°

c. 35–45°

d. 50–60°

90. Which of the following best demonstrates the rectum?

a. AP

b. lateral

c. RAO

d. RPO

91. For which barium enema position/projection is the central ray placed at the level of the ASIS and centered to the midaxillary plane?

a. lateral rectum

b. sigmoid colon

c. AP/PA

d. oblique

92. For the PA oblique axial projection of the colon, the body is rotated _____ .

a. 15°

b. 25 °

c. 35°

d. 45°

93. For the PA oblique axial projection of the colon, the tube is angled:

a. 30° cephalic

b. 30° caudal

c. 45° cephalic

d. 45° caudal

94. The AP axial oblique projection of the colon best demonstrates the:

a. rectosigmoid region

b. hepatic flexure

c. appendix

d. splenic flexure

95. For the AP axial oblique projection of the colon, the central ray passes:

a. through the pubic bone

b. just above the iliac crest

c. through the ASIS

d. 1–2 inches below the ASIS

96. On an air-contrast colon study, air is seen mostly filling the ascending colon with barium mostly filling the descending colon. This projection is most likely a:

a. PA

b. left lateral decubitus

c. lateral

d. right lateral decubitus

97. On an asthenic patient with an exceptionally long abdomen, it is not always possible to include the entire large intestine on a single 14 x 17 inch film placed lengthwise. Describe how positioning should be adapted to accommodate this patient.

Do You Remember?

98. If fluid is suspected in the right lung of a patient who cannot be placed upright, the right lateral decubitus chest should be performed.

a. true

b. false

99. On a Caldwell PA projection, the petrous ridges should completely fill the orbits.

a. true

b. false

100. "Scotty dogs" are best visualized in the _____ projection of the _____ spine.

a. AP, lumbar

b. oblique, lumbar

c. oblique, cervical

d. lateral, thoracic

101. The opening between the stomach and the duodenum is called the:

a. cardiac sphincter

b. duodenal sphincter

c. pyloric sphincter

d. ampulla of Vater

102. The sella turcica is a process on which bone?

a. temporal

b. parietal

c. ethmoid

d. sphenoid

103. The central ray for an RAO stomach should be placed at the level of:

a. T8

b. T10

c. L1

d. L4

104. Which two bones are separated by the lamdoidal suture?

a. temporal and occipital

b. parietal and occipital

c. the right and left parietal bones

d. temporal and parietal

105. The bony process on the skull that lies just posterior and inferior to the external auditory meatus is the:

a. styloid process

b. condyloid process

c. mastoid process

d. occipital condyle

106. Which of the following is *not* a paranasal sinus?

a. ethmoid

b. sphenoid

c. frontal

d. parietal

107. Patients undergoing an upper GI series should be NPO for approximately ____ hours before the examination.

a. 2–3

b. 5

c. 8–10

d. 24

STUDY TIP: CLASSROOM BEHAVIOR

While instructor Bob is teaching stomach positioning, Maria and Kathy are passing notes back and forth and seem to be enjoying some good jokes.

Instructor Bob:	Kathy, would you and Maria like to share your notes and some jokes with the class?
Kathy and Maria (in chorus):	No sir.
Instructor Bob:	Are you sure? It sounds like you have some interesting things to share.
Kathy:	Yes sir, we're sure. I'm really bored with positioning. I hate this subject.
Instructor Bob:	Hate it or not, this is my favorite subject and you have to learn it. Let's continue with the prep for the GI series ....

Certain behavior is inappropriate in any class, regardless of teacher or subject. Participating in such behavior will give the teacher the perception that you are not serious about learning.

- Do not engage in personal conversations during class. In particular, never laugh or giggle with a classmate while the teacher is lecturing.
- Do not read in class, in particular the newspaper.
- Never study for another teacher's examination during class.
- Never criticize a teacher's favorite subject.
- Do not attack an instructor's method of teaching or testing.
- Do not come to class without the necessary text and notes. Take notes and pretend to be serious about the subject at hand, even if you are uninterested.

> Your goal should be to be perceived as a serious, interested student by the teacher. Be sure your classroom behavior reflects this seriousness.

CHAPTER 17

Hepatobiliary System

LEARNING OBJECTIVES

At the completion of this chapter, the student should be able to:

1. List and describe the basic anatomic components of the hepatobiliary system.
2. Given drawings and radiographs, locate anatomic structures and landmarks.
3. Describe the expected location of the gallbladder for each of the four body habitus classifications.
4. Describe the physiology of the hepatobiliary system, including its role in digestion and the production of bile.
5. List the most common clinical indications for imaging the hepatobiliary system.
6. Explain why it is necessary to use radiographic contrast media to image the hepatobiliary system.
7. Describe patient preparation for each hepatobiliary imaging procedure for both typical and atypical patients, including the pediatric, geriatric and diabetic patient.
8. Describe the positioning used for an oral cholecystogram (OCG).
9. List or identify the central ray location and identify the extent of field necessary for each projection.
10. Explain the protective measures appropriate for each examination.
11. Recommend the technical factors for producing an acceptable radiograph for each routine OCG projection.
12. State the instructions given to the patient before and during the OCG procedure.
13. Explain the rationale for each of the following:
    a. Nonfat or low-fat diet 24 hours before an OCG
    b. Oral contrast administration 10–12 hours before an OCG
    c. Fat meal after contrast-filled radiographs of the hepatobiliary system
    d. Radiographs of the hepatobiliary system after a fat meal
    e. Upright and decubitus projections of the gallbladder
14. Given radiographs, evaluate positioning and technical factors.
15. State the purpose of postoperative cholangiogram.
16. State the goal of an endoscopic retrograde cholangiopancreatography (ERCP).
17. Describe the procedure for percutaneous transhepatic cholangiography (PTC).

Oral Cholecystogram (OCG) Routine Positions/Projections

Part	Routine
Gallbladder	(Oralcholecystogram) PA scout
	LAO
	Right lateral decubitus
	Upright PA

QUESTIONS

Anatomy and Physiology

For questions 1–13, identify the anatomy of the hepatobiliary system in Figure 17.1.

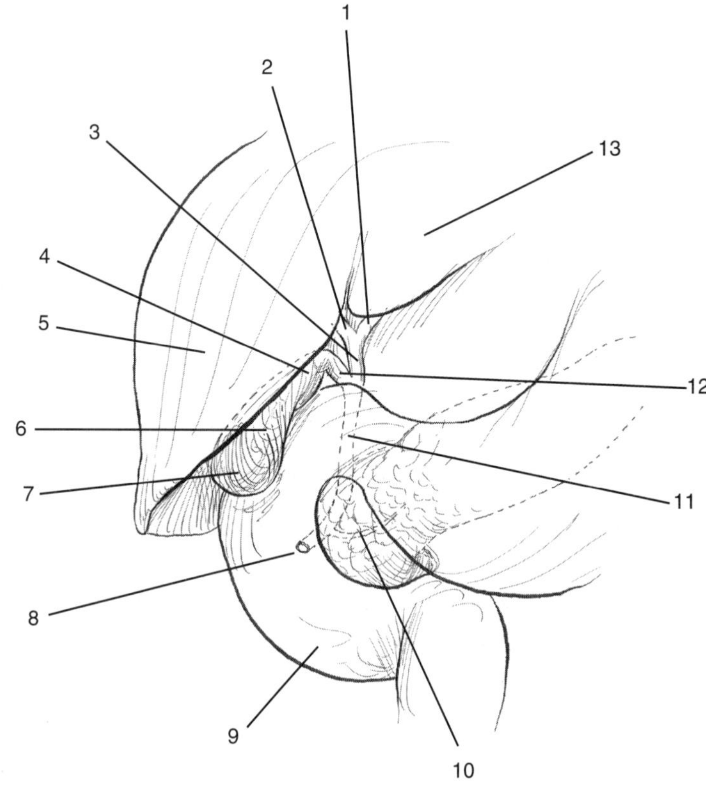

FIGURE 17.1 Diagram of hepatobiliary system, anterior view.

1. ____________________
2. ____________________
3. ____________________
4. ____________________
5. ____________________
6. ____________________
7. ____________________
8. ____________________
9. ____________________
10. ____________________
11. ____________________
12. ____________________
13. ____________________

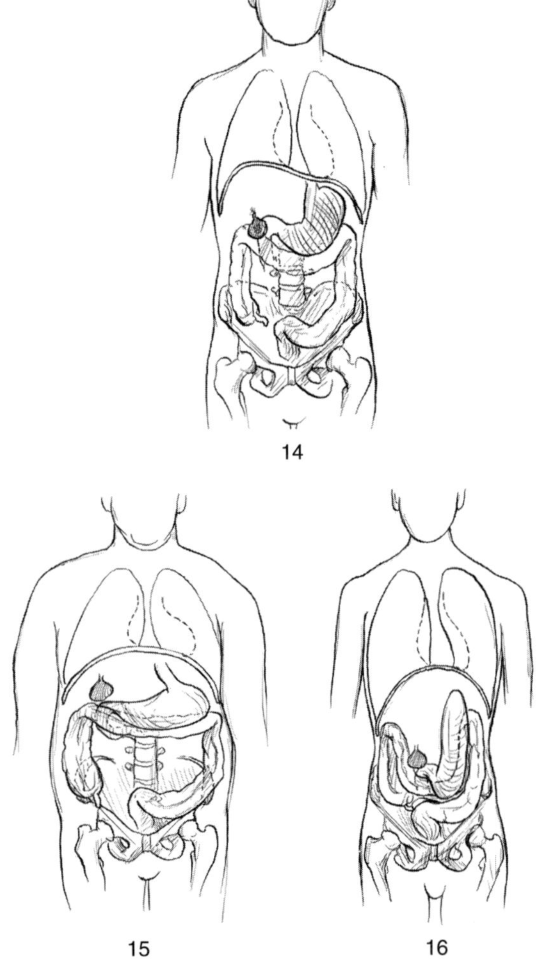

FIGURE 17.2 Diagram of body habitus with gallbladder position

For questions 14–16, identify the body habitus, given the positions of the gallbladder in Figure 17.2.

14. ______________________

15. ______________________

16. ______________________

17. Bilirubin is formed from the breakdown of

____________________________________.

18. When the sphincter of Oddi dilates (relaxes), bile enters the

____________________________________.

19. The role of bile salts in digestion is to

____________________________________.

20. The four lobes of the liver are called the ______________, ______________, ______________, and ______________.

21. The yellow pigment released during the destruction of red blood cells is called

____________________________________.

22. The liver is the primary organ responsible for destroying worn out red blood cells.

a. true

b. false

23. Females tend to develop gallstones more often than males.

a. true

b. false

24. An elevated bilirubin level is an indication for oral cholecystography.

a. true

b. false

25. The gallbladder is located near the upper border of the right lower quadrant in the sthenic-type patient.

a. true

b. false

26. The prefix chole- refers to:

a. liver

b. gallbladder

c. bile

d. cholesterol

27. Which of the following is a function of the gallbladder?

a. make bile

b. make bile salts

c. dilute bile

d. concentrate bile

28. The hepatic duct and the cystic duct join to form the:

a. papilla of Vater

b. common bile duct

c. pancreatic duct

d. right and left hepatic ducts

29. Blood leaving the stomach and small bowel travels to the liver by way of the:

a. hepatic vein

b. hepatic artery

c. central vein

d. hepatic portal vein

30. Which organ makes bile?

a. liver

b. gallbladder

c. pancreas

d. stomach

31. What is the chemical signal that causes the gallbladder to contract and release bile?

a. fat in the duodenum

b. low blood glucose

c. proteins in the duodenum

d. high blood glucose

32. In the _____ -type patient, the gallbladder is located very high and laterally.

a. hypersthenic

b. sthenic

c. hyposthenic

d. asthenic

33. Which hormone, secreted by the small intestine, stimulates the gallbladder to contract?

a. gastrin

b. cholecystokinin (CCK)

c. trypsin

d. amylase

34. The duct leading to and from the gallbladder is the:

a. hepatic duct

b. cholehepatic duct

c. common bile duct

d. cystic duct

35. The papilla of Vater is formed by the union of the pancreatic duct and the:

a. common bile duct

b. hepatic duct

c. cystic duct

d. sphincter of Oddi

36. Bile should *not* be found in the:

a. duodenum

b. hepatic duct

c. portal vein

d. cystic duct

37. Which duct connects the gallbladder to the common bile duct?

a. hepatic duct

b. papilla of Vater

c. pancreatic duct

d. cystic duct

Radiographic Procedures, Analysis, and Critical Thinking

For questions 38–41, identify the radiographic anatomy of the gallbladder in Figure 17.3.

38. ______________________

39. ______________________

40. ______________________

41. ______________________

42. The two most common indications for an OCG are ______________ and ______________.

43. For gallbladder radiography, thinner patients require a larger (steeper) oblique angle than broader patients.

a. true

b. false

44. The contrast medium used for OCG is essentially the same as that used for water-soluble contrast studies of the upper GI tract.

a. true

b. false

45. All types of hepatobiliary procedures use the same contrast medium.

a. true

b. false

46. The scout film for the OCG is taken with the patient in the _____ position.

a. prone

b. supine

c. oblique

d. upright

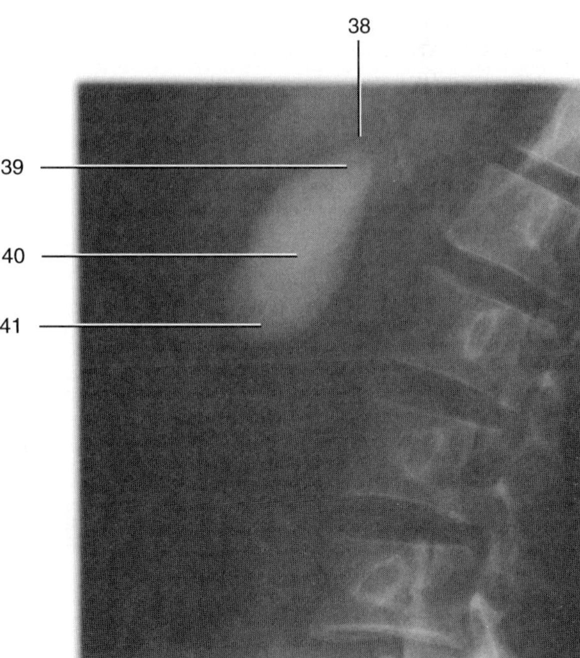

FIGURE 17.3 Radiograph of gallbladder, oral cholecystogram, oblique projection.

47. The patient should eat _____ the evening before an OCG.

a. nothing

b. a liquid meal

c. a high fat meal

d. a low fat meal

48. The best oblique position for radiographic visualization of the gallbladder is:

a. RAO, centered to the side up

b. RAO, centered to the side down

c. LAO, centered to the side up

d. LAO, centered to the side down

49. On a PA gallbladder radiograph, the central ray is placed at a level 2 inches below the last palpable rib. This positioning is accurate for _____ -type patients.

a. hyposthenic

b. hypersthenic

c. asthenic

d. sthenic

50. A patient is given 2 tablespoons of a substance containing large amounts of fat and films are taken 20 minutes later. This routine is part of a (an):

a. T-tube cholangiogram

b. percutaneous transhepatic cholangiogram (PTC)

c. endoscopic retrograde cholangiopancreatography (ERCP)

d. oral cholecystogram (OCG)

51. A lateral decubitus radiograph of the gallbladder is taken to demonstrate:

a. mobility of the gallbladder

b. function of the gallbladder

c. increased density of the gallbladder

d. layering of gallstones

52. For optimum visibility, the contrast medium for an OCG should be taken _____ hours before the examination.

a. 6

b. 8

c. 10–12

d. 18–24

53. Radiographs of the gallbladder are routinely taken on _____ inch films.

a. 8 x 10

b. 10 x 12

c. 11 x 14

d. 14 x 17

54. Which decubitus is most commonly part of a departmental protocol for gallbladder radiography?

a. dorsal

b. ventral

c. right lateral

d. left lateral

55. When filming with the patient upright, the position of the gallbladder will:

a. remain the same as in the recumbent position

b. drop 1–2 inches

c. drop 2–4 inches

d. drop 4–6 inches

56. Which of the following biliary examinations is the most accurate for detecting gallstones AND has the least risk for the patient?

a. percutaneous transhepatic cholangiography (PTC)

b. endoscopic retrograde cholangiopancreatography (ERCP)

c. oral cholecystogram (OCG)

d. sonography

57. During endoscopic retrograde cholangiopancreatography (ERCP), how does the contrast medium reach the biliary tree?

a. direct instillation

b. orally

c. IV injection

d. injection into the cystic duct during surgery

58. Which of the following is *always* a postoperative examination of the biliary tree?

a. percutaneous transhepatic cholangiography (PTC)

b. endoscopic retrograde cholangiopancreatography (ERCP)

c. oral cholecystogram (OCG)

d. T-tube cholangiogram

59. Which of the following uses a fiberoptic scope to diagnose hepatobiliary disorders?

a. percutaneous transhepatic cholangiography (PTC)

b. T-tube cholangiography

c. endoscopic retrograde cholangiopancreatography (ERCP)

d. operative cholangiography

60. Endoscopic retrograde cholangiopancreatography (ERCP) will demonstrate the:

1. biliary tree

2. pancreatic duct

3. liver

a. 1 and 2

b. 1 and 3

c. 2 and 3

d. 1, 2, and 3

61. Which of the following are performed by the direct injection of contrast into the biliary tree?

1. endoscopic retrograde cholangiopancreatography (ERCP)

2. percutaneous transhepatic cholangiography (PTC)

3. operative cholangiography

a. 1 and 2

b. 1 and 3

c. 2 and 3

d. 1, 2, and 3

62. Examination of the biliary system by direct injection through the liver is called:

a. operative cholangiography

b. percutaneous transhepatic cholangiography (PTC)

c. endoscopic retrograde cholangiopancreatography (ERCP)

d. T-tube cholangiography

63. A patient is experiencing severe diarrhea and vomiting and gallstones are suspected. Which of the following will likely be the first procedure ordered?

a. percutaneous transhepatic cholangiography (PTC)

b. oral cholecystogram (OCG)

c. endoscopic retrograde cholangiopancreatography (ERCP)

d. sonography

64. T-tube cholangiography is performed:

1. postoperatively

2. to visualize residual stones

3. on a patient with a cholecystectomy

a. 1 and 2

b. 1 and 3

c. 2 and 3

d. 1, 2, and 3

65. In which procedure is a contrast medium injected through a tube that has been placed in the patient for postoperative biliary drainage?

a. enteroclysis

b. operative cholangiography

c. T-tube cholangiography

d. endoscopic retrograde cholangiopancreatography (ERCP)

66. Which of the following procedures could be used to demonstrate stones in a gallbladder that is totally nonfunctional?

1. sonography

2. oral cholecystogram (OCG)

3. percutaneous transhepatic cholangiography (PTC)

a. 1 and 2

b. 1 and 3

c. 2 and 3

d. 1, 2, and 3

67. What is the optimum kilovoltage range when using iodine-based contrast media for oral cholecystography?

a. 50–55

b. 60–65

c. 70–75

d. 80–85

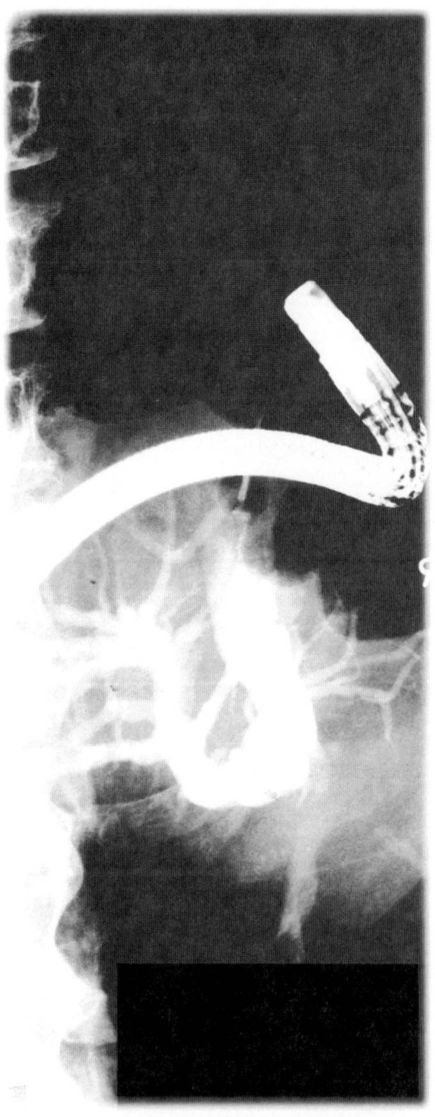

FIGURE 17.4 Radiograph of hepatobiliary system, ERCP, AP projection.

68. What clues on Figure 17.4 lead you to conclude that this radiograph is part of a ERCP exam rather than an oral cholecystogram or a PTC?

69. Describe the clinical history you should obtain from a patient arriving the morning of an oral cholecystogram (OCG).

70. If sonography is unable to demonstrate hepatobiliary physiology, why is it the first choice for imaging of this body system?

71. A physician examines the chart of a patient who is scheduled for an OCG and tells you to cancel the examinatoin because the patient's bilirubin is too high. Why was it necessary to cancel the examination?

72. A patient arrives in the emergency room presenting severe jaundice with vomiting and diarrhea for 3 days. An emergency sonogram is attempted but the patient is filled with too much fluid and gas to accurately diagnose hepatobiliary structure. What tests, if any, would likely be done next?

Do You Remember?

73. In a hypersthenic patient the stomach is elongated, lower, and more midline in position.

a. true

b. false

74. On a modified parietoacanthial (modified Waters) projection the orbitomeatal line should form a 37° angle with the plane of the film.

a. true

b. false

75. Which of the following would *not* be included as part of a departmental protocol for ribs?

a. PA chest

b. 45° oblique ribs

c. lateral ribs

d. AP ribs

76. If the epicondyles are placed parallel to the film and the hand is in the anatomic position, the resulting radiograph will demonstrate the:

a. lateral scapula

b. lateral humerus

c. AP internal rotation shoulder

d. AP humerus

77. For the lateral transcranial projection of the temporomandibular joints, the central ray is angled:

a. 15° cephalic

b. 15° caudal

c. 25° cephalic

d. 25° caudal

78. For the parietoacanthial (Waters) projection, the central ray emerges at the:

a. acanthion

b. canthion

c. glabella

d. nasion

79. For the tunnel view of the intercondylar fossa, the central ray is perpendicular to the:

a. patella

b. femur

c. tibia

d. intercondylar plane

80. Which of the following use a 72 inch SID?

1. lateral cervical spine

2. RAO sternum

3. PA chest

a. 1 and 2

b. 1 and 3

c. 2 and 3

d. 1, 2, and 3

81. The patient is on the left side and the central ray is angled 5° caudal, entering 2 inches below the iliac crest and 2 inches anterior to the posterior surface of the body. This position best describes the lateral:

a. sacrum

b. coccyx

c. lumbar spine

d. L5–S1 junction

82. For a lateral projection of the skull the _____ line is perpendicular to the film.

a. interpupillary

b. infraorbitomeatal

c. orbitomeatal

d. midsagittal

STUDY TIP: PLEADING FOR GRADES

Dean: I have got to get an A in this course. If I don't raise my GPA, I'll never get accepted to radiation therapy school.

Instructor Bob: Sorry, Dean, I've calculated your grade several times and it is a C.

Dean: How about these five questions from tests 1 and 2. They were terrible questions and very ambiguous. You should throw them out. And what about this essay question—I think I deserve more points.

Instructor Bob: Dean, you took those tests 3 months ago and we discussed the questions in class after the exam. And your essay question did not cover the necessary points to get a good grade. Why didn't you bring these to my attention earlier in the term.

Dean: I didn't need the points then. You know, my kids have been sick all semester and I have had to work extra hours at work the past month. I think I deserve a break.

Personal circumstances sometimes affect student performance. Although instructor Bob can give empathy and feel compassion for Dean's personal situations, he generally will not and cannot raise grades because of them.

- If the teacher made a math error in calculating your grade or did not see your answer because you put it on the back of the page, bring it to the teacher's attention immediately.
- Never wait until the end of a semester to question a grade or debate an answer to a question. This appears as if you are desperate for a higher grade and implies you were not interested enough to bring it to the attention of the teacher earlier in the term.
- Never plead for a grade using phrases such as "I must pass" or "I need an A." These imply that you want a grade that you may not merit.
- Grade changes must be based on performance, not charity. If you "must" get a higher grade, ask the teacher about the possibility of extra credit or perhaps retaking an examination that was given when you had a documented illness. Teachers are not required to grant such requests but many are willing to work with students on these issues.

> Pleading for grades is a waste of time and may even be counterproductive. Instead, discuss reasonable options with the teacher as to what you could do to increase your grade in the class.

CHAPTER 18

Urinary System

LEARNING OBJECTIVES

At the completion of this chapter, the student should be able to:

1. List and describe the basic anatomic components of the urinary system and identify the basic parenchymal unit of the kidney.
2. Given drawings and radiographs, locate anatomic structures.
3. Describe the physiology of the urinary system and describe its role in maintaining the body's homeostasis.
4. List four common clinical indications for imaging the urinary system.
5. Explain why it is necessary to use radiographic contrast media to image the urinary system.
6. List the two main categories of radiographic contrast media used in intravenous urography and the factors determining their use.
7. State the main difference between the contrast used in intravenous urography and retrograde cystography.
8. Discuss adverse patient reactions to radiographic contrast and list the medical responses necessary for each.
9. Describe typical patient preparation for each urinary procedure for both typical and atypical patients.
10. Describe the positioning used in imaging the urinary system.
11. List or identify the central ray location and identify the extent of field necessary for each projection.
12. Explain the protective measures appropriate for each examination.
13. Recommend the technical factors for producing an acceptable radiograph for each urinary procedure.
14. Identify the normal postinjection sequencing of radiographs during imaging of the urinary system.
15. Identify the hypertensive postinjection sequencing of radiographs during imaging of the urinary system.
16. State the instructions given to the patient before and during each urinary imaging procedure.
17. Explain the rationale for the following procedures/projections in urinary system imaging.
    a. Postinjection sequencing of radiographs following contrast media injection
    b. 30° RPO or LPO projections of the kidney
    c. Nephrotomograms
    d. Upright projections
    e. Postvoid projections
18. Given radiographs, evaluate positioning and technical factors.
19. Describe modifications of procedures for atypical or impaired patients to better demonstrate the anatomic area of interest.

Routine and Alternative Positions/Projections

Part	Routine	Alternative
Intravenous urogram (IVU)	AP abdomen (scout)	
	AP serial postinjection	Nephrotomograms
	Oblique	
	AP bladder	
		Upright postvoid AP
		Oblique bladder

QUESTIONS

Anatomy and Physiology

For questions 1–10, identify the anatomy of the urinary system in Figure 18.1.

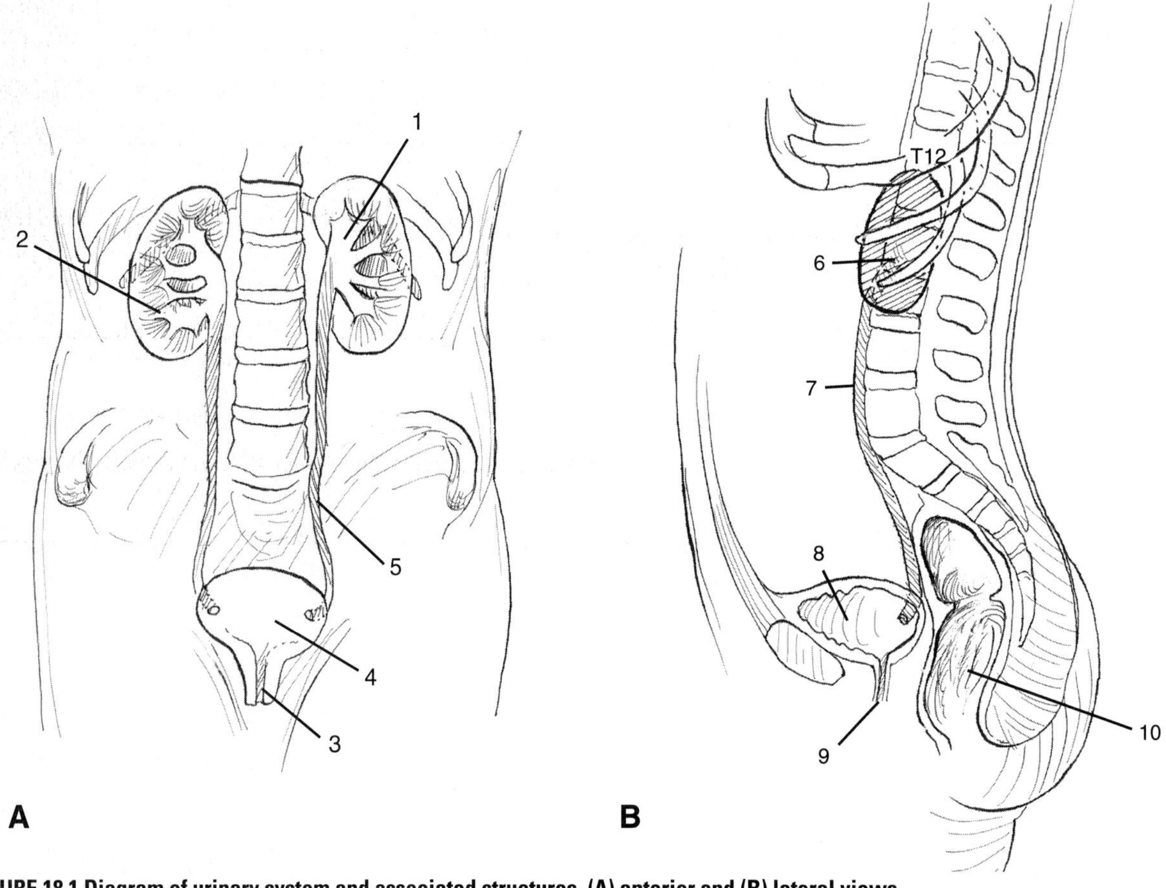

FIGURE 18.1 Diagram of urinary system and associated structures, (A) anterior and (B) lateral views.

1. ____________________

2. ____________________

3. ____________________

4. ____________________

5. ____________________

6. ____________________

7. ____________________

8. ____________________

9. ____________________

10. ____________________

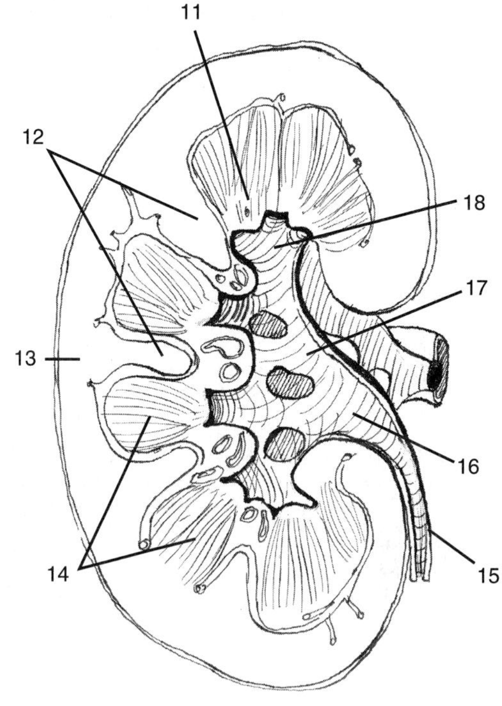

FIGURE 18.2 Diagram of kidney, coronal section.

For questions 11–18, identify the anatomy of the kidney in Figure 18.2.

11. ____________________

12. ____________________

13. ____________________

14. ____________________

15. ____________________

16. ____________________

17. ____________________

18. ____________________

For questions 19–24, identify the radiographic anatomy of the nephron in Figure 18.3.

19. Glomerulus

a. 1

b. 2

c. 3

d. 10

20. Proximal convoluted tubule

a. 1

b. 4

c. 7

d. 9

21. Collecting duct

a. 5

b. 6

c. 8

d. 9

22. Loop of Henle

a. 2

b. 4

c. 7

d. 9

23. Distal convoluted tubule

a. 2

b. 4

c. 9

d. 10

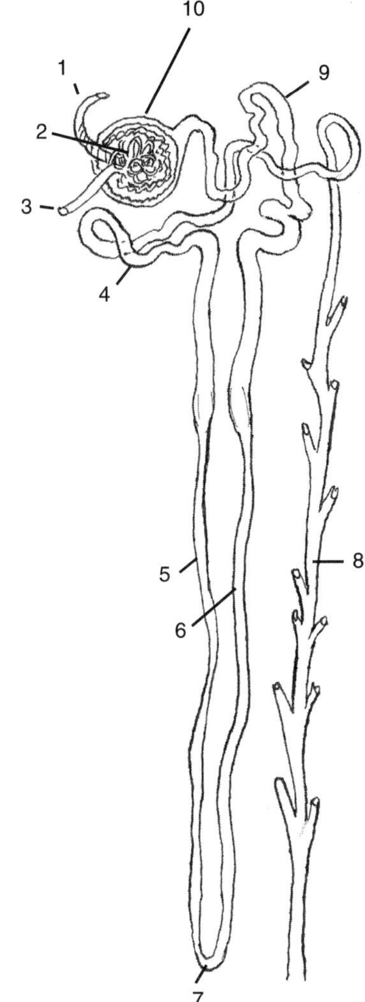

FIGURE 18.3 Diagram of nephron.

24. Afferent arteriole

a. 1

b. 2

c. 3

d. 8

25. After leaving the ureter, urine enters the _____________ through the _____________.

26. The term that means the opposite of retrograde is

______________________________.

27. Internally, the kidney is divided into two regions called the __________ and __________.

28. The inferior portion of the urinary bladder lies at the level of the

______________________________.

29. Women generally have more bladder infections than men because

______________________________.

30. Movement of urine in a reverse direction, from the bladder to the ureters, is called

______________________________.

31. In preparing for an IVU, diabetic patients are normally kept without liquids longer than non-diabetic patients to increase their level of dehydration.

a. true

b. false

32. The kidneys and ureters lie in the retroperitoneal space.

a. true

b. false

33. Blood enters the renal corpuscle through the efferent arteriole.

a. true

b. false

34. The structural and functional unit of the kidney is called the glomerulus.

a. true

b. false

35. Urine flows from the collecting tubules to the calyces to the renal pelvis before leaving the kidney.

a. true

b. false

36. The right kidney is normally situated higher than the left kidney.

a. true

b. false

37. Which glands lie on top of each kidney?

a. urethral

b. ovaries

c. testes

d. adrenals

38. The prefix pyelo- refers to:

a. kidney

b. renal pelvis

c. nephron

d. renal pyramid

39. The top of the left kidney normally lies at the level of:

a. T8

b. T10

c. T12

d. L2

40. The medial concave surface of the kidney is the:

a. papillae

b. pyramid

c. pelvis

d. hilus

41. The act of expelling urine is known as:

a. defecation

b. deglutition

c. micturition

d. incontinence

42. The junction of the ureters and the bladder is the:

a. uterovesical junction

b. urethrovesical junction

c. ureterovesical junction

d. trigone

43. The structural and functional unit of the kidney is the:

a. calyx

b. nephron

c. glomerulus

d. cortex

44. The ureters extend from the kidneys to the:

a. urinary bladder

b. adrenal gland

c. urethra

d. external environment

45. Which urinary organ has both an internal and an external sphincter?

a. kidney

b. ureter

c. bladder

d. urethra

46. The urethra serves as the passageway for urine from the bladder to the:

a. kidney

b. renal pelvis

c. external environment

d. ureter

For questions 47–50, match the term with its definition.

Definition	Term
47. _____ inability to control voiding	**a.** cystitis
48. _____ bladder infection	**b.** polyuria
49. _____ excessive urination	**c.** incontinence
50. _____ lack of urination	**d.** anuria
	e. hematuria

51. The trigone is located in the:

a. kidney

b. ureter

c. bladder

d. urethra

52. The cluster of blood capillaries surrounded by Bowman's capsule is called the:

a. nephron

b. corpuscle

c. renal pelvis

d. glomerulus

Radiographic Procedures, Analysis, and Critical Thinking

For questions 53–57, identify the radiographic anatomy on the IVU in Figure 18.4.

53. ______________________

54. ______________________

55. ______________________

56. ______________________

57. ______________________

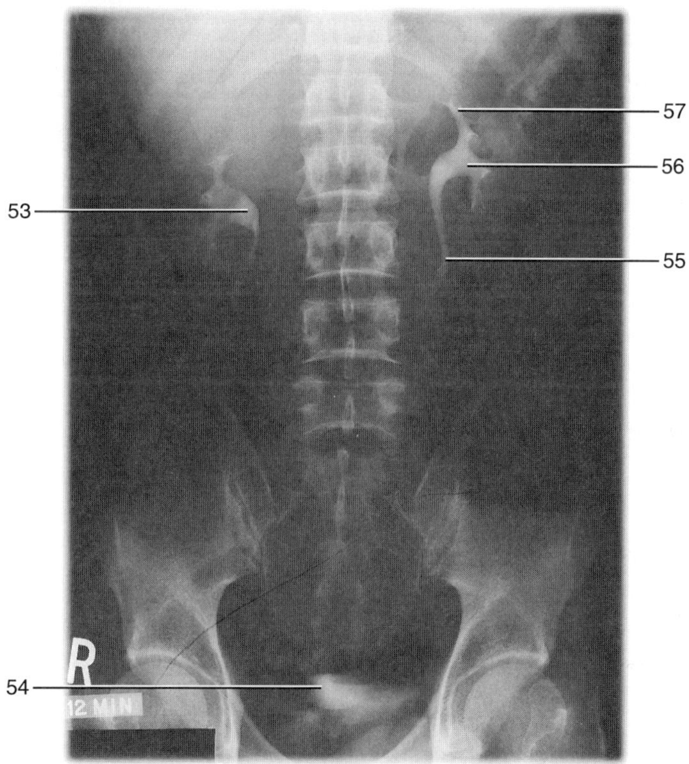

FIGURE 18.4 Radiograph of IVU, AP projection.

For questions 58–62, identify the radiographic anatomy on the IVU in Figure 18.5.

58. ______________________

59. ______________________

60. ______________________

61. ______________________

62. ______________________

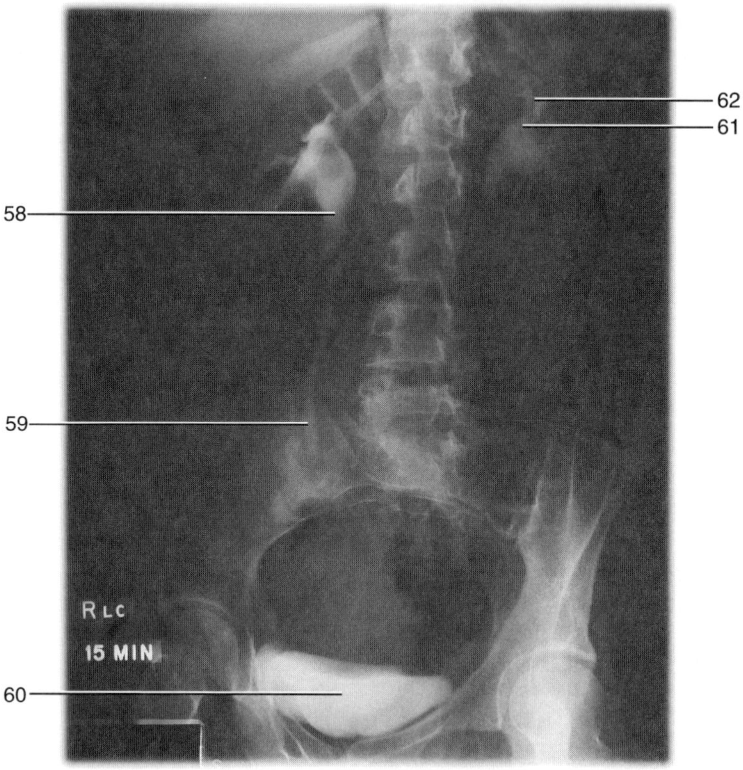

FIGURE 18.5 Radiograph of IVU, oblique projection.

63. Occasionally, a radiographer must determine patient position by looking for clues on the radiograph. Determine the patient position on Figure 18.5 and discuss how you arrived at the answer.

64. For filming of the urinary tract, respiration is normally suspended following

____.

65. The two distinct phases of renal function during an IVU are the ______________ and ______________.

66. Oblique kidney projections during an IVU examination require a patient rotation of approximately ______________ degrees.

67. If an 11 x 14 inch cassette is placed crosswise to obtain an AP projection of the kidneys, the central ray should be placed at the level:

a. of the xiphoid process

b. between the xiphoid process and the iliac crest

c. at the iliac crest

d. 2 inches above the xiphoid process

68. An AP upright postvoid film taken on a 14 x 17 inch cassette should be centered:

a. at the level of the ASIS

b. at the level of the iliac crest

c. 1 inch above the iliac crest

d. 1 inch below the iliac crest

69. Compression is used to:

a. increase patient comfort

b. increase the speed of contrast flow through the nephron

c. slow the speed of contrast flow through the nephron

d. obstruct the flow of contrast and increase filling of the calyces

70. For the average patient, the urinary bladder will be adequately filled _____ minutes after IV contrast injection.

a. 5

b. 10

c. 30

d. 45

71. Which position best demonstrates mobility of the kidneys?

a. supine

b. RPO

c. lateral decubitus

d. upright

72. To place the right kidney parallel to the plane of the film, it is necessary to rotate the patient:

a. 30° RPO

b. 45° RPO

c. 30° LPO

d. 45° LPO

73. Which examination best demonstrates a narrowing of the urethra?

a. cystography

b. voiding urethrography

c. retrograde urography

d. IVU

74. Which examination best demonstrates the *functioning* ability of the urinary system?

a. IVU

b. retrograde urography

c. voiding cystourethrography

d. cystography

75. Which examination is usually performed by a physician in an operating room?

a. IVU

b. retrograde urography

c. cystography

d. voiding cystourethrography

76. Tomography is often performed during IVU examinations because it:

a. gives the patient less dose than overhead films

b. can be done faster than overhead films

c. removes overlying gas and fecal shadows

d. requires less contrast medium

77. The central ray for an AP projection of the urinary bladder should be directed:

a. to the symphysis pubis

b. 2 inches above the symphysis pubis

c. to the iliac crest

d. to the ASIS

78. During which urinary procedure is a 60-second radiograph required?

a. nephrotomography

b. retrograde urography

c. hypertensive IVU

d. IVU

79. The optimum kVp range for examinations utilizing iodinated contrast media is:

a. 60–70

b. 70–75

c. 80–90

d. 90–100

80. Nephrotomograms are usually taken:

a. before contrast is injected

b. 1–6 minutes after contrast is injected

c. 5–15 minutes after contrast is injected

d. after the postvoid film has been checked

81. The contrast medium for cystography is:

a. gravity injected into the bladder through a catheter

b. force-injected into the bladder through a catheter

c. injected intravenously

d. introduced into the bladder via a suprapubic injection

82. The central ray for an IVU scout radiograph is centered to the level of the:

a. xiphoid process

b. ASIS

c. lower margin of the ribs

d. iliac crest

83. Evaluation of the kidneys and ureters by direct catheterization of the ureter is called:

a. IV urography

b. infusion tomography

c. retrograde urography

d. nephrotomography

84. For the oblique projection of the urinary bladder, the central ray is directed:

a. 1/2 inch medial to the side up ASIS

b. 1/2 inch medial to the side down ASIS

c. 2 inches medial to the side up ASIS

d. 2 inches medial to the side down ASIS

85. Which of the following are considered *mild* reactions to injected iodinated contrast media?

1. vomiting

2. metallic taste

3. dyspnea

a. 1 and 2

b. 1 and 3

c. 2 and 3

d. 1, 2, and 3

86. Which of the following is considered a *severe* reaction to injected iodinated contrast media?

a. hypotension

b. hives

c. vomiting

d. tachycardia

87. An unexpected, life-threatening reaction to injected iodinated contrast media is known as:

a. anaphylaxis

b. analepsis

c. allergy

d. anergy

88. The timing of filming during an IVU begins when the:

a. radiologist enters the room

b. radiologist leaves the room

c. injection is started

d. injection is completed

89. All commonly used urographic contrast media:

a. are ionic

b. are nonionic

c. contain iodine

d. both b and c

90. Compared to ionic contrast media, nonionics:

1. produce fewer adverse effects

2. are more expensive

3. contain more iodine

a. 1 and 2

b. 1 and 3

c. 2 and 3

d. 1, 2, and 3

A 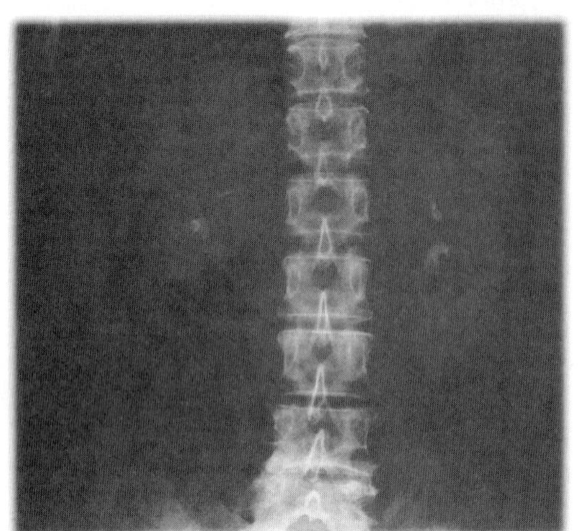

B 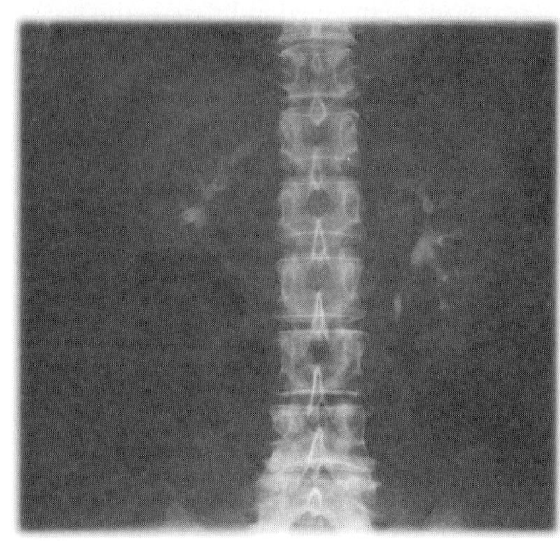

FIGURE 18.6 Radiograph of IVU, AP projection, (A) timed film #1 (B) timed film #2.

91. A radiographer forgot to mark the IVU radiographs in Figure 18.6 and is trying to determine which radiograph is the 5-minute film and which is the 10-minute film. Describe the radiographic clues that would help make this determination.

92. On an asthenic patient with an exceptionally long abdomen, it is not always possible to include the entire urinary system on a single 14 x 17 film. Describe at least two adaptations in positioning that could be done to accommodate this patient.

93. When taking a clinical history before an IVU, list three risk factors that you would notify the radiologist or supervising technologist about before proceeding with the examination.

94. A radiographer is performing an IVU, takes the first film after 5 minutes and observes no contrast in the collecting system of the kidney. Closer inspection reveals contrast in the bladder. Explain this apparent discrepancy.

95. A physician examines the chart of a patient who is scheduled for an IVU and tells you to cancel the examination because the patient has a BUN of 67. Why is it necessary to cancel the IVU with this level of BUN?

Do You Remember?

96. With the patient in the supine position, which of the following would be mostly filled with air on a double-contrast examination?

1. descending colon

2. pylorus of the stomach

3. transverse colon

a. 1 and 2

b. 1 and 3

c. 2 and 3

d. 1, 2, and 3

97. A physician has requested the following examinations for a patient. In what *order* should they be performed?

1. IV urogram

2. barium enema

3. upper GI

a. 1, 2, 3

b. 3, 2, 1

c. 2, 3, 1

d. 1, 3, 2

98. Patient preparation for an upper GI includes which of the following?

1. cleansing enemas

2. NPO after midnight

3. no tobacco products in the morning

a. 1 and 2

b. 1 and 3

c. 2 and 3

d. 1, 2, and 3

99. If recumbent, a patient should be placed into the _____ position for a right lateral skull.

a. RAO

b. LAO

c. LPO

d. RPO

100. The central ray for a PA projection of the cranium exits at the:

a. vertex

b. glabella

c. nasion

d. acanthion

101. The patient's head is resting on the nose and chin, and the median sagittal plane is perpendicular to the plane of the film. The central ray exits between the lips and is directed perpendicular to the midpoint of the film. This position demonstrates the:

a. nasal bones

b. mandibular rami

c. temporomandibular joints

d. orbits

102. A patient's lower leg measures 16 inches from joint to joint. To obtain a radiographic examination of the lower leg, the radiographer should:

a. use two 14 x 17 films, turned obliquely, for the AP and lateral

b. obtain both the AP and lateral on one split 14 x 17 film

c. include the leg with the knee joint on 14 x 17 films and take the ankle joint on 8 x 10 films

d. include an AP of the joint closest to the injury on one 14 x 17 film and a lateral of the opposite joint on another 14 x 17 film

103. The head of the radius articulates with the:

a. scaphoid

b. capitellum

c. trochlea

d. styloid process of the ulna

104. If the infraorbitomeatal line is perpendicular to the film, how many degrees tube angle is used for the AP axial (Townes) projection of the cranium?

a. 8

b. 15

c. 23

d. 37

105. What line should be perpendicular to the plane of the film for the open-mouth odontoid position of the cervical spine?

a. mastoid tip and upper incisors

b. mastoid tip and lower incisors

c. upper incisors and occipital bone

d. gonion and EAM

STUDY TIP: SUCCESS REQUIRES PERSISTENCE

Gina: I give up. I have taken notes exactly the way you outlined and studied the way that you told me to. I'm still not doing well. Maybe I really don't want to be a radiographer anyway.

Instructor Bob: Hey, everyone feels that way once in a while. You have been improving and I think with a little more persistence, you can get the kind of grades you want.

Gina: I just don't have any more hours in a day to give. I have a family you know.

Instructor Bob: Success may not require any more additional effort, just more of the same. Changes in grades take time. Remember, persistence is often more important than genius. Persistence requires a strong, positive mental attitude and some clear goals. Have you really changed your mind about becoming a radiographer?

Gina: No, I really want this degree badly—I was just venting.

Instructor Bob: That's OK. I know you are motivated but only persistence will keep you on the track to the degree. Let's go over that exam to see what you missed.

- Nothing can take the place of persistence. To succeed in any educational program, you must have it.
- Persistence requires that one have a clear goal in mind and a strong desire to reach that goal. If you don't know where you want to go and don't want to get there, failure will undoubtedly occur regardless of innate intelligence.

> Motivation and persistence are siblings. Whereas motivation is essential to show you the path, persistence is the fuel to carry you to the goal.

SECTION VII

SPECIAL RADIOGRAPHY

CHAPTER 19

Mobile and Intraoperative Radiography

LEARNING OBJECTIVES

At the completion of this chapter, the student should be able to:

1. List and describe basic principles of mobile radiography.
2. Describe additional fundamentals of mobile radiography when performed intraoperatively.
3. List and explain the stages of perioperative radiography.
4. Explain the surgical suite setup and special considerations.
5. List and explain principles of aseptic technique.
6. List and describe principles of radiation protection with respect to mobile and intraoperative radiography.
7. List and describe surgical specialties and the radiographic procedures typically performed for each.

QUESTIONS

1. The three phases of perioperative radiography are ______________, ______________, and ______________.

2. If it is necessary for a radiographer to leave the operating room to obtain a radiologist reading, he or she must

______________________________________.

3. Complete surgical attire includes a gown, ______________, and ______________.

4. The method used to achieve and maintain a sterile field is known as

______________________________________.

5. The two most common cardiac procedures requiring intraoperative radiography are ______________ and ______________.

6. The most common thoracic surgical procedure using intraoperative radiography is

______________________________________.

7. During mobile fluoroscopy, the primary source of radiation exposure to health care personnel comes from

______________________________________.

8. The distance needed to avoid accidental contact with a sterile field is called the

______________________________________.

9. Should alarm signals be emitted, it is the mobile radiographer's responsibility to reset or troubleshoot nonradiographic equipment that may be in the patient's room.

   a. true

   b. false

10. Because of the acute nature of mobile radiography, it is usually acceptable for the radiographer to leave tubes and other artifacts in place during filming.

    a. true

    b. false

11. Grid cassettes should be used for mobile AP abdomen projections.

    a. true

    b. false

12. All items in the surgical suite are considered sterile.

    a. true

    b. false

13. The sterile corridor can only be entered by the intraoperative radiographer while the cassette is being positioned.

    a. true

    b. false

14. Due to the nature of mobile radiography, gonadal shielding is not possible or necessary.

    a. true

    b. false

15. Mobile radiographers should wear their radiation monitoring device outside the lead apron.

a. true

b. false

16. When opened, the edges of a sterile package are considered sterile.

a. true

b. false

17. The horizontal and vertical surfaces of an instrument table are considered sterile.

a. true

b. false

18. The most common mobile projection is the:

a. PA chest

b. AP chest

c. lateral chest

d. decubitus chest

19. Which decubitus is normally performed as part of a mobile acute abdomen series?

a. dorsal

b. ventral

c. left lateral

d. right lateral

For questions 20–24; match the following procedures with the correct operative phase.

a. preoperative

b. intraoperative

c. postoperative

d. not an operative procedure

20. _____ PA chest to rule out pneumonia before a gastrostomy

21. _____ AP femur in the recovery room

22. _____ AP abdomen to demonstrate biliary stones during surgery

23. _____ PA chest x-ray to confirm tuberculosis on an AIDS patient

24. _____ sonography of kidney to localize tumor prior to surgery

25. Sterile means free from:

a. all infectious organisms

b. most infectious organisms

c. all organisms

d. most organisms

26. The area between the instrument table and the draped patient is the:

a. safe margin

b. aseptic zone

c. sterile corridor

d. aseptic instrument zone

27. When is a nonsterile radiographer permitted to reach over a sterile field?

a. only when positioning the cassette under the patient

b. only when handing the cassette to the physician/nurse

c. only before the incision has been made

d. never

28. Placement of catheters such as Hickman, central line, or Groshung is an intraoperative radiographic procedure performed during:

a. neurosurgery

b. gynecologic surgery

c. orthopedic surgery

d. oncologic surgery

29. Open reduction internal fixation is a procedure requiring intraoperative radiography during:

a. neurosurgery

b. gynecologic surgery

c. orthopedic surgery

d. oncologic surgery

30. Which of the following would be performed in a "cysto" room?

a. laminectomy

b. percutaneous nephrolithotomy

c. coronary artery bypass

d. arterial-venous graft

31. Explain why the term "mobile" is more appropriate than the term "portable" when describing x-ray units that can be moved around.

32. Describe several types of nonradiology equipment that the radiographer must be familiar with to efficiently perform mobile radiography.

33. Compare positioning of a standard PA projection of the chest with a mobile AP chest, describing some positioning differences and limitations due to the mobile procedure.

34. Compare positioning of a standard AP projection of the femur with a postoperative, mobile AP femur, describing some positioning differences and limitations due to the mobile procedure.

35. Describe the procedure by which a cassette is transferred to a sterile cover.

36. Describe the primary ways by which the mobile radiographer can limit radiation exposure to other health care providers.

37. A radiographer brushes against a sterile instrument table when positioning a cassette for an open reduction of the humerus. Describe the actions the radiographer should take.

Do You Remember?

38. For the parieto-orbital oblique (Rhese) projection, the forehead, nose, and cheek should be touching the table.

a. true

b. false

39. In the anatomic position, which carpal is found in the distal row on the medial side?

a. scaphoid

b. hamate

c. capitate

d. trapezium

40. In the RAO position for a barium enema, the _____ portion of the large intestine is best demonstrated.

a. transverse colon

b. ileocecal valve

c. right colic flexure

d. left colic flexure

41. The upright position is used in paranasal sinuses examinations in order to:

a. demonstrate fluid in the sinuses

b. minimize distortion

c. project the petrous ridges below the level of the maxillary sinuses

d. demonstrate deviation of the nasal septum

42. On an AP (Caldwell) projection for paranasal sinuses, the petrous ridges should:

a. completely fill the orbits

b. fill the upper third of the orbits

c. fill the lower third of the orbits

d. be free from superimposition with the orbits

43. The sphenoid sinus is clearly demonstrated on which of the following projections?

1. PA Caldwell

2. lateral

3. submentovertical

a. 1 and 2

b. 1 and 3

c. 2 and 3

d. 1, 2, and 3

44. A radiographer obtains an AP hip and observes that the lesser trochanter is not visualized on the film. This suggests that the:

a. leg was not internally rotated

b. toes were not pointing straight up

c. patient probably has an intertrochanteric fracture

d. patient was correctly positioned

45. The glenohumeral joint is more commonly referred to as the:

a. acromioclavicular joint

b. shoulder joint

c. elbow joint

d. sternoclavicular joint

46. What anatomic feature distinguishes cervical vertebra from thoracic or lumber vertebrae?

a. zygapophyseal joints

b. articular facets

c. transverse foramina

d. neural arches

47. Which projection best demonstrates zygapophyseal joints?

1. lateral thoracic spine

2. lateral cervical spine

3. oblique lumbar spine

a. 1 and 2

b. 1 and 3

c. 2 and 3

d. 1, 2, and 3

STUDY TIP: ARE GRADES IMPORTANT?

Juan: I feel miserable getting that "C" grade. I know I can do better and I really tried.

Instructor Bob: Maybe you could have done better but the course is over now and it is too late to improve the grade.

Juan: Everyone will be disappointed. I feel like a failure.

Instructor Bob: Juan, it's great that you want to make good grades. I certainly would not want to discourage that. But you really know the course material and have used it effectively in the clinic. There is more to learning than the grade.

Juan: I suppose you are right.

Instructor Bob: It's best that you not keep focusing negatively on that grade. Instead, why don't we go to lunch with Pat and Kathy and talk about strategies to improve your grade next semester.

- Overemphasizing grades can lead to excess stress and possible test anxiety.
- Underemphasizing grades can lead to low achievement.
- Never focus on bad test scores or other grades for long periods and never blame your performance on others.
- Accept responsibility for your grades. If you are not happy with them, analyze the reasons for your low grades and take action to improve them through the effective use of study or test-taking strategies.

Grades are an important source of motivation for most students. Use caution in overemphasizing or underemphasizing their worth.

Crossword Puzzle and Word Search Activities

CHAPTER 1

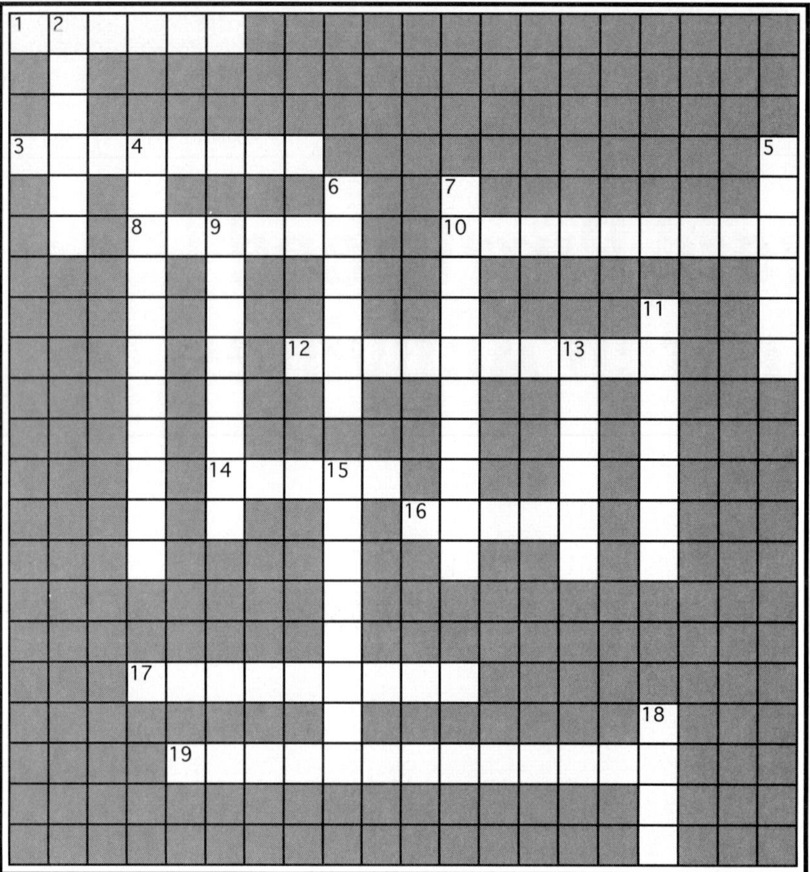

ACROSS

1 Away from the head of the body.
3 To turn palm of hand upward.
8 Lying face up.
10 Any reclining position.
12 Central ray skims a body part.
14 Angling central ray along longitudinal axis of body.
16 Palm of the hand.
17 Recumbent with a horizontal beam.
19 Opposite side of the body or part.

DOWN

2 To move away from the central axis of the body.
4 On the same side as the body or part.
5 To straighten a joint.
6 Toward the median plane of the body.
7 Path of central ray.
9 Closer to the origin of a part.
11 Posterior surface of foot.
13 Turning foot inward.
15 Forward or front part of the body.
18 To decrease the angle of a joint.

CHAPTERS 2 AND 3

```
R M E D I A S T I N U M W W N N
H A I Z F I S N Y E V N T F M H
Q B N C T R A C H E A S D G D Q
S S G E H I L U M X H N A O Z E
C J L P U Q W U M H K R I Z V E
B G A I S R Y L V M H U A F C D
R W R G T Y Y A L P P Y A P A Z
O S Y L V V K S A S E L Z X F P
N U N O L O W I M L R N W N Y P
C W X T C G D N N J I H L X C G
H R E T R O P E R I T O N E A L
I X K I I Y T O G L O K O S R K
D A Y S I Q M G M M N Z U D I S
P H A R Y N X C P K E H I B N X
U G L U C O S E Z H U G Q R A R
P T S A L V E O L I M F S T S E
```

pharynx
glucose
diaphragm
larynx
mediastinum
epiglottis
retroperitoneal
bronchi
alveoli
carina
hilum
peritoneum
aneurysm
kub
trachea

CHAPTER 4

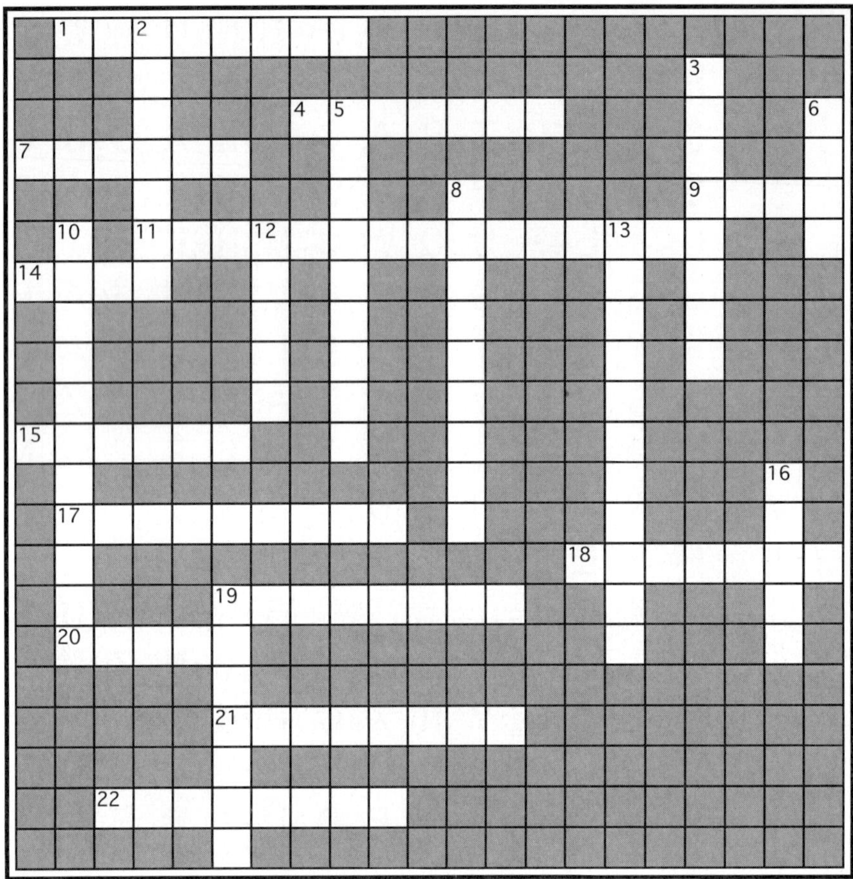

ACROSS

1 The pea-shaped carpal is the _____.
4 The medial end of the clavicle is called the _____ extremity.
7 The scapula has three _____.
9 The forearm consists of the radius and the _____.
11 The _____ joint is found between middle and distal phalanges.
14 A metacarpal has a base, shaft, and _____.
15 The Gaynor-Hart method is used to demonstrate the _____ canal.
17 The hand contains 14 _____.
18 The head of the humerus articulates with the _____ cavity.
19 The navicular bone is also called the _____.
20 Carpals are classified as _____ bones.
21 The beak-like process on the proximal ulna is called the _____ process.
22 The lesser _____ projects anteriorly from the proximal humerus.

DOWN

2 The large rough process on the distal radius is the _____ process.
3 The West-Point method is used to demonstrate the _____.
5 The lesser multangular is also called the _____.
6 The capitulum of the humerus articulates with the _____ of the radius.
8 The acute flexion position of the elbow is used to demonstrate the _____ process.
10 The five _____ comprise the palm of the hand.
12 The Coyle method is used to demonstrate trauma to the _____.
13 The two _____ of the humerus are easily palpable on its distal end.
16 The Lawrence position is called the AP _____.
19 The angled view of the scaphoid is called the _____ method.

CHAPTER 5

```
I L I U M C O N D Y L E R W V V
C C X T S I M E N I S C U S S T
Q U U V A A F I B U L A R I S L
K W N B W L C M Q C I A B A U N
T L M E O D U R C F T U G S O Y
I U I J I I P S O N P E A T O K
S S B G I F D A A I T V S G C W
E T C E A G O L T T L H U R R C
S A G H R M P R E E G I U L U A
A R X V I O E S M U L M A C C L
M S C U S U S N H R E L C C I C
O A B R A B M I T F D R A T A A
I L O S H A F T T I A N B I T N
D D P H A L A N X Y C K Z B E E
H T W K I N O M I N A T E I H U
X H M T R O C H A N T E R A N S
```

calcaneus
condyle
cruciate
cuboid
cuneiform
dorsoplantar
femur
fibula
hughston
ilium
inominate
ischium
ligament
meniscus
patella
phalanx
pubis
sacroiliac
sesamoid
settegast
shaft
talus
tarsal
tibia
trochanter
tuberosity

CHAPTER 6

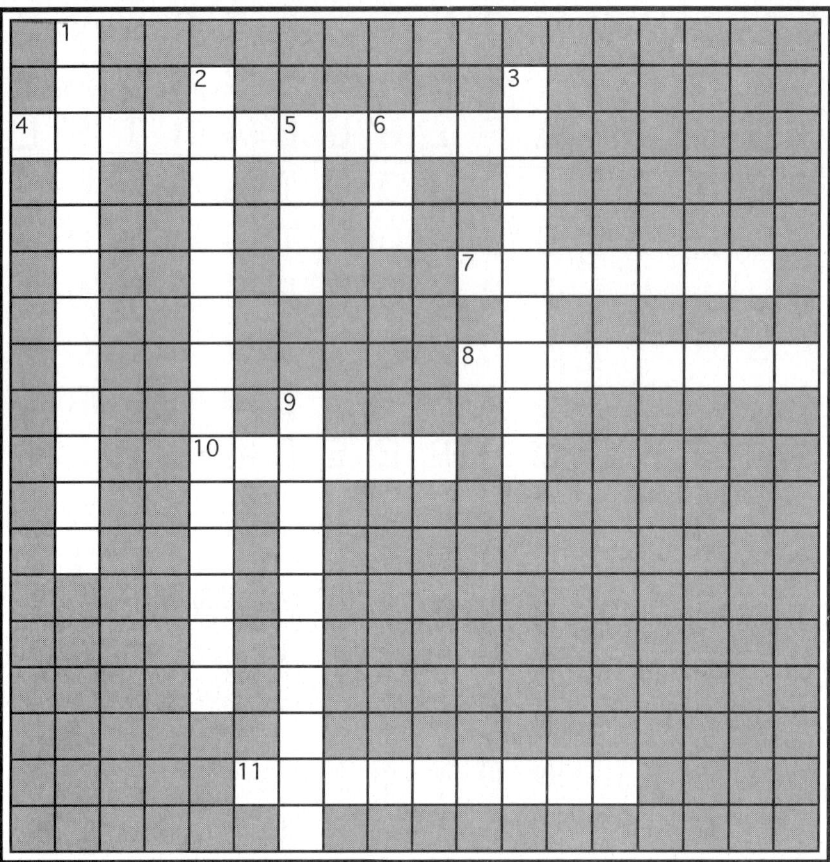

ACROSS

4 Behind the sternum.
7 Inferior portion of sternum.
8 Ribs not attaching to the sternum.
10 Number of pairs of ribs.
11 Superior portion of sternum.

DOWN

1 Collapse of part or all of a lung.
2 Joint where rib meets vetebral body.
3 Also called the corpus.
5 Ribs that attach directly to the sternum.
6 Best oblique position for the sternum.
9 Collection of blood in the pleural cavity.

CHAPTERS 7, 8, AND 9

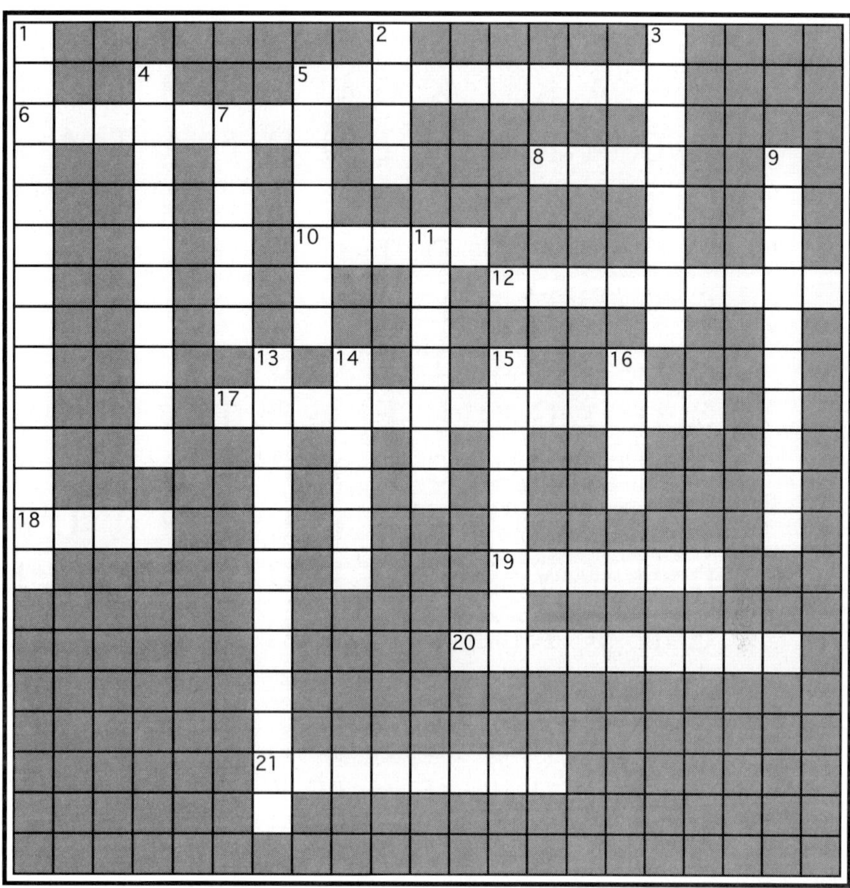

ACROSS

5 The _____ is the large, flat portion of the sacrum.
6 The primary feature of C1 is the anterior _____.
8 The vertebral arch is also known as the neural _____.
10 The prominenet bony ridge on the sacrum is called the sacral _____.
12 The seventh cervical vertebra is called the vertebra _____.
17 The superior and inferior articulating processes form a _____ joint.
18 The large lateral portions of the sacrum are called _____.
19 The final segment of the vertebral column is the _____.
20 Abnormal lateral curvature of the spine is called _____.
21 The wagging jaw AP is called the _____ method.

DOWN

1 The inferior vertebral notch of one vertebra and superior vertebral notch of another form an _____ foramen.
2 The two main parts of a vertebra are the vetebral arch and the _____.
3 Hunchback deformity is called _____.
4 The two articulations on each side of a thoracic vertebra are called _____.
5 The _____ lies between the vertebral body and the lamina.
7 The thoracic spine has a _____ curvature.
9 The _____ foramina are in the cervical vertebrae only.
11 The laminae unite posteriorly to form the _____ process.
13 Whiplash injuries are caused by _____.
14 The bulky structures that contain the articular facets of C1 are the lateral _____.
15 _____ vertebra have attachments for ribs.
16 The odontoid process is also called the _____.

CHAPTER 11

```
G X B R A C H Y C E P H A L I C
A L A K Z K D W X X M I F N Z T
A C A N T H I O M E A T A L A C
D I V B A E A D E A X I U E H W
T O G E E D I U E P X W M J M O
L R L C R L Y H T J J O J B E J
R G A I E T L C D L T A R L S N
G O D G O L E A R I X U X A O E
B N O N U C G X B T Q R Z C C S
S I W O A S E R U S P I U A E L
D O T Y S S O P H M I C E N P P
G N K K M A I T H E R L O T H I
V J R V R C V O S A C E J H A J
X Q P F C U P J N T L P B I L E
Z Q N O S C Y U E Q J I P O I H
B I Y B L M I N I O N E C N C X
```

glabella
vertex
auricle
infraorbitomeat
brachycephalic
acanthion
gonion
tragus
inion
doliocephalic
nasion
occiput
acanthiomeatal
mesocephalic

CHAPTERS 12 AND 13

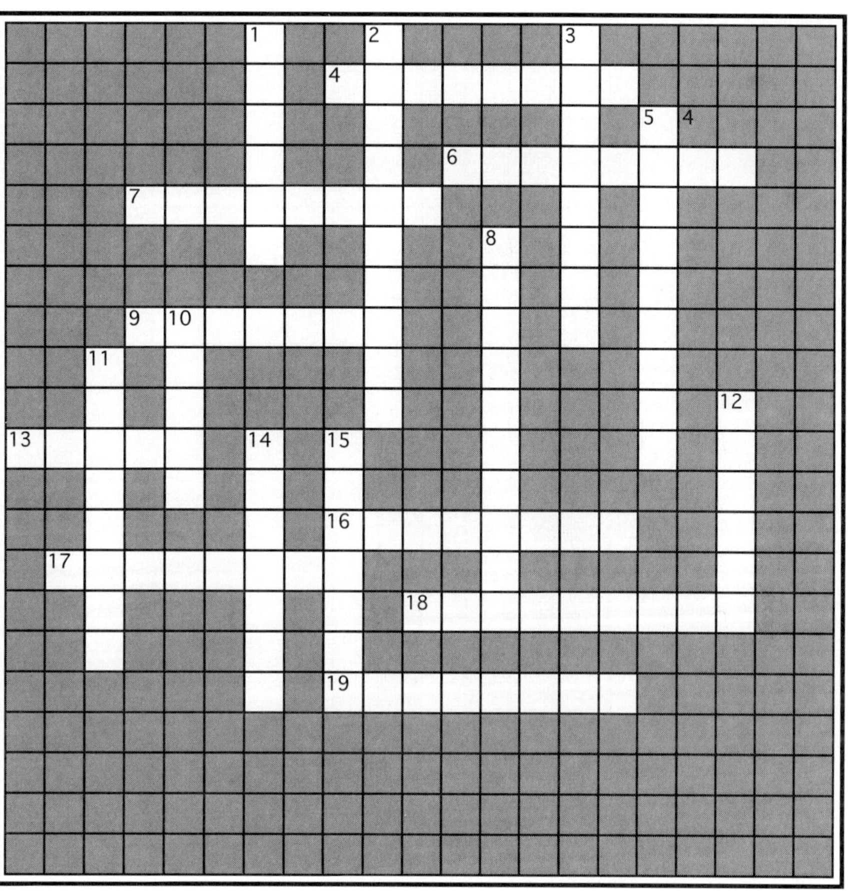

ACROSS

4 The _____ bone contains the tear apparatus.
6 The squamous suture joins the _____ and temporal bones.
7 The _____ bone contains the foramen rotundum and ovale.
9 The _____ bone forms the forehead.
13 The large lateral portions of the sphenoid bone are called the greater _____.
16 The carotid and jugular foramina are found in the _____ bone.
17 Both the mandible and the maxillae have _____ processes.
18 The two halves of the mandible join at the mandibular _____.
19 The _____ suture joins the two parietal bones.

DOWN

1 The _____ is also called the AP axial projection.
2 The depression found at the base of the zygomatic process is the _____ fossa.
3 The _____ bones form most of the lateral cranium.
5 The _____ processes form part of the lateral wall of the nasal cavity.
8 The transverse portion of the ethmoid bone is called the _____ plate.
10 The _____ is also called the parietoorbital oblique projection.
11 The processes which articulate with C1 are the occipital _____.
12 The _____ is also called the parietoacanthial projection.
14 The _____ process projects downward from the temporal bone.
15 The _____ portion of the temporal bone contains the organs of hearing.

CHAPTERS 15 AND 16

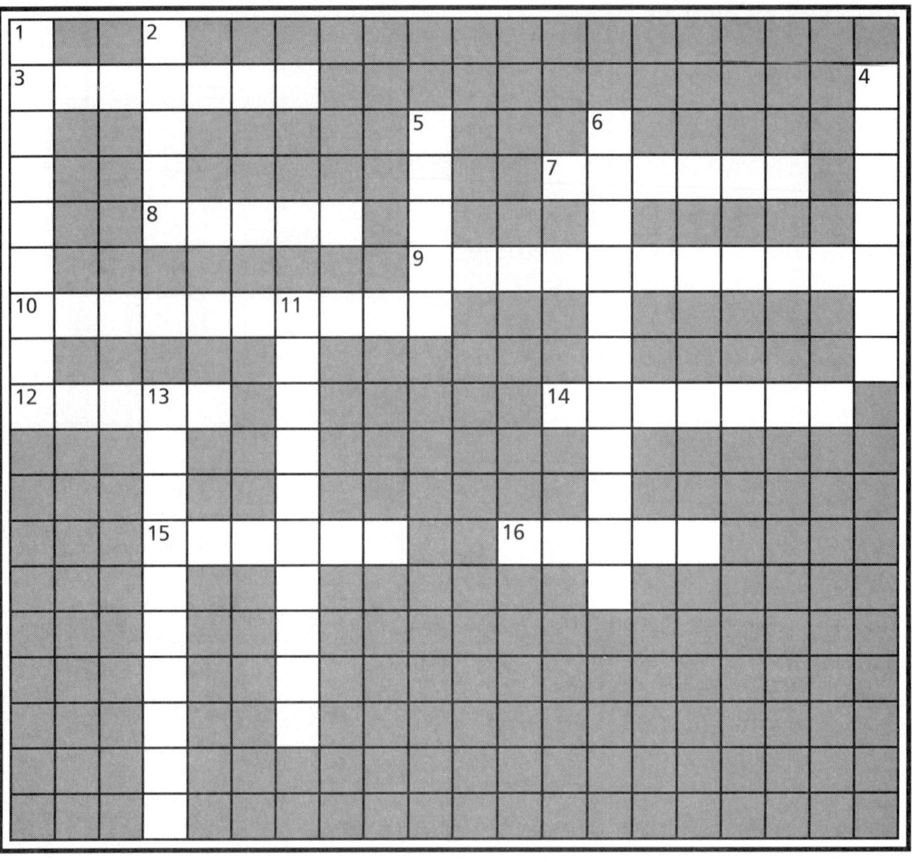

ACROSS

3 The _____ sphincter allows food to enter the duodenal bulb.
7 The ampulla is part of the _____.
8 The _____ is the first segment of the large intestine.
9 Chewing is also known as _____.
10 The _____ colon lies between the two flexures.
12 Deep folds in the stomach lining are called _____.
14 The esophagus enters the stomach at the _____ orifice.
15 The inner lining of the digestive tract is the _____.
16 Hemorrhoids are dilated _____.

DOWN

1 A circular ring of muscle is a _____.
2 The right _____ flexure lies near the liver.
4 The _____ is the middle portion of the small intestine.
5 Semisolid, partially digested food is called _____.
6 Rhythmic muscular contractions of the digestive tract is called _____.
11 The _____ prevents food from entering the trachea.
13 The GI tract is also called the _____ canal.

CHAPTERS 17 AND 18

B	Y	U	E	L	I	V	E	R	S	Y	G
D	B	L	U	B	S	A	U	E	R	L	A
I	I	J	R	A	R	V	H	A	W	R	L
B	L	E	E	H	I	T	N	N	N	E	L
M	I	C	T	U	R	I	T	I	O	N	B
R	A	E	E	R	R	S	B	E	S	A	L
I	R	R	R	U	I	U	Q	U	B	L	A
U	Y	Q	P	X	R	G	J	R	O	W	D
H	H	C	Y	I	U	R	O	I	W	F	D
Q	R	L	L	T	K	I	D	N	E	Y	E
E	A	I	D	C	Z	K	C	E	E	A	R
C	B	L	N	E	P	H	R	O	N	F	X

liver
biliary
urinary
bilirubin
urine
trigone
kidney
renal
ERCP

bile
calyx
urethra
gallbladder
ureter
IVU
micturition
nephron

Final Examination

1. Which plane divides the body into anterior and posterior portions?

   a. sagittal

   b. transverse

   c. coronal

   d. frontal

2. Which plane is parallel to the table top when the patient is positioned for a lateral lumbar spine?

   a. transverse

   b. sagittal

   c. coronal

   d. mid-axillary

3. Which region lies bilaterally in the lowest part of the abdomen?

   a. inguinal

   b. lumbar

   c. hypochondriac

   d. hypogastric

4. Movement of the arm toward the central axis of the body is:

   a. flexion

   b. abduction

   c. extension

   d. adduction

5. The costal margin lies at the level of:

   a. T7

   b. T10

   c. L3

   d. L5

6. Which landmark lies at the level of T2–T3?

   a. manubrial notch

   b. thyroid cartilage

   c. sternal angle

   d. mentum

7. The single most important factor in preventing the transfer of pathogens from radiographer to patient is:

a. changing into clean surgical scrubs when arriving for work

b. wearing gloves

c. using universal precautions for every patient

d. hand washing

8. A patient is lying on her right side and the x-ray beam is placed horizontally to exit at the spinous process of L4. This position is called:

a. AP left lateral decubitus

b. PA left lateral decubitus

c. AP right lateral decubitus

d. PA right lateral decubitus

9. On a PA chest radiograph a radiographer observes that the sternoclavicular joints are not symmetrical in relation to the vertebral column. Which of the following conclusions may be reached?

a. the patient was slightly tilted

b. the lung apices were likely not included in their entirety on the film

c. the patient was rotated

d. the patient was probably correctly positioned

10. Whenever possible, chest x-rays are performed in the upright position in order to:

a. demonstrate pneumothorax

b. provide greater comfort to the patient

c. raise the diaphragm to its highest possible position

d. minimize distortion/magnification of the heart and great vessels

11. Which of the following are true regarding the trachea?

a. it transports both food and air

b. it is anterior to the esophagus

c. both a and b

d. neither a nor b

12. Which of the following is the best region of the radiograph to examine in order to detect rotation on a lateral chest?

a. sternoclavicular joints

b. hemidiaphragms

c. posterior ribs

d. hilum

13. To remove the scapulae from the lung fields for a PA chest, the patient is instructed to:

a. roll the shoulders forward

b. take in a deep breath and let it all out

c. take in a deep breath

d. place the chin up as high as possible on the cassette holder

14. In which of chest position/projection is the pulmonary apices demonstrated below the clavicular shadows?

a. PA

b. lateral

c. decubitus

d. lordotic

15. An oblique chest radiograph is requested to demonstrate a suspicious mass in the left primary bronchus. The patient should be placed in the _____ position at an angle of _____ degrees.

a. RAO, 30

b. RAO, 45

c. LAO, 30

d. LAO, 45

16. Routine PA and lateral projections of the chest are taken at _____ kVp.

a. 60–70

b. 70–80

c. 90–100

d. 100–120

17. A radiographer counts 8 posterior ribs visualized above the diaphragm on a PA chest radiograph. Which of the following is a correct conclusion?

a. should be retaken with deeper inspiration

b. should be retaken with less inspiration

c. should be retaken with shoulders rolled forward

d. film is satisfactory

18. A patient with severe emphysema normally requires:

a. a reduction in kVp

b. a decubitus film

c. a lordotic film

d. both obliques

19. The central ray location for most supine abdominal radiography is:

a. ASIS

b. iliac crest

c. 1.5 inches above the iliac crest

d. 1.5 inches below the iliac crest

20. What is the correct breathing instruction for a KUB?

a. hold breath on full expiration

b. hold breath on full inspiration

c. shallow breathing during the exposure

d. hold breath after small amount of inspiration

21. A patient for an abdominal series presents with severe dizziness, nausea and vomiting. Routine films for this patient should include:

a. upright abdomen, PA upright chest and supine abdomen

b. upright abdomen and PA upright chest

c. left lateral decubitus, AP chest and supine abdomen

d. right lateral decubitus, AP chest and supine abdomen

22. The term ileus refers to:

a. middle portion of small intestine

b. final portion of small intestine

c. one of the pelvic bones

d. bowel obstruction

23. The largest organ in the right upper quadrant is the:

a. stomach

b. gallbladder

c. liver

d. spleen

24. If a patient has a tear or rupture in the duodenal mucosa, free air on an upright abdomen will likely form:

a. under the liver

b. under the diaphragm

c. above the diaphragm

d. between the stomach and the spleen

25. The optimum kVp range for non-contrast abdominal projections is:

a. 60–70

b. 70–80

c. 90–100

d. 100–120

26. Which of the following is the least useful landmark for abdominal radiography, since it varies in position from patient to patient?

a. ASIS

b. pubic bone

c. iliac crest

d. umbilicus

27. The thumb has _____ phalanges.

a. 1

b. 2

c. 3

d. 4

28. For obliques of the wrist, the body part is angled ___ degrees.

a. 15

b. 20

c. 30

d. 45

29. Which projection affords the least superimposition of the shafts of the radius and ulna?

a. AP

b. PA

c. lateral

d. lateral oblique

30. In which projection of the elbow is the epicondylar line/plane placed parallel to the film?

a. AP

b. lateral

c. medial oblique

d. lateral oblique

31. Which of the following projections best demonstrates the radial styloid process?

a. lateral hand

b. AP elbow

c. AP wrist

d. lateral oblique elbow

32. A patient's fully extended arm is placed on the table with the hand pronated and the film centered 1 inch below the epicondyles. This projection is a (an) ___ of the elbow

a. AP

b. PA

c. medial oblique

d. lateral oblique

33. Which of the following is the most important factor to consider when deciding whether to utilize a grid for humerus radiography?

a. size of film needed

b. size of body part

c. severity of injury

d. all of the above

34. Which of the following must be included on a lateral projection of the humerus?

1. S-C Joint
2. glenoid fossa
3. elbow joint

a. 1 and 2

b. 1 and 3

c. 2 and 3

d. 1, 2, and 3

35. Which of the following could safely be done on a patient with a shoulder dislocation?

1. AP neutral rotation, shoulder
2. scapular Y projection
3. transthoracic shoulder

a. 1 and 2

b. 1 and 3

c. 2 and 3

d. 1, 2, and 3

36. The Grashey position of the shoulder is performed to better demonstrate the:

a. coracoid process

b. lesser tubercle

c. glenoid cavity/fossa

d. greater tubercle

37. The central ray should enter at the _____ for an AP projection of the shoulder.

a. coracoid process

b. coronoid process

c. acromion process

d. greater tuberosity

38. Which of the following are true for an AP axial projection of the clavicle?

1. the central ray should be angled cephalad

2. patient should be supine

3. the arm should be flexed and abducted

a. 1 and 2

b. 1 and 3

c. 2 and 3

d. 1, 2, and 3

39. For the AP projection for the scapula, the patient's arm is:

a. flexed

b. internally rotated

c. adducted

d. abducted

40. Which position/projection of the clavicle should not be used when fracture is evident?

a. supine

b. prone

c. erect

d. axial

41. Which of the following articulates with the proximal row of carpals?

a. metacarpals

b. ulna

c. radius

d. greater multangular

42. The correct central ray location for a frog-leg lateral hip projection is:

a. femoral neck

b. femoral head

c. crease of the groin

d. level of the greater trochanter

43. Which of the following are correct regarding the tangential patella (Hughston method)?

1. patient is prone

2. tube is angled 45° cephalad

3. center to the patellofemoral joint

a. 1 and 2

b. 1 and 3

c. 2 and 3

d. 1, 2, and 3

44. Which of the following should be clearly demonstrated on an AP projection of the foot?

1. navicular

2. calcaneous

3. medial cuneiform

a. 1 and 2

b. 1 and 3

c. 2 and 3

d. 1, 2, and 3

45. For tunnel views of the knee, the central ray is placed at a right angle to the:

a. patella

b. long axis of the femur

c. long axis of the tibia

d. mid-sagittal plane

46. The tibial tuberosity is best demonstrated on the:

a. AP knee

b. AP lower leg

c. tangential patella

d. lateral knee

47. Which of the following ankle projections demonstrates the lateral malleolus free from bony superimposition?

a. AP

b. lateral

c. 45° internal oblique

d. 15° internal oblique

48. Which of the following are parts of a trauma hip series?

1. AP

2. axiolateral (Danelius-Miller)

3. frog-leg lateral

a. 1 and 2

b. 1 and 3

c. 2 and 3

d. 1, 2, and 3

49. There are _____ phalanges in the left foot.

a. 9

b. 12

c. 13

d. 14

50. Which bones lie on the medial aspect of the foot?

1. internal cuneiform

2. navicular

3. cuboid

a. 1 and 2

b. 1 and 3

c. 2 and 3

d. 1, 2, and 3

51. For the AP projection of the foot, the central ray is angled _____ degrees.

a. 5

b. 10

c. 15

d. 20–25

52. For the mediolateral projection of the foot, the plantar surface of the foot is:

a. 45° to the film

b. 15° to the film

c. parallel to the film

d. perpendicular to the film

53. The sustentaculum tali is on the medial aspect of the:

a. talus

b. navicular

c. calcaneous

d. cuboid

54. What is the correct central ray location for AP oblique projections of the sacroiliac joints?

a. 1 inch medial to the elevated ASIS

b. at the elevated ASIS

c. 1 inch lateral to the elevated ASIS

d. 1 inch superior to, and 1 inch medial to the elevated ASIS

55. For the Clements-Nakayama modification of the lateral hip, the central ray should be angled posteriorly _____ degrees.

a. 5

b. 10

c. 15

d. 25

56. Which structure articulates with the head of the femur?

a. glenoid fossa

b. tibial plateau

c. tibial condyles

d. acetabulum

57. Which of the following utilize a breathing technique?

1. AP ribs

2. RAO sternum

3. transthoracic shoulder

a. 1 and 2

b. 1 and 3

c. 2 and 3

d. 1, 2, and 3

58. The tubercle of a rib articulates with the:

a. sternum

b. transverse process of a vertebra

c. tubercle of an adjacent rib

d. body of a vertebra

59. What kVp range is optimal for ribs below-the-diaphragm?

a. 60–65

b. 70–75

c. 75–80

d. 80–90

60. Which of the following positions/projections best demonstrates fractures of the posterior portion of the left ribs?

a. AP

b. LPO

c. RPO

d. left lateral

61. The last _____ pairs of ribs are called floating ribs.

a. 2

b. 4

c. 6

d. 7

62. For the oblique sternum projection, the central ray should enter _____ inches to the _____ of the spine

a. 2, right

b. 4, right

c. 2, left

d. 4, left

63. To demonstrate the sternoclavicular articulation with minimum superimposition,

a. tube should be angled 15° cephalad

b. weights should be used

c. patient should be in the upright position

d. the patient should be obliqued 15°

64. Compared to chest radiography, upper rib films should be taken at a:

a. higher kVp

b. lower kVp

c. higher MAS

d. lower MAS

65. Which landmark is used to determine the central ray location for an AP cervical spine?

a. hyoid bone

b. thyroid cartilage

c. suprasternal notch

d. top of ear attachment

66. To clearly demonstrate the intervertebral disk spaces on an AP cervical spine:

a. the central ray is placed perpendicular to the film

b. the central ray is directed 15-20° caudal

c. the central ray is directed 15-20° cephalad

d. flexion and extension laterals are taken

67. Which projection best demonstrates the intervertebral foramina of the cervical spine?

a. AP oblique

b. AP

c. flexion lateral

d. lateral

68. A lateral cervical spine is performed using 180 cm (72") SID in order to:

a. improve contrast.

b. reduce exposure factors.

c. decrease magnification.

d. decrease motion

69. The patient is placed in a lateral position with the arm closest to the film raised and the hand placed on the head. The shoulder farthest from the film is depressed and the central ray enters just superior to the suprasternal notch. This describes the:

a. lateral cervical spine

b. lateral thoracic spine

c. flexion lateral

d. swimmers position

70. When radiographing the odontoid process in the open-mouth position, the upper incisors should be placed in a line perpendicular with the:

a. mastoid tip

b. external auditory meatus

c. top of the ear

d. mandibular condyle

71. Which of the following projections best demonstrate the spinal apophyseal joints?

1. lateral C-spine

2. lateral T-spine

3. oblique L-spine

a. 1 and 2

b. 1 and 3

c. 2 and 3

d. 1, 2, and 3

72. The second cervical vertebra is called the:

a. atlas

b. axis

c. dens

d. body

73. What is the optimal tube angle and direction for PA oblique projections of the cervical spine?

a. 15–20°, caudal

b. 15–20°, cephalic

c. 25–30°, caudal

d. 25–30°, cephalic

74. For the _____ projection, the chin is raised as much as possible.

a. open mouth

b. lateral

c. flexion lateral

d. extension lateral

75. All of the following are utilized when positioning for a lateral cervical spine except:

a. 72 inch SID

b. patient holds weights to depress shoulders

c. take on deep inspiration

d. center to C4

76. The _____ spine is characterized by foramina in its transverse processes.

a. cervical

b. thoracic

c. lumbar

d. sacral

77. The large foramen in the thoracic vertebrae through which the spinal cord passes is called the:

a. transverse foramen.

b. foramen magnum

c. vertebral foramen

d. intervertebral foramen

78. For an oblique of the thoracic spine, the body should be rotated _____ degrees from the plane of the film.

a. 20

b. 30

c. 45

d. 70

79. The midcoronal plane is perpendicular to the cassette and the central ray enters at a level three inches below the sternal angle. This best describes which of the following?

a. AP thoracic spine

b. AP lumbar spine

c. lateral thoracic spine

d. swimmers thoracic spine

80. For the AP thoracic spine, kyphosis can be reduced somewhat by:

a. inverting the feet

b. flexing the knees

c. abducting the thighs

d. extending the legs

81. The radiographer must not excessively collimate an AP thoracic spine projection because _____ may be present.

a. lordosis

b. scoliosis

c. kyphosis

d. spondylolisthesis

82. Oblique projections of the thoracic spine should clearly demonstrate the:

1. intervertebral foramina

2. disk spaces

3. zygapophyseal joints

a. 1 and 2

b. 1 and 3

c. 2 and 3

d. 1, 2, and 3

83. A lateral thoracic spine radiograph must demonstrate:

a. T1–T12

b. T1–T10

c. T7–T12

d. T4–T12

84. A breathing technique is sometimes used to blur out the ribs for a lateral thoracic spine projection. The exposure time should be at least:

a. 1/4 second

b. 1/2 second

c. 1 second

d. 4 seconds

e. 15 seconds

85. The _____ of the thoracic spine are not well demonstrated on the lateral projection due to superimposition from the ribs.

a. disk spaces

b. intervertebral foramina

c. transverse processes

d. spinous processes

86. Wedge filters are sometimes used for the _____ projection of the thoracic spine.

a. AP

b. oblique

c. lateral

d. swimmers

87. On a lateral thoracic spine, the top of the film should be placed _____ inch(es) above the top of the shoulder.

a. 0

b. 1

c. 2

d. 4

88. The most inferior segment of the vertebral column is formed by the fusion of 4-5 vertebrae known collectively as the:

a. sacrum

b. ala

c. lamina

d. coccyx

89. Which of the following forms the largest portion of the posterior wall of the bony pelvis?

a. sacrum

b. coccyx

c. L5

d. ilium

90. The two laminae of a vertebra unite in the midline posteriorly to form the:

a. articular facet

b. apophyseal joint

c. spinous process

d. transverse process

91. Which structure of a lumbar vertebra lies most posteriorly?

a. pedicle

b. spinous process

c. transverse process

d. body

92. Which structure comprises the "ear" of a Scotty dog?

a. spinous process

b. transverse process

c. inferior articulating process

d. superior articulating process

93. The LPO position of the lumbar spine demonstrates essentially the same structures as the:

a. LAO

b. RAO

c. RPO

d. lateral

94. The _____ projection of the lumbar spine demonstrates the disk spaces with the least amount of bony superimposition.

a. AP

b. AP oblique

c. PA oblique

d. lateral

95. For the AP projection of the sacrum, the central ray is directed:

a. 10° caudal

b. 10° cephalic

c. 15° caudal

d. 15° cephalad

96. On an AP coccyx radiograph, the coccyx should be projected:

a. above the pubic bone

b. on the inferior sacrum

c. on the pubic symphysis

d. below the pubic bone

97. In order to more clearly visualize the L5-S1 joint space in the AP axial projection, the tube should be angled _____ degrees _____.

a. 15, cephalad

b. 15, caudal

c. 35, cephalad

d. 35, caudal

98. For an AP oblique projection of the lumbar spine in the RPO position, the sagittal plane is placed _____ inches medial to the _____ ASIS.

a. 2, right

b. 2, left

c. 4, right

d. 4, left

99. In the mid-lumbar spine, zygapophyseal joints generally form a _____ degree angle to the midsagittal plane.

a. 15

b. 30

c. 45

d. 60

100. The optimal kVp range for AP and oblique lumbar spine radiographs is:

a. 65–75

b. 75–80

c. 80–85

d. 85–90

101. Before attempting cervical spine obliques on a trauma patient, the radiographer should first take a/an:

a. AP pelvis

b. open-mouth view

c. lateral C-spine

d. AP or PA chest

102. How many vertebra must be visualized on a trauma lateral cervical spine projection?

a. minimum of 4

b. minimum of 5

c. minimum of 6

d. 7

103. If the occipital bone is superimposed on the odontoid process when attempting a trauma open mouth position, the:

a. head is flexed too far

b. head is rotated to the left

c. head is extended too far

d. central ray is not angled properly

104. Which of the following has become an essential modality in imaging of the trauma spine?

a. CT

b. MRI

c. ultrasound

d. radionuclide imaging

105. On a trauma swimmers lateral radiograph, the right humeral head overlies C7. What would be the most appropriate action?

a. repeat the film, angling the tube caudal

b. repeat the film, increasing the kVp

c. repeat the film using a deeper inspiration

d. turn in the film for reading without repeating it

106. A short, broad skull where the petrous ridges form an angle of approximately 54 degrees to the midline of the body is known as:

a. dolichocephalic

b. mesocephalic

c. brachycephalic

d. megacephalic

For questions 107 - 111, match the surface landmark with its description

	Surface landmark	Description
107. _____	vertex	**a.** smooth flat surface between the eyebrows
108. _____	gonion	**b.** most superior surface of cranium
109. _____	mental point	**c.** tip of the chin
110. _____	glabella	**d.** junction of upper lip and inferior nose
111. _____	acanthion	**e.** angle of the mandible

112. The _____ line connects the tip of the chin with the external auditory meatus.

a. acanthiomeatal line

b. mentomeatal line

c. supraorbitomeatal line

d. infraorbitomeatal line

113. Which of the following is not associated with the eth,oid bone?

a. pterygoid process

b. lateral mass

c. perpendicular plate

d. crista galli

114. Which of the following are terms asssociated with the ear?

1. TEA

2. EAM

3. pinna

a. 1 and 2

b. 1 and 3

c. 2 and 3

d. 1, 2, and 3

115. When possible, skull radiography is performed upright because:

1. it is more comfortable for the patient

2. it results in less magnification

3. it demonstrates air-fluid levels

a. 1 and 2

b. 1 and 3

c. 2 and 3

d. 1, 2, and 3

116. If the IOML is perpendicular to the film for a PA Caldwell projection of the skull, how many degrees caudal would you angle the tube?

a. 7

b. 8

c. 15

d. 23

117. The cribriform plate is located in the _____ bone.

a. vomer

b. palatine

c. sphenoid

d. ethmoid

118. Which process on the mandible fits into the temporomandibular fossa?

a. coronoid

b. coracoid

c. condyloid

d. zygomatic

For questions 119 - 123, match the process with the bone on which it is found.

	Process	Bone
119. _____	posterior clinoid process	**a.** temporal bone
120. _____	styloid process	**b.** mandible
121. _____	coronoid process	**c.** sphenoid bone
122. _____	pars petrosa	**d.** frontal bone
123. _____	superciliary arch	**e.** lacrimal bone

124. What structure is found at the junction of the coronal and sagittal sutures?

a. inion

b. lambda

c. gonion

d. bregma

125. The positioning accuracy of which projections is evaluated by observing the position and symmetry of the petrous ridges?

1. parietoacanthial (Waters)
2. semiaxial AP (Townes)
3. PA Caldwell

a. 1 and 2

b. 1 and 3

c. 2 and 3

d. 1, 2, and 3

126. The positioning accuracy of a lateral skull projection is evaluated by observing the position and symmetry of the:

1. mandibular condyles
2. orbital plates
3. petrous ridges

a. 1 and 2

b. 1 and 3

c. 2 and 3

d. 1, 2, and 3

127. For which projection is the central ray placed perpendicular to the IOML?

a. PA Caldwell

b. semiaxial AP (Townes)

c. submentovertex

d. parietoacanthial (Waters)

128. A patient is placed into an RAO position with the midsagittal plane parallel to the film. Which projection does this describe?

- **a.** parietoacanthial (Waters)
- **b.** semiaxial AP (Townes)
- **c.** submentovertex
- **d.** lateral

129. In which projection is the patients head fully extended?

- **a.** parietoacanthial (Waters)
- **b.** semiaxial AP (Townes)
- **c.** submentovertex
- **d.** lateral

For questions 130 - 134, match the projection with the part demonstrated.

	Projection	Part demonstrated
130. _____	axiolateral (Law)	**a.** mandible
131. _____	oblique axial (May)	**b.** temporal bone
132. _____	parietoacanthial (Waters)	**c.** zygomatic arch
133. _____	axioposterior oblique (Mayer)	**d.** nasal bones
134. _____	panorex	**e.** sella turcica

135. In the posterior profile projection (Stenvers) of the temporal bone, the head is rotated ____ degrees from a true PA and the central ray is directed ____ degrees cephalic.

- **a.** 15, 15
- **b.** 45, 12
- **c.** 30, 30
- **d.** 45, 45

136. The acanthiomeatal line is used as a positioning aide for which of the following?

- **a.** axioposterior oblique (Mayer)
- **b.** axiolateral (Law)
- **c.** axiolateral transcranial (Schuller)
- **d.** parieto-orbital oblique (Rhese)

137. Where does the central ray exit for parietoacanthial (Waters) of the facial bones?

- **a.** acanthion
- **b.** nasion
- **c.** glabella
- **d.** inner canthus

138. Open and closed mouth projections are taken to demonstrate what anatomy?

- **a.** orbits
- **b.** TMJ
- **c.** nasal bones
- **d.** temporal bones

139. Which sinus appears just inferior to the sella turcica on a lateral projection?

a. frontal

b. maxillary

c. ethmoid

d. sphenoid

140. Which structures are usually in contact with the table for the parieto-orbital oblique (Rhese) projection?

a. forehead, nose and chin

b. nose, zygoma and chin

c. forehead, zygoma and nose

d. forehead and lips

141. Which of the following is not generally part of a department routine for orbits?

a. modified parietoacanthial (Waters)

b. parieto-orbital oblique (Rhese)

c. PA Caldwell

d. lateral

142. A trauma patient is unable to tilt their head for a mandible exam. The correct tube angle for an axiolateral mandible would be:

a. 10–15° caudal

b. 10–15° cephalic

c. 25–35° caudal

d. 25–35° cephalic

143. If the orbitomeatal line is perpendicular to the film for a trauma AP projection (reverse Caldwell), how many degrees cephalad should the tube be angled?

a. 7

b. 8

c. 15

d. 23

144. On a trauma AP axial (Townes) projection, a large metallic artifact is seen overlying the vertex of the skull. Which of the following should be done?

a. repeat the film as soon as patient condition permits

b. do not repeat the film, since this region is not essential for a Townes projection

c. do not repeat the film if this region is demonstrated on the other trauma radiographs

d. do not repeat the film unless requested to do so by the attending physician

145. Which of the following are acceptable methods for assessing the level of consciousness of a patient prior to a trauma skull exam?

1. call their name using normal voice volume

2. shake the patient and check for a response

3. touch the patient on the arm observe any response

a. 1 and 2

b. 1 and 3

c. 2 and 3

d. 1, 2, and 3

146. Peristalsis begins in the:

a. mouth

b. esophagus

c. stomach

d. small intestine

147. Which of the following is part of the alimentary canal.

1. pylorus

2. jejunum

3. cecum

a. 1 and 2

b. 1 and 3

c. 2 and 3

d. 1, 2, and 3

148. Food is prevented from entering the bronchi by the:

a. epiglottis

b. glottis

c. larynx

d. hyoid cartilage

149. Which of the following is closest in position to the esophageal sphincter?

a. pylorus

b. pharynx

c. duodenum

d. fundus

150. The digestive function of the parotid gland is to produce:

a. bile

b. chyme

c. saliva

d. pepsin and stomach acid

151. Compared to a sthenic patient, the hypersthenic body type will have a stomach located:

a. lower and more medial

b. lower and more lateral

c. higher and more medial

d. higher and more lateral

152. The kVp range for esophagus examinations is:

a. 60–69

b. 70–79

c. 80–89

d. over 90

153. Double contrast exams are frequently performed on the:

1. stomach

2. small intestine

3. large intestine

a. 1 and 2

b. 1 and 3

c. 2 and 3

d. 1, 2, and 3

154. For esophagus obliques, the patient is turned ____ degrees and the central ray is placed at the level of:

a. 30–40, T6

b. 30–40, T4

c. 50–60, T6

d. 50–60, T4

155. Filming for small bowel series generally occurs at _____ minute intervals.

a. 5–10

b. 10–20

c. 30–60

d. 120

156. During a double-contrast GI series, air is found in the pylorus portion of the stomach when the patient is placed into which positions?

1. recumbent LPO
2. supine
3. recumbent RAO

a. 1 and 2

b. 1 and 3

c. 2 and 3

d. 1, 2, and 3

157. Barium sulfate:

1. causes very few adverse reactions
2. is not absorbed by the small intestine
3. causes minor allergic reactions such as itching and hives in 5% of patients

a. 1 and 2

b. 1 and 3

c. 2 and 3

d. 1, 2, and 3

158. On an air-contrast barium enema, air is seen mostly filling the descending colon with barium mostly filling the ascending colon. This projection is most likely a:

a. PA

b. left lateral decubitus

c. lateral

d. right lateral decubitus

159. In the PA axial or butterfly position of the colon, the tube is angled ____ degrees in the _____ direction.

a. 35, cephalad

b. 35, caudal

c. 45, cephalad

d. 45, caudal

160. In order for barium to flow at a reasonable rate, the enema bag should be placed _____ inches above the table.

a. 12–24

b. 24–36

c. 36–42

d. greater than 42

161. The kVp for double contrast enema exams is _____ that for single contrast barium studies.

a. 10 kVp more than

b. 20 kVp more than

c. 10 kVp less than

d. the same as

162. Common patient preparation for a barium enema examination includes:

1. laxatives 1-2 days prior to the exam

2. NPO after midnight

3. low residue diet for 1-2 days prior to the exam

a. 1 and 2

b. 1 and 3

c. 2 and 3

d. 1, 2, and 3

163. During an enema, barium flow normally continues until the:

a. barium reaches the terminal ileum

b. barium reaches the cecum

c. patient complains of fullness

d. barium begins to leak around the retention catheter

164. Barium is contraindicated for exams of the large intestine when:

1. the patient has had recent colon surgery

2. cancer is suspected

3. perforation of the colon is suspected

a. 1 and 2

b. 1 and 3

c. 2 and 3

d. 1, 2, and 3

165. For the AP and oblique projections of the large intestine, the central ray enters:

a. at the ASIS

b. at the lower margin of the ribs

c. at the iliac crest

d. 1–2 inches above the iliac crest

166. The flexures of the colon are best demonstrated by the _____ position/projection(s).

a. AP

b. oblique

c. lateral

d. oblique axial

167. For the lateral projection of the large intestine, the central ray enters:

a. at the ASIS

b. at the iliac crest

c. at the lower margin of the ribs

d. 1–2 inches above the iliac crest

168. Abnormal enlargement and dilation of the veins in the rectal plexus is known as:

a. intussusception

b. hiatal hernia

c. hemorrhoids

d. diverticulosis

169. During an enema, barium leaving the descending colon would next enter the:

a. appendix

b. right colic flexure

c. left colic flexure

d. cecum

170. The Chassard-Lapine position is taken primarily to demonstrate abnormalities of the:

a. rectum

b. rectosigmoid junction

c. right colic flexure

d. appendix

171. Which of the following exams are used to demonstrate invasive, obstructive biliary tract tumors?

1. oral cholecystogram

2. percutaneous transhepatic cholangiogram

3. ERCP

a. 1 and 2

b. 1 and 3

c. 2 and 3

d. 1, 2, and 3

172. Which of the following questions should be asked of a patient prior to taking any films for an oral cholecystogram?

1. does the patient have a GB?

2. did the patient take the oral contrast?

3. did the patient have breakfast?

a. 1 and 2

b. 1 and 3

c. 2 and 3

d. 1, 2, and 3

173. Which organs are involved with making or storing bile?

1. liver

2. pancreas

3. gallbladder

a. 1 and 2

b. 1 and 3

c. 2 and 3

d. 1, 2, and 3

174. When ingested fat enters the duodenum the:

a. liver secretes bile

b. liver makes bile

c. gallbladder releases bile

d. gallbladder concentrates bile

175. Compared to a sthenic patient, the asthenic body type will have a gallbladder located:

a. lower and more medial

b. lower and more lateral

c. higher and more medial

d. higher and more lateral

176. The patient should _____ the evening before an oral cholecystogram.

a. take laxatives

b. refrain from tobacco products

c. skip dinner

d. eat a low fat meal

177. For a PA projection of the gallbladder, the central ray is placed at the level of the last palpable rib for _____ type patients.

a. hyposthenic

b. hypersthenic

c. asthenic

d. sthenic

178. Following the oral cholecystogram, a post-fat meal is sometimes given to:

a. concentrate the contrast media

b. cause the contrast to enter the gallbladder

c. cause the contrast to leave the gallbladder

d. cause the contrast to mix with bile in the gallbladder

179. Filming for an oral cholecystogram includes:

1. PA

2. RAO

3. upright PA

a. 1 and 2

b. 1 and 3

c. 2 and 3

d. 1, 2, and 3

180. During percutaneous transhepatic cholangiography, how does the contrast medium reach the biliary tree?

a. direct instillation

b. orally

c. intravenous injection

d. injection into the cystic duct during surgery

181. Which of the following has largely replaced the oral cholecystogram?

a. ultrasound

b. ERCP

c. radionuclide imaging

d. MRI

182. When the sphincter of Oddi dilates (relaxes), bile enters the:

a. cystic duct

b. gallbladder

c. hepatic duct

d. duodenum

183. Which of the following is not a lobe of the liver?

a. right

b. quadrate

c. middle

d. caudate

184. The optimum kVp range for radiologic urinary examinations is:

a. 60–70

b. 70–75

c. 80–90

d. 90–100

185. The oblique positions for an IVU, require a patient angle of _____ degrees.

a. 5

b. 30

c. 45

d. 70

186. Which of the following is the most serious reaction to injected urographic contrast media?

a. dyspnea

b. a hot flush feeling in the face

c. a metallic taste in the mouth

d. urticaria

187. On an AP projection, which kidney is parallel to the film?

a. right

b. left

c. both right and left

d. neither right nor left

188. Retrograde pyelography does not demonstrate the:

a. kidney pelvis

b. ureters

c. nephrons

d. renal calculi

189. When would barium be given as a contrast medium for urography?

a. patients who are allergic to iodine

b. patients who have experienced a previous severe reaction to urographic contrast

c. patients experiencing complete renal failure

d. never

190. The trigone is a region bounded by the two ureteral openings and the:

a. urethra

b. urinary bladder

c. renal pelvis

d. glomerulus

191. The term which means the opposite of antegrade is:

a. perigrade

b. retrograde

c. intragrade

d. intergrade

192. The structural and functional unit of the kidney is called the:

a. glomerulus

b. calyx

c. nephron

d. pyramid

193. A compression band is often placed across the patient's abdomen during an IVU to:

a. slow the speed of contrast flow through the nephron

b. increase the speed of contrast flow through the nephron

c. increase patient comfort

d. obstruct the flow of contrast and increase filling of the calyces

194. To demonstrate function of the urethra, the patient is often asked to _____ during filming.

a. void

b. perform the Valsalva maneuver

c. drink 4–5 glasses of water

d. defecate

195. In order to remove gas and fecal shadows from IVU films:

a. patients should be asked to hold their breath on deep inspiration

b. patients are given laxatives the night before the exam

c. lateral and upright films are taken

d. linear tomography is performed

196. For oblique projections of the urinary bladder, the central ray is directed:

a. 1/2 inch medial to the side up ASIS

b. 1/2 inch medial to the side down ASIS

c. 2 inches medial to the side up ASIS

d. 2 inches medial to the side down ASIS

197. Perioperative radiography is that which occurs _____ surgery.

a. before

b. after

c. during

d. before, during and after

198. When radiographers leave the surgical suite to obtain a reading, they must:

a. clearly announce to the surgical team they are leaving the OR suite

b. wear a long-sleeved gown over the scrub clothes

c. remove surgical scrubs before leaving the suite

d. don fresh surgical scrubs when they return to the suite

199. The region between the draped patient and the instrument table is known as the:

- **a.** unsafe region
- **b.** aseptic zone
- **c.** sterile corridor
- **d.** aseptic instrument zone

200. If a radiographer brushes against the sterile instrument table when positioning a cassette in the operating suite, he/she should:

- **a.** notify the surgical team immediately
- **b.** notify the surgical team only if that part of the table is going to be used by the surgeon
- **c.** notify the charge nurse after the procedure has been completed
- **d.** ignore the incident to avoid embarrass-ment